Cañadell's Pediatric Bone Sarcomas

Mikel San-Julian
Editor

Cañadell's Pediatric Bone Sarcomas

Epiphysiolysis before Excision

Second Edition

Springer

Editor
Mikel San-Julian
University of Navarra
Department of Orthopaedic Surgery
Pamplona
Spain

ISBN 978-3-319-24218-7 ISBN 978-3-319-24220-0 (eBook)
DOI 10.1007/978-3-319-24220-0

Library of Congress Control Number: 2015957397

Springer Cham Heidelberg New York Dordrecht London

Printed on acid-free paper

Springer International Publishing AG Switzerland is part of Springer Science+Business Media (www.springer.com)

Foreword

Over the past several decades, great advances have been made in the diagnosis and treatment of malignant bone tumors in children. Improvements in imaging, chemotherapy, and surgical treatment have increased the 5-year survival from historical rates of 10–20 % to current rates of 60–70 %. This has led to increasing interest in preserving a functional limb. Limb salvage surgery in the pediatric population creates unique challenges which are addressed in this book by Cañadell. These include the smaller size of a young patient's skeleton, particularly the problems associated with the growth potential of the unaffected leg and eventual limb length discrepancy.

Sparing of the growth plate is an early feature of diaphyseal and meta-diaphyseal osteosarcoma. Capitalizing on this characteristic, Jose Cañadell has developed an innovative technique to preserve the epiphysis while resecting primary bone malignancies lying adjacent to the growth plate of skeletally immature patients. Using external fixation devices, controlled distraction of the epiphysis from the growth plate permits iatrogenic separation of the epiphysis from the affected region, achieving a safe margin. Cañadell's local control rates attest to the success of the procedure as an oncologically sound technique. The Cañadell technique has been developed through rigorous examination of the behavior of osteosarcoma, as well as an interrogation of the best modalities for assessing tumor invasion of the growth plate. Combining an innovative treatment philosophy with a sound knowledge of the behavior of osteosarcoma and basic bone and growth plate biology, as well as an extensive experience with ancillary investigations and adjuvant therapies, Cañadell has developed a robust surgical technique for the management of a challenging tumor in selected patients.

This book is the culmination of Cañadell's endeavors over more than three decades. It traces the steps that he has taken to validate the safety and efficacy of the Cañadell technique as we know it today. Carefully grouped into rationale chapters, this book guides those with a particular interest in musculoskeletal oncology through a technique that they may find valuable when the goal is epiphyseal sparing surgery. The diagrams are clear and the stepwise description of the technique is logical. The selection of histological and anatomic imaging frames has been careful and clearly highlights the important elements underpinning the success of this technique. As a special feature of this book, Cañadell has even included a question and answer section at the end which aims to test whether the educational objectives of his book are being met.

Jose Cañadell's book of techniques is unique and innovative and justifies its place on the shelves of institutions which are focused on advancing the treatment of musculoskeletal tumors.

Rochester, MN, USA Franklin H. Sim, MD

Foreword to the First Edition

Sparing of the growth plate is an early feature of diaphyseal and meta-diaphyseal osteosarcoma. Capitalising on this characteristic, Jose Cañadell has developed an innovative technique to preserve the epiphysis while resecting primary bone malignancies lying adjacent to the growth plate of skeletally immature patients. Using external fixation devices, controlled distraction of the epiphysis from the growth plate permits iatrogenic separation of the epiphysis from the affected region. Subsequent resection is enhanced by a safe distal margin and Cañadell's local control rates attest to the success of the procedure as an oncologically sound technique. The Cañadell technique has been developed through rigorous examination of the behaviour of osteosarcoma, as well as an interrogation of the best modalities for assessing tumour invasion of the growth plate. Combining an innovative treatment philosophy with a sound knowledge of the behaviour of osteosarcoma and basic bone and growth plate biology, as well as an extensive experience with ancillary investigations and adjuvant therapies, Cañadell has developed a robust surgical technique for the management of a challenging tumour in selected patients.

This book is the culmination of Cañadell's endeavours over the last two decades. It traces the steps that he has taken to validate the safety and efficacy of the Cañadell technique as we know it today. Carefully grouped into rationale chapters, this book guides those with a particular interest in musculoskeletal oncology through a technique that they may find valuable when the goal is epiphyseal sparing surgery. The diagrams are clear and the stepwise description of the technique is logical. The selection of histological and anatomic imaging frames has been careful and clearly highlights the important elements underpinning the success of this technique. As a special feature of this book, Cañadell has even included a question and answer section at the end which aims to test whether the educational objectives of his book are being met.

Jose Cañadell's book of techniques is unique and innovative and justifies its place on the shelves of institutions which are focused on advancing the treatment of musculoskeletal tumours.

Rochester, MN, USA Franklin H. Sim

Preface

In the last 40 years, the outcome for patients affected by malignant bone tumors has improved dramatically. Better knowledge of the disease, improvement of imaging methods, new surgical techniques and particularly the advent of chemotherapy have brought about an unsuspected success in this kind of patient.

Forty years ago, preserving the life of these patients was the only aim of physicians, while nowadays preserving the limb and its function and avoiding complications are the challenges for the orthopedic surgeon, because the survival rates continue to improve. Forty years ago, anybody who tried to preserve a joint near a bone tumor would have been considered a fool. Nowadays, this is a desire common to everybody who treats these patients.

Since 1984, we have used a technique in our Department which has become increasingly popular among orthopedic surgeons interested in bone tumors: physeal distraction (epiphysiolysis) before excision in order to preserve the joint in metaphyseal bone tumors in children. This little book is a concise summary of why we use this technique in selected cases.

The review of histopathological pieces for this second edition indicates that Cañadell's technique is of broader application than the authors realized at the time of writing the first edition of the book. As times goes on, the indications for the technique have been enlarged, since the results continued being so good. Recently published results from many other experienced centers confirm the positive results achieved at the authors' center.

In the time since the publication of the first edition of this book, Dr Cañadell has died; his remarkable contributions in the treatment of pediatric bone sarcomas and the value of this legacy are presented in this book.

Mikel San-Julian

Preface to the First Edition

In the last 30 years, the outcomes achieved with patients affected by malignant bone tumours have improved dramatically. Better knowledge of the disease, improvement of imaging methods, new surgical techniques and particularly the advent of chemotherapy have brought about unanticipated therapeutic successes in this kind of patient.

Thirty years ago, physicians were content if they could preserve the life of these patients; nowadays, however, survival rates continue to improve and the challenge for the orthopaedic surgeon is to preserve the limb and its function and to avoid complications. Thirty years ago, anybody who tried to preserve a joint near a bone tumour would have been considered a fool. Nowadays, this is a realistic goal for everybody who treats these patients.

Since 1984, we have been using in our orthopaedics department a technique which has become increasingly popular among surgeons specialized in bone tumours: physeal distraction (epiphysiolysis) before excision to preserve the joint in metaphyseal bone tumours in children.

This little book describes the technique and provides a synopsis of why we use it and how we select which patients to use it with.

Pamplona, Spain — José Cañadell

Pamplona, Navarra, Spain — Mikel San-Julian

Acknowledgments

We would like to express our gratitude to everyone who has contributed directly or indirectly to this book, especially to all the team at the Department of Orthopaedic Surgery and Traumatology at the University Clinic of Navarra, whose daily work in the outpatients department, in the operating room and in the laboratory, in conjunction with rigorous research projects, has helped to improve the techniques described and widen their indications.

Our thanks also go to all the specialists from other departments, in particular the departments of radiology, pediatrics, and pathology, who have collaborated with us in this venture, helping us to broaden our perspectives. While this book and the work it outlines is clearly the result of a multidisciplinary effort, there are certain individuals without whom the development of these techniques might never have happened. One of these individuals is Dr. Luis Sierrasesúmaga, Director of the Department of Pediatrics. With his dedication to excellence in research and to the highest standards of treatment and care of children with cancer, he has inspired and supported us throughout our endeavors.

We also wish to thank the nursing personnel: Maite Moyano, Pilar Lacasa, Ana Villanueva, Natividad Iribarren, Carmen Sánchez, Isabel San-Martin, Lucía Martinez, Roncesvalles Murillo, Maria J. Percaz, Elena Ibarburu, Mónica Suescun, Isabel Lerga, Begoña Gonzalez, Miriam C. Fernández, and many others, who at all times have been such a dependable and invaluable source of help both to doctors and patients.

Lastly, we would like to mention Paz Gúrpide (†) for providing the outline for this book, Javier Gardeta for his presentation of the iconography, and David Burdon for his help with translation of the text.

Contents

Contributors

Jesús Dámaso Aquerreta, MD, PhD Department of Radiology, Clínica Universidad de Navarra, Pamplona, Navarra, Spain

Alberto Benito, MD, PhD Department of Radiology, Clínica Universidad de Navarra, Pamplona, Navarra, Spain

QiQing Cai, MD, PhD Department of Bone and Soft Tissue Cancer, HeNan Cancer Hospital, ZhengZhou, HeNan Province, People's Republic of China

José Cañadell†, MD, PhD Department of Orthopaedic Surgery, University of Navarra, Pamplona, Navarra, Spain

Màrius Aguirre-Canyadell, MD, PhD Department of Orthopaedic Surgery and Traumatology, Orthopaedic Oncology Unit, Hospital Universitari Vall d'Hebron, Universitat Autònoma De Barcelona, Barcelona, Spain

Jose A. Cara, MD, PhD Servicio Médico San Pedro, Department of Orthopaedic Surgery, San Pedro de Alcántara, Málaga, Spain

ZhaoQiang Chen, MD, PhD Department of Orthopedic Oncology, TianJin Hospital, TianJin Medical University, TianJin, People's Republic of China

Enrique de Alava, MD, PhD Department of Pathology, Virgen del Rocio University Hospital, Sevilla, Spain

Julio de Pablos, MD, PhD Department of Osrthopaedic Surgery, Hospital San Juan de Dios, Pamplona, Navarra, Spain

Antonio Marcelo G. de Souza, MD, PhD Orthopaedic Oncology Service, Cancer Hospital of Pernambuco, Recife, Brasil

P.D. Sander Dijkstra, MD, PhD Department of Orthopaedic Surgery, Leiden University Medical Center, Leiden, The Netherlands

Charles E. Dumont Department of Orthopaedics, Orthopaedie Zentrum Zuerich, Zuerich, Switzerland

G. Ulrich Exner Department of Orthopaedics, Orthopaedie Zentrum Zuerich, Zuerich, Switzerland

Francisco Forriol, MD, PhD Department Clinical Sciences, School of Medicine, University San Pablo, Madrid, Spain

Moira Garraus, MD, PhD Department of Pediatrics, Hospital San Joan de Deu, Barcelona, Spain

YongCheng Hu, MD, PhD Department of Orthopedic Oncology, TianJin Hospital, TianJin Medical University, TianJin, People's Republic of China

Miguel Angel Idoate, MD, PhD Department Pathology, University of Navarra Avda. Pio XII, Pamplona, Navarra, Spain

Fernando Lecanda, PhD Program in Solid Tumors and Biomarkers, Center for Applied Medical Research (CIMA), Pamplona, Spain

Maria Dolores Lozano, MD, PhD Department of Pathology, Clínica Universidad de Navarra, Pamplona, Navarra, Spain

Isabel Martin, MD, PhD Centro de salud de La Rochapea, Pamplona, Spain

Mathew J. Most, MD Division of Orthopedic Oncology, Department of Orthopedics and Physical Rehabilitation, UMass Memorial Health Care, Worcester, MA, USA

Ana Patiño-García, MD, PhD Department of Pediatrics, University Clinic of Navarra, IdiSNA, Navarra Institute for Health Research, Pamplona, Navarra, Spain

Mikel San-Julian, MD, PhD Department of Orthopaedic Surgery, University of Navarra, Pamplona, Navarra, Spain

Luis Sierrasesúmaga, MD, PhD Department of Pediatrics, University Clinic of Navarra, Pamplona, Navarra, Spain

Franklin H. Sim, MD Department of Orthopedic Surgery, Mayo Clinic, Rochester, MN, USA

Antonie H.M. Taminiau, MD, PhD Department of Orthopaedic Surgery, Leiden University Medical Center, Leiden, The Netherlands

Jesús Vazquez[†]**, MD, PhD** Department of Pathology, University of Navarra, Pamplona, Spain

Blanca L. Vazquez-García, MD Department of Orthopaedic Surgery, Complejo Hospitalario de Navarra, Pamplona, Navarra, Spain

Roberto Vélez, MD, PhD Department of Pathology, University of Navarra, Pamplona, Spain

Zhen Wang, MD, PhD Department of Orthopedic Oncology, XiJing Hospital, the Fourth Military Medical University, Xi'an, ShanXi Province, People's Republic of China

SongFeng Xu, MD, PhD Department of Orthopedics, General Hospital of Ji'Nan Military Region, Ji'Nan, ShanDong Province, People's Republic of China

WeiTao Yao, MD, PhD Department of Bone and Soft Tissue Cancer, HeNan Cancer Hospital, ZhengZhou, HeNan Province, People's Republic of China

XiuChun Yu, MD, PhD Department of Orthopedics, General Hospital of Ji'Nan Military Region, Ji'Nan, ShanDong Province, People's Republic of China

Marta Zalacain-Díez, PhD Pediatrics Laboratory, University Clinic of Navarra, Pamplona, Navarra, Spain

Chapter 1
History of Surgery for Limb Bone Tumors

Francisco Forriol

Abstract In this chapter, we take a look at the long history of developments in the treatments of bone tumors. Early in the twentieth century, only certain small, localized cancers that could be removed by surgery were curable. Then came radiation, which was used after surgery to control the growth of small tumors that could not be widely removed. The introduction of neoadjuvant and preoperative (induction) chemotherapy was the next big step forward. For some patients it was possible to combine treatments: adjuvant multi-agent chemotherapy, limb-salvage surgery and radiotherapy. Meanwhile, the development of new imaging techniques permitted better diagnosis and assessment of disease. As diagnostic and therapeutic techniques improve, patients with musculoskeletal sarcomas can expect increased survival, decreased complications and side effects, and an improved quality of life.

Keywords Bone tumors • Chemotherapy • Radiotherapy • Limb salvage – surgery

1.1 Introduction

The history of tumor treatment is a long story. Tumors were recognized back in the times of Hippocrates, who adopted the terms "carcinos" and "carcinoma", based on the Greek word for a crab. Later, the Roman physician Celsus translated the term into "cancer", and Galen used the word "oncos" (swelling, in Greek) to describe tumors. We can distinguish different phases of this history on the basis of discoveries and the introduction of new technologies. Early in the twentieth century, only small, localized cancers that could be removed by surgery were curable. At a second stage, radiation was used after surgery to control small tumor growths that could not be surgically removed. A big step then came with the introduction of chemotherapy

In memoriam of José Cañadell (1923–2014), a master and pioneer in the treatment of malignant bone tumors.

F. Forriol, MD, PhD
Department of Clinical Sciences, School of Medicine, University San Pablo – CEU, Campus de Monteprincipe, Boadilla del Monte, Madrid 28668, Spain
e-mail: fforriol@mac.com

M. San-Julian (ed.), *Cañadell's Pediatric Bone Sarcomas: Epiphysiolysis before Excision*, DOI 10.1007/978-3-319-24220-0_1

agents; standard current treatment consists of multiagent therapy, with both neoadjuvant, preoperative or induction chemotherapy, and adjuvant chemotherapies associated with surgery and radiotherapy in some cases. The parallel development of new imaging techniques permitted better diagnosis and assessment of the disease.

The overall incidence of osteosarcoma is 1.5–2.5 per million persons per year, while for chondrosarcoma it is 1–1.2 per million per year, and for Ewing sarcoma 0.5–1 per million per year. For this reason, centers have been established that specialize in the interdisciplinary treatment of bone tumors, and research often involves multidisciplinary and multicenter studies. Large cooperative groups have successfully completed international clinical trials. The Vienna Bone Tumor Registry was founded in 1962 [167], while randomized protocols have been developed on the basis of the Cooperative Osteosarcoma Study COSS [6, 210] and the Cooperative Ewing Sarcoma Study CESS [102], or the Scandinavian Sarcoma Group (SSG), the European Osteosarcoma Intergroup (EOI) and the Children's Oncology Group (COG) in the USA [195].

1.1.1 Histological Classification

The nineteenth century saw the birth of scientific oncology, with the advent of the modern microscope and new histological techniques. Rudolf Virchow, the founder of cellular pathology, provided the scientific basis for modern cancer study, correlating microscopic pathology with disease. He analyzed the tissues that were resected during surgery and laid the foundations for modern practice, in which the pathologist has an essential role in determining both the diagnosis and the prognosis of cancerous disease. The first screening test for diagnosing tumors was that developed by George Papanicolau in 1923 for the early diagnosis of cervical cancer.

James Ewing (1866–1943) was the first person to describe the sarcoma which bears his name, a primary malignant bone tumor. He initially reported the sarcoma as a "bone endothelioma", in the belief that it derived from the blood vessels in the bone, but he later reclassified it as an "endothelial myeloma". He also described Ewing sarcoma of the soft tissues. He was the first professor of pathologic anatomy at Cornell University. In 1906, Ewing and his team published their findings about lymph sarcoma in dogs, showing how the disease could be transmitted from one animal to another during coitus. He was a co-founder, in 1907, of the American Association for the Control of Cancer. In 1913, he began to work in collaboration with James Douglas, an engineer interested in the therapeutic potential of radium. Ewing was the first Director of Research and President of the Medical Board of the General Memorial Hospital which would later become known as the Memorial Sloan Kettering Cancer Center, in New York. Under his leadership this center developed a new approach to treating cancer. His photograph was featured on the front cover of Time magazine in 1931, with the caption "Cancer Man Ewing" [93].

Another leading figure in the history of treatment for bone tumors was William Fischer Enneking (1926–2014) to whose team we owe much of our knowledge about the natural history of orthopedic tumors. Whilst a doctor at the University of Florida, he started work with Howard Hatcher, a specialist interested in diagnosing and treating musculo-skeletal tumors and diseases. In the surgical field, he performed one of the first limb salvage operations and developed a course in musculo-skeletal pathology. Enneking studied many whole-mount surgical specimens and was thereby able to determine the natural progression of bone tumors, which led to improved surgical procedures with better oncologic outcomes. High-grade sarcomas progress in a centripetal fashion. Bone sarcomas start either within the medullary space or near the surface of the bone. Surface tumors can be either periosteal or parosteal, originating from either the periosteum or the bone surface.

As malignant tumors progress, they do not respect natural barriers. They have a tendency to destroy the medullary cancellous bone and may extend up the medullary space involving marrow and generating apparent skip lesions [64]. During the process of tumor progression, the tumor outgrows its blood supply and spontaneous necrosis occurs. Such necrosis reflects aggressive tumor behavior, and it is important to note that it should not be confused with the necrosis that occurs as a chemotherapeutic response. The American Joint Committee on Staging End Results Classification System and their tumor Grades I, II or III are based on the number of mitoses per high-powered field [63, 66, 166]. The extent of necrosis is graded to the percentage of residual viable tumor [93, 94]. Wunden et al. [213] found that chemotherapy-induced tumor necrosis is also the most important indicator of event-free survival for patients who have had operative treatment of Ewing sarcoma. Spontaneous necrosis is slight in untreated bone tumors and rarely exceeds 25 % in osteosarcomas [167] and 20 % in Ewing sarcomas [51].

Progressively a malignant tumor grows within the medullary space, and the cortex is ultimately destroyed, frequently leading to soft tissue extension. An osteosarcoma or Ewing sarcoma involving the distal part of the long bones will initially respect the cartilaginous barriers, growth plate or articular cartilage; later, however, penetration through these structures occurs [184].

Enneking et al. [62, 63, 66] defined surgical margins by developing staging systems for both benign and malignant tumors. When the host is unable to contain a bone sarcoma, an inflammatory and vascular zone – typically an infiltrative margin and a pseudocapsule, that is, a zone that is contaminated by microscopic islands of tumor – develops in the margin between the normal tissue and tumor. Margins should be wide according to Enneking's definition, meaning that both the tumor and the biopsy scar surrounded by an unviolated cuff of healthy tissue must be removed en bloc [34, 62, 125, 148], marginal resections should be avoided, and intralesional or piecemeal surgery is clearly not sufficient. In addition, Enneking et al. [62–64, 66] formulated a means of classifying surgical procedures on the basis of the surgical plane of dissection in relation to the tumor and the method of accomplishing the removal, and gave surgeons a common language to distinguish between intralesional, marginal, intracompartmental or radical (extracompartmental) procedures.

In most cases where the osteosarcoma appears to be localized, tumor cells have already been disseminated without clinical or radiological manifestations [128, 153, 187, 193, 197]. Bone sarcomas can metastasize, and 80 % of osteosarcomas have either micrometastatic or macrometastatic disease at the time of presentation [120], while about 20 % of patients with Ewing sarcoma present with clinically apparent primary metastases [147] and the bone itself is a potential metastatic site. This explains the high local failure rate: between 5 and 25 % [50, 59, 132, 180], when there is known microscopic tumor spread. Metastases confined to the lungs and or pleural space have been associated with a fair outcome, while involvement of bone or bone marrow is reported to imply an intermediate prognosis.

Until nearly the end of the twentieth century, diagnosing cancer often required exploratory surgery and pathological analysis of the resected tissue. Biopsy of musculoskeletal lesions should be carefully planned and performed after radiographic staging studies are completed [164]. Bone and soft tissue biopsy is challenging; core needle biopsy appears to be more accurate than fine needle aspiration, and incisional biopsy appears to be more accurate than either of these techniques. The advantages of a percutaneous technique compared with an incisional one are the low risk of contamination and the minimally invasive nature. However, if the result of a percutaneous biopsy is nondiagnostic, a small incisional biopsy should be performed. Incorporation of ultrasonography or computed tomography for guidance is easy and safe and can be useful for increasing the accuracy of the biopsy [196].

1.1.2 The Support of the Image Diagnosis

During the late 1970s and the 1980s, limb salvage surgery became a very popular technique. This was the result of several advances, one of the most important being that the imaging of bone and soft-tissue tumors improved as a result of the use of computed tomography (CT) scans, radioisotope scans, and magnetic resonance imaging (MRI). Tumors could be visualized precisely, and this allowed for adequate removal. Imaging tests such as ultrasound (sonography), computed tomography (CT scans), magnetic resonance imaging (MRI scans), and positron emission tomography (PET scans) have replaced many exploratory surgical procedures. CT scans and ultrasound can also be used to guide biopsy needles into tumors. With the use of CT and MRI, it is possible to evaluate the bone tumor size more precisely. The surgeon can then plan the resection preoperatively and decrease the need for removal of extensive amounts of normal tissue. In this way, by reducing the amount of normal tissue resected, functional outcomes are improving without sacrificing acceptable oncologic results.

Ernest Amory Codman (1869–1940) described, originally in the context of osteosarcoma, the eponymous triangular area that appears on radiographic images at the point where the periosteum, raised by a bone tumor, joins the bone cortex. A graduate of Harvard Medical School, Codman was a close friend of the neurosurgeon Harvey Cushing. After traveling around Europe and working in Vienna with Eduard Albert, he devoted his final year of training at the Massachusetts General Hospital, in Boston, to the use of the recently described Röntgen rays. He worked as a radiologist ("skiagrapher") at the Boston Children's Hospital, and in 1911 he opened his own hospital, the Codman Hospital. He collected 148 cases of bone sarcoma which enabled him to establish 25 clinical, radiographic and histological criteria to define this kind of tumor. He was a pioneer in many areas of medicine, wrote the first atlas of normal skeletal radiography, the first articles on repair of the rotator cuff in the shoulder and the first book on shoulder pathology, but he is perhaps best remembered for his studies on the clinical and radiographic diagnosis of osteosarcoma and his pioneering evidence-based medical work. He created the first cancer register in the USA and was the first to describe the chondroblastoma: a primary tumor of cartilaginous origin which is known as Codman's tumor [22, 42].

Of imaging techniques, computed tomography (CT) has an important role in the local and extraskeletal staging of a bone tumor and in detecting pulmonary metastases. Magnetic resonance imaging (MRI) precisely outlines both the extra- and intraosseous extension of a tumor and reveals possible skip metastases. MRI has been proposed and tried as a non-invasive method for assessing the response of Ewing sarcoma to preoperative chemotherapy, but the changes identified by static imaging, with or without gadolinium enhancement, are not useful for determining the tumor response [70, 80, 90, 213]. MRI has been found to overestimate the extent of residual disease [213]. Later dynamic and angiographic MRI techniques may provide a more accurate estimate of the extent of tumor necrosis following chemotherapy [68, 113, 202]. Scintigraphy and dynamic contrast-enhanced MR images are useful in objective presurgical prediction of tumor response and regression to preoperative chemotherapy. Early detection of local recurrences and metastases is a further advantage of MRI and also of dynamic positron emission tomography (PET) with its high sensitivity.

1.2 The Hard Way of Radiotherapy

In 1896, the German physicist Wilhelm Conrad Röntgen presented his historic lecture entitled "*On a New Kind of Rays*". Röntgen named the ray the "X-ray", with "x" being the algebraic symbol for an unknown quantity. In 1901, his work was to earn him the first Nobel Prize ever awarded in physics. Within months, systems were being devised to use X-rays for diagnosis, and within 3 years radiation was being applied to treat cancer. Like X-rays, radium emits ionizing radiation, but of a shorter wavelength. Marie Curie, through the Curie Institute in Paris, publicized the potential of radium for treating and curing cancer. The public confused the two sources of radioactivity for a long time, since both are used medically. Radiation therapy began with radium and with relatively low-voltage diagnostic machines. A major breakthrough took place when it was discovered that daily doses of radiation over several weeks greatly improved the patient's chance of being cured. But at the same time it was discovered that radiation could cause cancer as well as cure it. Radium's reputation as a quasi-miracle elixir was promoted in the 1920s with an enthusiasm that is hard to recapture in the knowledge of the damage it inflicted on so many who worked with it, including Marie Curie herself. Many early radiologists used the skin of their arms to test the strength of radiation from their radiotherapy machines, looking for a dose that would produce a "pink reaction" – an erythema – which looked like sunburn. They called this the "erythema dose," and this was considered an estimate of the proper daily fraction of radiation. It is no surprise that many of them developed leukemia from regularly exposing themselves to radiation.

The more rapid cell turnover is, the greater the effect of radiation is [38]. This is what enables postoperative radiation therapy to reduce the incidence of local recurrences of soft tissue sarcomas [138]. One of the main problems with radiotherapy is that ionizing radiation cannot differentiate between normal and pathologic tissue. With regard to bone, the growth plate has relatively high cell turnover, and radiation can decrease or stop bone growth [165].

Radiation therapy is generally used for patients who have refused definitive surgery, require palliation, or have lesions in axial locations. Radiotherapy takes on greater importance in the treatment of tumors of the axial skeleton and facial bones, and is more frequently used in Ewing sarcoma and peripheral primitive neuroectodermal tumors of the bone. In comparison with these, osteosarcoma is not a particularly radiosensitive tumor, although there was a time when the recommended management of this tumor was local radiotherapy to the primary tumor followed by amputation 6 months later, provided that the chest remained clear of metastasis and that the primary tumor remained under control. However, this approach made no difference to survival, though some patients who had developed lung metastases and in whom the primary tumor had remained under control were spared the loss of a limb. Sweetham et al. [193, 194] performed a retrospective survey of the cases of tibial and femoral osteosarcoma treated at major centers in the United Kingdom between 1952 and 1959 to assess the outcome of treatment by surgery and radiotherapy. Radiotherapy followed by amputation produced better results, in terms of survival, than amputation alone. For the largest age group, patients under 20 years, only 22 % survived 5 years. The survival rate of the group treated by radiotherapy alone was lower than that of the group treated by amputation or that of the group treated by a combination of radiotherapy and amputation.

The results of postoperative radiation therapy, described by Suit et al. [189, 190] and Lindberg [119], indicate that it effectively lowers the risk of local recurrence of sarcomas in the distal limb, but as Morton et al. [138] described, such treatment has not been as successful for more proximal lesions of the arm and thigh. Patients treated by operation and radiation therapy alone develop systemic metastases, particularly in the lungs [138]. Eilber et al. [60] reported than pre- and post- operative radiotherapy was highly effective at reducing the high recurrence rate in patients who did not undergo amputation surgery [189]: in patients who were treated with nonamputative excision of all gross tumor and postoperative radiation therapy, the expected local recurrence rate of 30–50 % was reduced to approximately 17 % [76, 189, 190]. A pilot study in 1976 of preoperative chemotherapy and radiation followed by surgical resection indicated that in most patients local tumor control and limb salvage could be accomplished with little morbidity and an even lower local recurrence rate than 17 % [138]. Definitive local radiation for Ewing sarcoma is recognized as necessary, and such treatment has involved high doses of radiation [25, 67, 88, 104, 213]. Because of problems with high doses, operative treatment has been investigated as an alternative that could allow a reduction in the dose of, or obviate the need for, local radiation therapy.

Intra-operative radiation therapy (IORT) was first established as a treatment modality for locally advanced tumors, and its use in the treatment of osteosarcoma was described by Abe and Yamamuro [1]. IORT minimizes the amount of tissue that is exposed to radiation because normal tissues can be moved out of the way during surgery and shielded, allowing a higher dose of radiation to the tumor. Osteosarcoma is one of the most radioresistant tumors, but IORT uses high-dose single irradiation, and total necrosis of irradiated bone has been confirmed histologically [105, 145, 198]. The radiation can be given directly to the tumor or to the nearby tissues after tumor resection. IORT and brachytherapy are more commonly used in abdominal or pelvic cancers and in cancers that tend to recur, or to treat microscopic residual disease [28, 52].

Advances in radiation physics and computer technology during the last quarter of the twentieth century made it possible to focus radiation more precisely with the techniques of conformal radiation therapy (CRT) and intensity modulated radiation therapy (IMRT), both of which use CT images and computers to establish the location of a tumor on a very precise 3-D map [52]. Other approaches to improvement include the use of chemical modifiers or radiosensitizers, which are substances that make cancer more sensitive to radiation, and the search for substances that may help protect normal cells from radiation.

1.2.1 Immunotherapy

Von Haberer [18] began the quest for "nature's solutions" for cancer, but it was William Coley as a young surgeon at New York Memorial Hospital who, disillusioned with conventional approaches, first tried to stimulate the patient's own immune system as a cancer treatment. Serendipitously, he came across the case of an immigrant patient who presented on his left cheek a sarcoma that had been operated on twice, and which recurred below his left ear. The wound after surgery could not be closed, and the tumor progressed until a final operation was only partially able to remove the tumor. After the last operation the wound became severely infected with *Streptococcus pyogenes* and the patient developed a high fever. Surprisingly after each attack of fever the ulcer improved, the tumor shrank, and finally disappeared completely. Coley found the patient 7 years later in excellent health without any trace of cancer [91]. Coley suspected that the infection was responsable for the cure. He resolved to infect his next ten patients [43, 44]. Bloodgood [18] agreed that Coley's serum with the toxins of *Streptococcus* and *Bacillus prodigiosus* should be employed in all inoperable cases and also before and after the operation in operable sarcoma cases.

Coley's toxins [44] inspired researchers to start experimental immunological studies [157]. The dendritic cell therapy devised by Steinmann in 1973 yielded clinical applications in 1995 [55, 188]. Research continued into ways of treating tumors by boosting the immune system using biological agents, particularly monoclonal antibodies. The first agents of this kind were rituximab (Rituxan) and trastuzumab (Herceptin) for treating lymphomas and breast cancer, but growth factors like gefitinib (Iressa), imatinib (Gleevec) and cetuximab (Erbitux) and angiogenic factors like bevacizumab (Avastin) have also come into use. In the nineteenth century, before hormones were discovered, Thomas Beatson found that rabbit breasts stopped producing milk after ophrectomy and studied the use of this principle for treating breast cancer. His research laid the foundations for the hormone therapy currently used with breast cancer patients, such as tamoxifen and aromatase inhibitors.

1.2.2 The Big Change: Chemotherapy

During World War II, naval personnel who had been exposed to mustard gas were found to have undergone toxic changes in their bone marrow cells. During that same period, the US Army was studying a number of chemicals related to mustard gas to develop more effective agents for war and also develop protective measures. A compound called nitrogen mustard was studied and found to work against lymphoma. This agent was the first of a list of more effective agents, called alkylating agents, which killed rapidly growing cancer cells by damaging their DNA. Sidney Farber, in Boston, demonstrated that aminopterin, which blocked a critical chemical reaction needed for DNA replication, produced remissions in children with acute leukemia. Aminopterin was the predecessor of methotrexate, which heralded the era of chemotherapy.

Another major step forward was the discovery of the advantage of using multiple chemotherapy drugs. Doxorubicin, cisplatin, high-dose methotrexate and ifosfamide are considered the most active agents against osteosarcoma, and most successful protocols have been built around combinations of several of these drugs [15].

Metastatic cancer was first cured in 1956 when methotrexate was used to treat a rare tumor called choriocarcinoma. In the 1960s, chemotherapy drugs cured many patients with Hodgkin disease, childhood acute lymphoblastic leukemia and testicular cancer.

Chemotherapy was first introduced for malignant bone tumor treatment on a large scale in the 1970s, and now is the cornerstone treatment for this disease. Adriamycin (doxorubicin) was shown to have some activity [19], but the response rate varied greatly between studies. Gottlieb et al. combined Adriamycin with dacarbazine (DTIC) (ADIC), with DTIC and vincristine (VADIC), and with DTIC and vincristine and cyclophosphamide (CYVADIC), which resulted in a 59 % response rate if bone sarcomas were excluded [150, 151]. The 5-year survival rate in the historical series presented before 1970 [50, 153, 193] was about 20–25 %; there was little difference between the survival rate of patients treated by immediate primary amputation and those treated by radiotherapy with amputation or those in whom radiotherapy was abandoned when early metastases occurred [27].

In 1976, in an attempt to increase the duration of response and to reduce toxicity, the EORTC Soft Tissue and Bone Sarcoma Group embarked on a randomized study comparing the efficacy of the four-drug CYVADIC combination [150]. Jaffe and Rosen with their co-workers [96, 99, 112, 158, 162], were the first to report satisfactory results in osteosarcomas that responded well to high-dose methotrexate and Adriamycin. With this treatment, the 5-year survival rate increased to 60 % in Ewing sarcoma and to 70–75 % in non-metastatic osteosarcoma, in contrast to 15 % and 20 % respectively, observed in the historical control groups. The first results combining chemotherapy showed an increase in the numbers of patients who remained free from metastases after surgery [45–47, 96, 152, 192]. Postoperative adjuvant therapy with high dose methotrexate and citrovorum rescue and/or Adriamycin reduced the incidence of pulmonary metastases from osteosarcomas [45–47, 96–99, 159–163].

The current standard consists of neoadjuvant and adjuvant chemotherapy. Neoadjuvant chemotherapy was introduced by Rosen et al. [163], and was found to induce necrosis in the primary tumor, facilitate surgical resection and eradicate micrometastases [5, 7, 15]. It has contributed to an improved prognosis in osteogenic sarcoma [44, 45, 96, 97, 99, 152, 159–163, 192] and also in Ewing tumors [12, 48]. Skeletal sarcomas seem to respond to preoperative continuous intra-arterial infusion of Adriamycin [54, 87]. In 1976, Morton et al. [138] showed that the effectiveness of intra-arterial Adriamycin was confirmed by the histologic evidence of tumor necrosis present in post-Adriamycin biopsies. Moreover, intra-arterial Adriamycin, followed by radiation therapy, resulted in dramatic tumor regression. Histologically, the degree of tumor necrosis was up to 88 %, and almost 40 % of the specimens contained no viable tumor cells.

The response to neoadjuvant chemotherapy is an important prognostic factor, and the drugs for adjuvant chemotherapy should be selected on the basis of the degree of tumor necrosis induced by neoadjuvant chemotherapy [10, 16, 102, 133, 148, 149, 160].

Eilber et al. [60] describe preoperative therapy before contamination of tissue planes by any type of surgery. They chose Adriamycin because of the high response rate obtained in bone tumors and also because of its known potential to sensitize the tissues to subsequent radiation therapy. Radiation of a tumor with an intact blood supply before surgical excision could possibly improve the radiation effect at the tumor margins and, therefore, improve the overall local recurrence rate. Campanacci and Laus [30] treated 248 high-grade central bone osteosarcomas by amputation or disarticulation; in 5.2 % the tumor recurred at the amputation site. In the view of Campanacci et al. [29], adjuvant chemotherapy does not have a significant effect on local recurrences, which should be treated by radical operation or, if this is not possible, by irradiation; chemotherapy may be used as an adjuvant. Bleyer et al. [17], in 41 consecutive patients with newly diagnosed osteogenic sarcoma between 1952 and 1977, found that the chemotherapy group had a significant increase in both survival and disease-free survival compared to the historical group who had not received chemotherapy. With adjunct chemotherapy only one of the seven patients had developed pulmonary metastases 9 months after diagnosis.

Today, research is necessary to improve the activity and reduce the side effects of chemotherapy with new drugs and new combinations of drugs. In addition, research is needed into new delivery techniques and novel approaches to targeting drugs more specifically at the cancer cells. Examples include the use of colony-stimulating factors, chemoprotective agents and approaches that reduce drug resistant clones. However, establishing treatment protocols has not been straightforward, and many failures have been reported, although published survival rates are now improving. Giving cisplatin intra-arterially did not improve results [71]. A controlled trial adding granulocyte colony stimulating factor (G-CSF) to doxorubicin and cisplatin, led by the European Osteosarcoma Intergroup, failed to achieve a survival advantage [116]. A French trial suggested that similar results may be obtained with ifosfamide instead of doxorubicin [114], and an American trial suggested that the addition of ifosfamide or liposomal muramyl tripeptide, an immunomodulator, to standard three-drug chemotherapy with doxorubicin, cisplatin, and high-dose methotrexate did not seem to confer any advantages.

1.2.3 Surgery in Malignant Tumors of the Limbs

Oncologic orthopedic surgery was long confined to amputation in order to remove malignant tissue and to avoid recurrence and metastases. However, specialists sought ways to preserve limbs and maintain satisfactory function, and thereby to avoid the psychological and cosmetic problems caused by amputation [5, 79]. Advances in imaging techniques and in biomedical engineering, an understanding of the optimal margins for resection determined by Enneking's tumor staging [62], and the use of chemotherapy, have led to a major shift away from amputation towards limb-salvage surgery [7, 15]. However, it should be noted that Jaffe et al. [97] reported that only 10 % of patients with osteosarcoma were cured exclusively with chemotherapy, and highlighted the significance of surgery in osteosarcoma treatment.

Billroth, in Germany, Handley, in London and Halsted, in Baltimore, were the first tumor surgeons. William Stewart Halsted, professor of surgery in Johns Hopkins, described radical breast amputation for breast cancer at the end of the nineteenth century. The work of such specialists led to "cancer operations" designed to remove the entire tumor along with the lymph nodes in the region where the tumor was located. Stephen Paget, in England, concluded that cancer cells spread by way of the bloodstream to all organs in the body but were able to grow only in a few organs. This understanding of metastasis became a key element in recognizing the limitations of cancer surgery. When anesthesia became available in 1846, surgery advanced so fast that the next 100 years became known as "the century of the surgeon." During the final decades of the twentieth century, surgeons developed greater technical expertise in minimizing the amounts of normal tissue removed during cancer operations. Less invasive ways of destroying tumors without removing them are being studied, such as cryosurgery [129], which uses liquid nitrogen spray. Lasers can be used to cut through tissue or to vaporize cancers of the cervix, larynx, liver, rectum, skin, and other organs. Radiofrequency ablation transmits radio waves to a small antenna placed in the tumor to kill cancer cells by heating them.

1.2.3.1 Amputation

Amputation was the main, standard therapeutic option for patients with osteosarcoma before the 1970s, when non-amputative surgical procedures such as local excision or even the wider en bloc resection resulted in an unacceptable 60–90 % incidence of local tumor recurrence [21]. The 5-year survival in osteosarcoma in the first half of the twentieth century was less than 20 % [49], and most patients died of lung metastases [127, 128]. Extending the operative field to amputation of the limb one joint above the tumor was adopted, and this reduced the incidence of local recurrence to 5–25 % [50, 60, 69, 132, 146]. Amputation to achieve local tumor control of skeletal and soft tissue sarcomas was based on clinical experience using surgery as the primary treatment modality. Various complications are caused by amputations: wound necrosis, infection, overgrowth of bone in children, neuroma, stump pain and phantom limb pain [5].

Rotationplasty as a functional amputation procedure was first described in 1930 for treating shortening after tuberculous ankylosis of the knee joint [20], and was later popularized by Van Nes [203] for congenital defects of the femur. Rotationplasty was designed for the reconstruction of bone defects around the knee following above-knee amputation. The distal femur with tumor is removed and the distal part of lower leg and ankle are preserved. Then, the tibia and the foot are rotated 180° and attached to the femoral stump. The rotated ankle, at the appropriate height of the contralateral knee, acts as a functional knee joint, so that the patient can function with a below-knee artificial prosthesis [108, 215]. Good long term results were reported for survival, function and cosmetic and social acceptance [83, 89, 108], but the situation is, of course, cosmetically challenging. The technique is also available for tumors of the proximal femur [209] and, in the arm, for primary malignant tumors of the elbow or shoulder [208].

A special type of lower limb tumor is that which affects the pelvis. Hemipelvectomy is the only operation applicable in most malignant tumors of the pelvic girdle, and this is the operation which affords the best chance of curing malignant bone and soft tissue tumors of the upper thigh. The first attempt at hemipelvectomy was by Billroth; according to Ravitch and Wilson [155, 156] this failed attempt was casually reported by Savariaud in 1902 [175] whilst he was reporting his own unsuccessful attempt at hemipelvectomy. In 1895, Girard [77, 78] of Bern performed the first hemipelvectomy with survival of the patient [78]. By the time of his 1902 report, Savariaud was able to find 13 cases in all, one of them carried out by Salistcheff, of

Tomsk, in Russia, in 1900. Only four of these patients had survived the operation. Ransohoff [154], of Cincinnati, in 1909, performed a hemipelvectomy for tuberculosis of the hip, often called the first successful such operation in the USA. He lost “not more than a few ounces of blood” and was given an infusion of salt water. However, his patient died more than a month later of unrelieved sepsis. In the UK, Lee and Alt [115] presented their experience of seven operations, with no deaths. The largest individual experience was that of Sir Gordon Gordon-Taylor [81], with 102 pelvis amputations.

1.2.3.2 Limb Salvage Techniques

Limb-saving procedures in bone tumor patients involve resection of the bony lesion with a wide margin of soft tissue and reconstruction by cadaver allogenic grafts or prostheses [4, 23, 33, 35, 58, 111, 121, 138, 164, 170, 199, 200, 205, 216]. Some authors report attempted reimplantation of the affected bone after extracorporeal treatment, such as soaking in ethanol [191], autoclaving [8, 74], or irradiation [201].

Limb-sparing techniques were first devised during the early 1970s, but were developed in the 1990s for most malignant bone tumors. The modern tools of anesthesiology enable safe limb-saving intervention. These procedures can be offered to patients only when life expectancy is comparable with that of ablative surgery. Treatment results for 925 osteosarcoma patients in a COSS study, and 975 Ewing sarcoma patients in an EICESS study, justify limb-salvage surgery when the correct indications are present; 5-year survival rates are similar to or better than those for amputation [9, 130, 177]. Greenberg et al. [84] and Christ et al. [40], in separate studies, compared the functional and psychological assessment of osteosarcoma survivors treated by amputation and limb sparing. In general, most survivors were in good mental and physical health and the emotional disturbance among these patients was no different from that in the general population. On the other hand, patients with initial amputations had substantial difficulty maintaining an optimal level of limb function.

Early attempts, at the beginning of the twentieth century, at limb salvage in bone tumors were developed in lower leg tumors by Ferdinand Sauerbruch, in Germany [174]. In the same year, the inter-scapulo-thoracic resection of the shoulder girdle was developed by Tikhov in Tomsk, Russia. A similar method was described by Linberg (Smolensk, Russia) in 1928 [118]. Ernest Juvara (1870–1933), a Romanian doctor, developed a technique (which bears the name of Vittorio Putti) for arthrodesis in the treatment of malignant bone tumors, performed by resecting the tumor and performing arthrodesis in the affected joint.

There are two options for knee reconstruction after resection of the upper end of the tibia and lower end of the femur: arthrodesis and arthroplasty. There are several options for reconstruction after limb-sparing tumor resections in the limbs, and the choice is conditioned by the patient’s age (adult or growing child) and the tumor site and size. During the procedure, various techniques may be used, some of which are temporary and others definitive. Great care must be taken during surgery in order to avoid complications. Some techniques require one operation, while others involve a long process involving many different techniques. The development of these limb-sparing techniques has only been possible subsequent to finding the means to cure patients' diseases. The options for reconstruction after limb-salvage tumor resection include arthrodesis, endoprosthetic replacement, allografts, autografts, rotation-plasty or physeal distraction and bone distraction.

1.2.3.3 Graft Indications in Bone Tumor Surgery

In 1908 Lexer [117] reported his first four clinical bone tumor cases in which he used massive allografts derived from tissue procured from amputation. Methods of bone and cartilage preservation and storage were slowly adapted [26]. Bauer [11], in 1910, showed that bone could be preserved by refrigeration for as long as 3 weeks and then, in dogs, could be transplanted as allografts. At the same time, Kaush [103] established that boiled bone was far inferior to autogeneic bone. Albee and Gallie both used stored bone [3, 72], chilled or boiled, for clinical surgery. A hospital bone bank was organized by Inclan [95] in Havanna, Cuba, in 1942, who procured human bone at operation and preserved it in blood or saline solution at between 2 and 5 °C before implanting it [206]. Duthie [57] established the first bone bank in the UK, in Edinburgh, in 1953, while at the same time Sanchis-Olmos [173] founded the first Spanish tissue bank in Madrid. Merle d'Aubigné established the French equivalent in Hopital Cochin, Paris, in 1955. Three centers reported variable outcomes with the use of allografts for limb salvage following tumor resection: Ottolenghi from Argentina [144], Parrish [145] in the United States, and Volkov [204] in the Soviet Union. The use of allografts increased after a series of reports by Mankin et al. [122–124, 126, 183], and today bone banks have been established around the world in specialized bone tumor centers.

Autografts are performed using vascularized or nonvascularized fibula grafts to fill diaphyseal bone defects after wide tumor resection. The fibula is more suitable for reconstruction of the upper limbs than for that of the lower limbs. The vascularized fibula can be inserted into the allograft, such as the tibia, in order to reinforce its total bone grafting capacity [37]. A previous method for autografting was to remove the bone tumor from the resected bone and then sterilize the bone by autoclaving, irradiation [201] or pasteurization [136] before reimplantation.

Allografts have been used commonly since the 1970s for reconstruction of the remaining bone after limb-sparing tumor resection. Reconstructive options for such large defects include structural allograft transplantation [23, 36, 41, 61, 65, 92, 124, 139, 169, 214], endoprosthetic arthroplasty [14, 23, 85, 86, 134, 142, 200, 212], and composite reconstruction using allografts and metal prostheses [13, 56].

The most important late complications are graft collapse and instability, or osteoarthritis of the joint. Several studies have reported high rates of fracture, non-union, infection, and other major complications that often require removal or revision of the allograft [53, 60, 61, 65, 75, 92, 126, 139, 172]. The majority of allograft complications occur within the first 2 years of therapy. Mankin et al. [126] reported on delayed union of the graft (32 %), a complication that can be partly explained by long-term chemotherapy, graft fracture (12–20 %) and infection (11 %).

1.2.3.4 Prostheses in Tumor Surgery

In the context of radical excision surgery, there has been development of special segmental bone and joint replacement systems, which are usually referred to as tumor endoprotheses or megaprotheses [79]. The term *megaprosthesis* seems to have been first used in the International Workshop on Design and Application of Tumor Prostheses, held at the Mayo Clinic in 1981. Endoprostheses are frequently considered to be the gold standard treatment after resection of tumors that involve a joint, particularly the knee and hip; but, even with the most modern devices, prosthetic survival without re-operation is still only 60 % at 5 years.

The first noteworthy report – it included a 2-year follow up study – on a metal hip joint was published in 1943 by Austin Moore and Harald Bohlman [135] in the United States. Total femur reconstruction was first described by Buchman [24] in the mid-twentieth century. The first tumor endoprostheses were mostly based on a custom made monoblock of cast steel alloys. There followed various developments in terms of the materials used: titanium and cobalt–chrome–molybdenum alloys; various acrylic polymers were subjected to trials and found to fail as a result of wear and were abandoned.

Prosthesis design has also evolved from a monoblock and fixed hinge model to modular endoprostheses and rotating platforms, with improved geometry to enhance fixation and stability [39, 178, 179]. Modular endoprostheses, which are currently standard and have predominated in surgical practice since 1980, consist of a number of different components in readily available sets. Various combinations of components can be assembled in the operating room in order to best address the specific bone defect of the patient.

In the former USSR, the first tumor prosthesis was implanted in 1967 by Sivash and Trapeznikov. By 1972 John Scales [176], in Stanmore, England, was using titanium endoprostheses for massive replacement after tumor surgery. Scales used intramedullary stem fixation with PMMA, and was also the first surgeon to introduce extending prostheses with a growing mechanism. The first custom-made knee prosthesis for tumors was implanted in 1975 in Vienna, followed by a total of 15 cases between 1976 and 1982 with different types of cementless stem fixation with two plates and a fixed hinge [106]. The design was then changed, and from this, in 1982, arose a modular system, which was published as the Kotz modular femur-tibia reconstruction system (KMFTR) [107]. In the United States, in 1977, Ralph Marcove used total femur and total knee replacement in osteosarcoma cases [127]. In Italy, Mario Campanacci published an account of the total resection of the distal femur or proximal tibia for bone tumors in 1979 [33]. Modular ceramic prostheses for the humerus have been in use since 1972 [168]. More recently, the combination of allograft and prosthetic components (APC) has been advocated as an optional solution [13, 56].

Limb salvage surgery of the proximal tibia is one of the most demanding reconstructions owing to difficulties with soft tissue coverage [100, 181, 182], a high rate of infection (12–36 %) [13, 41, 56, 85, 100, 140], and the need to restore the knee extensor mechanism [14, 23, 85, 124, 139, 142], all of which lead to high failure rates (27–55 %) [41, 56, 92, 211]. As an alternative, the use of proximal tibia osteoarticular allografts after tumor resection may restore bone stock and help reconstruct the extensor mechanism [41, 92, 122, 139].

Relative to the use of allografts, prosthetic reconstruction offers some advantages, such as, maintenance of motion and immediate functional restoration [2, 14, 23, 134, 139, 140, 142, 200, 211]. Although high survival rates have been reported with current modular-type reconstruction [134, 140], the complication rate increases more rapidly with time compared with conventional endoprostheses, which is of great importance considering the young age of most osteo- and Ewing- sarcoma patients. In the large series published by Mittelmayer [134], aseptic loosening (27 %) and infection and fracture (54–54 %) of the implant were the most frequent complications leading to a need for intervention. Deep infection and aseptic loosening are the most frequent causes of failure [82].

For peri-acetabular tumors, Enneking and Dunham [63], Steel [186], Zatsepin [214] and Nilsonne et al. [143] preferred resection of the involved part of the pelvis and a reconstructive procedure in which the femur was put in contact with the remaining part of the pelvis [207]. The aim of the procedure was arthrodesis or prosthesis reconstruction, so that the results would be long-lasting and full weight-bearing would be possible. The disadvantage was, and is, the inevitable discrepancy in leg length, with a less than satisfactory functional and cosmetic result. Johnson [101] described a procedure in which the osseous gap was filled with cement in combination with a total hip replacement.

1.2.3.5 Malignant Bone Tumors in Growing Patients

The metaphysis is the predominant site of malignant bone tumors in children. For many years, when the adjacent metaphysis was involved in a malignant tumor, the physis was resected to obtain complete tumor excision with clear margins. This inevitably resulted in a discrepancy of limb length or dysfunction of the joint [73]. In some cases, preservation of the epiphyseal portion of the bone and the joint surface may be achieved by physeal distraction. However, this applies only to patients in whom the epiphysis is still open [31, 171]. Using Cañadell's technique, the epiphysis of the tumor-bearing bone can be preserved so that the function and growth capability of the involved joint are maintained. The indications for the Cañadell technique are that (1) the tumor should be localized in the metaphysis; (2) the growth plate should be open; and (3) the tumor should not affect the physis, which should be confirmed by radiography, arteriography, CT or MRI preoperatively and pathological analysis of the resection after the operation [31]. MRI is considered to be the gold standard technique for determining the invasiveness of metaphyseal tumors [131, 171].

Skeletal reconstruction in skeletally immature children and adolescents is particularly challenging in that it must be dynamic in order to accommodate future growth. Expandable prostheses were developed in an effort to control the limb length discrepancy following limb-sparing surgery, but multiple surgical interventions were required to carry out the lengthening procedure [86, 109, 110]. Automatic modules were only used in distal femur locations. Noninvasive extendable lengthening devices, for instance those driven by an electromagnetic field from outside the body, are now available and broaden the indications for limb salvage in young patients [2, 86]. However, a conventional prosthesis can also be applied, followed by lengthening using an external fixator [32].

The use of osteosynthesis techniques (intermedullary pins and plates) is usual in tumor surgery, taking into consideration the special biomechanical characteristics of large bone defects and of the grafts used in limb sparing. The external fixator is of particular interest, usually being used as a temporary solution before tumor resection surgery (to prevent pathologic fractures), during resection surgery (to maintain bone length or perform physeal distraction) or after surgery to combat complications (infection, graft fracture) or correct deformities (dysmetry) [32, 35, 170].

1.3 Conclusion

History shows us that experience is our best teacher. Despite difficulties along the path of development, we have been able to find new ways of improving treatment and life expectancy. As diagnostic and therapeutic techniques improve, patients with musculoskeletal sarcomas can expect increased survival, decreased complications and side effects, and an improved quality of life. Much work remains to be done, and bone tumor surgeons need to keep pushing to better their patients' quality of life and to keep working to increase the survival rate with more accurate and convenient systems of diagnosis and treatment. We are now witnessing the introduction of targeted therapies including monoclonal antibodies and small signaling pathway inhibitors and drugs that act on specific immune checkpoints. Additionally, the search is on for new biomaterials to deliver drugs specifically and effectively into cancer cells. Moreover, research on expression profiling and proteomics can increasingly help us to distinguish more aggressive cancers from less aggressive ones, information that could also be useful for cancer screening. Further knowledge is needed about oncogenes and tumor suppressor genes. Finally, from the technical point of view, work is needed on systems that can remove tumors completely without surgical trauma.

References

1. Abe M, Takahashi M, Yabumoto E, Adachi H, Yoshii M, Mori K. Clinical experiences with inteaoperative radiotherapy of locally advanced cancers. Cancer. 1980;45:40–8.
2. Abudu A, Grimer RJ, Tillman R, Carter SR. The use of prostheses in skeletally immature patients. Orthop Clin North Am. 2006;37:75–84.
3. Albee FH. Bone graft surgery. Philadelphia: WB Saunders; 1915.
4. Alman BA, De-Bari A, Krajbich JI. Massive allografts in the treatment of osteosarcoma and Ewing sarcoma in children and adolescents. J Bone Joint Surg Am. 1995;77-A:54–64.
5. Ando K, Heymann M-F, Stresing V, Mori K, Rédini F, Heymann D. Current therapeutic strategies and novel approaches in osteosarcoma. Cancers. 2013;5:591–616.
6. Andreou D, Bielack SS, Carrle D, Kevric M, Kotz R, Winkelmann W, et al. The influence of tumor-and treatment-related factors on the development of local recurrence after adequate surgery. An analysis of 1355 patients treated on neoadjuvant Cooperative Osteosarcoma Study Group protocols. Ann Oncol. 2011;22:1228–35.
7. Arndt CA, Crist WM. Common musculoskeletal tumors of childhood and adolescence. N Engl J Med. 1999;341:342–52.
8. Asada N, Tsuchiya H, Kitaoka K, Mori Y, Tomita K. Massive autoclaved allografts and autografts for limb salvage surgery. A 1–8 year follow-up of 23 patients. Acta Orthop Scand. 1997;68:392–5.
9. Ayerza MA, Farfalli GL, Aponte-Tineo L, Muscolo L. Does increased rate of limb-sparing surgery affect survival osteosarcoma? Clin Orthop Relat Res. 2010;468:2854–9.
10. Bacci G, Ferrari S, Bertoni F, Ruggieri P, Picci P, Longhi A, et al. Long-term outcome for patients with nonmetastatic osteosarcoma of the extremity treated at the Istituto Ortopedico Rizzoli according to the Istituto Ortopedico Rizzoli Osteosarcoma-2 protocol: an updated report. J Clin Oncol. 2000;18:4016–27.
11. Bauer F. Über Knochentransplantation. Z Chirurg. 1910;37:20.
12. Bernstein M, Kovar H, Paulussen M, Randall RL, Schuck A, Teot LA, et al. Ewing's sarcoma family of tumors: current management. Oncologist. 2006;11:503–19.
13. Biau DJ, Dumaine V, Babinet A, Tomeno B, Anract P. Allograftprosthesis composites after bone tumor resection at the proximal tibia. Clin Orthop Relat Res. 2007;456:211–7.
14. Bickels J, Wittig JC, Kollender Y, Neff RS, Kellar-Graney K, Meller I, et al. Reconstruction of the extensor mechanism after proximal tibia endoprosthetic replacement. J Arthroplasty. 2001;16:856–62.
15. Bielack SS, Kempf-Bielack B, Delling G, Exner GU, Flege S, Helmke K, et al. Prognostic factors in high-grade osteosarcoma of the extremities or trunk: an analysis of 1,702 patients treated on neoadjuvant cooperative osteosarcoma study group protocols. J Clin Oncol. 2002;20:776–90.
16. Bilbao JI, Martín Algarra S, Martínez de Negri J, Lecumberri F, Longo J, Sierrasesúmaga L, et al. Osteosarcoma: correlation between radiological and histological changes after intra-arterial chemotherapy. Eur J Radiol. 1990;11:98–103.
17. Bleyer WA, Haas JE, Feigl P, Greenlee TK, Schaller RT, Morgan A, et al. Improved three-year disease-free survival in osteogenic sarcoma. Efficacy of adjunctive chemotherapy. J Bone Joint Surg (Br). 1982;64-B:233–8.
18. Bloodgood J. The conservative treatment of giant-cell sarcoma, with the study of bone transplantation. Ann Surg. 1912;56:210–39.
19. Bonadonna G, Monfardini S, deLena M, Fossatti-Bellani F, Buretta G. Phase I and preliminary phase II evaluation of Adriamycin (NSC-12127). Cancer Res. 1970;30:2572–82.
20. Borggreve J. Kniegelenkersatz durch das in der Beinlangachse um 180 Grad gedrehte Fussgelenk. Arch Orthop Unfallchir. 1930;28:175–8.
21. Bowden L, Booher RJ. The principles and techniques of resection of soft parts of sarcoma. Surgery. 1958;44:963–77.

22. Brand RA. Ernest Amory Codman MD, 1869–1940. Clin Orthop Relat Res. 2009;467:2763–5.
23. Brien EW, Terek RM, Healey JH, Lane JM. Allograft reconstruction after proximal tibial resection for bone tumors: an analysis of function and outcome comparing allograft and prosthetic reconstructions. Clin Orthop Relat Res. 1994;303:116–27.
24. Buchman J. Total femur and knee joint replacement with a vitallium endoprosthesis. Bull Hosp Joint Dis. 1965;26:21–34.
25. Burgert Jr EO, Nesbit ME, Garnsey LA, Gehan EA, Herrmann J, Vietti TJ, et al. Multimodal therapy for the management of nonpelvic, localized Ewing's sarcoma of bone: intergroup study IESS-II. J Clin Oncol. 1990;8:1514–24.
26. Burwell RG. History of bone grafting and bone substitutes with special reference to osteogenic induction. In: Urist MR, O'Connor BT, Burwell RG, editors. Bone grafts, derivates and substitutes. Oxford: Blutterworth-Heinemann; 1994. p. 3–101.
27. Cade S. Osteogenic sarcoma. A study based on 133 patients. J R Coll Surg Edinb. 1955;1:79.
28. Calvo FA, Sierrasesúmaga L, Martin I, Santos M, Voltas J, Berian JM, Cañadell J. Intraoperative radiotherapy in the multidisciplinary treatment of pediatric tumors. A preliminary report on initial results. Acta Oncol. 1989;28:257–60.
29. Campanacci M, Bacci G, Paganini P, Giunti A. Multiple-drug chemotherapy for the primary treatment of osteosarcoma of the extremities. J Bone Joint Surg (Br). 1980;62-B:93–101.
30. Campanacci M, Laus M. Local recurrence after amputation for osteosarcoma. J Bone Joint Surg (Br). 1980;62-B:201–7.
31. Cañadell J, Forriol F, Cara JA. Removal of metaphyseal bone tumours with preservation of the epiphysis. Physeal distraction before excision. J Bone Joint Surg (Br). 1994;76-B:127–32.
32. Cañadell J, San-Julian M, Cara J, Forriol F. External fixation in tumour pathology. Int Orthop. 1998;22:126–30.
33. Capanna R, Morris HG, Campanacci D, Del Ben M, Campanacci M. Modular uncemented prosthetic reconstruction after resection of tumours of the distal femur. J Bone Joint Surg (Br). 1994;76-B:178–86.
34. Cara del Rosal JA, Cañadell J. Biopsy technique in the treatment of osteosarcoma. Int Orthop. 1994;18:375–8.
35. Cara JA, Cañadell J. Limb salvage for malignant bone tumors in young children. J Pediatr Orthop. 1994;14:112–8.
36. Cara JA, Lacleriga A, Cañadell J. Intercalary bone allografts. 23 tumor cases followed for 3 years. Acta Orthop Scand. 1994;65:42–6.
37. Ceruso M, Falcone C, Innocenti M, Delcroix L, Capanna R, Manfrini M. Skeletal reconstruction with a free vascularized fibula graft associated to bone allograft after resection of malignant bone tumor of limbs. Handchir Mikrochir Plast Chir. 2001;33:277–82.
38. Chapman JA, Deakin DP, Green JH. Slipped upper femoral epiphysis after radiotherapy. J Bone Joint Surg (Br). 1980;62-B:337–9.
39. Choong PF, Sim FH, Pritchard DJ, Rock MG, Chao EY. Megaprostheses after resection of distal femoral tumors. A rotating hinge design in 30 patients followed for 2–7 years. Acta Orthop Scand. 1996;67:345–51.
40. Christ CH, Lane JP, Christ AE. Long-term psychosocial adaptation of osteosarcoma survivors. Oncology. 1993;335:1.
41. Clohisy DR, Mankin HJ. Osteoarticular allografts for reconstruction after resection of a musculoskeletal tumor in the proximal end of the tibia. J Bone Joint Surg Am. 1994;76-A:549–54.
42. Codman EA. The registry of bone sarcoma as an example of the end-result idea in hospital organization. Bull Amer Coll Surg. 1924;8:34–8.
43. Coley BL, Higinbotham NL. Indications for hemipelvectomy. Surgery. 1958;44:766.
44. Coley WB. Treatment of inoperable malignant tumors with toxins of erisipelas and the bacillus prodigiosus. Trans Am Surg Assoc. 1894;12:183–212.
45. Cortes EP, Holland JF. Glidewell 0. Amputation and adriamycin in primary osteosarcoma: a 5 years report. Cancer Treat Rep. 1978;62:271–7.
46. Cortes EP, Holland JF, Wang JJ, Sinks LF, Blom J, Senn H, et al. Amputation and Adriamycin in primary osteosarcoma. N Engl J Med. 1974;291:998–1000.

47. Cortes EP, Holland JF, Wang JJ, Sinks LF. Doxorubicin in disseminated osteosarcoma. JAMA. 1972;221:1132–8.
48. Cotterill SJ, Ahrens S, Paulussen M, et al. Prognostic factors in Ewing's tumor of bone: analysis of 975 patients from the European Intergroup Cooperative Ewing's Sarcoma Study Group. J Clin Oncol. 2000;18:3108–14.
49. Coventry MB, Dahlin DC. Osteogenic sarcoma. A critical analysis of 430 cases. J Bone Joint Surg Am. 1957;39:741–57.
50. Dahlin DC, Coventry MB. Osteogenic sarcoma: a study of 600 cases. J Bone Joint Surg Am. 1967;49-A:101–10.
51. de Stéfani E, Carzoglio J, Deneo Pellegrini H, Olivera L, Cendan M, Kasdorf H. Ewing's sarcoma: value of tumor necrosis as a predictive factor. Bull Cancer. 1984;71:16–21.
52. Delaney G, Jacob S, Featherstone C, Barton M. The role of radiotherapy in cáncer treatment: estimating optimal utilization from a review of evidence-based clinical guidelines. Cancer. 2005;104:1129–37.
53. Dick HM, Malinin TI, Mnaymneh WA. Massive allograft implantation following radical resection of high-grade tumors requiring adjuvant chemotherapy treatment. Clin Orthop Relat Res. 1985;197:88–95.
54. DiPietro S, dePalo G, Gennari L, Molinari R, Damascelli B. Cancer chemotherapy by intra-arterial infusión with Adriamycin. J Surg Oncol. 1973;5:521–30.
55. Dohnal AM, Graffi S, Witt V, Eichstill C, Wagner D, Ul-Haq S, et al. Comparative evaluation of techniques for the manufacturing of dendritic cell-based vaccines. J Cell Mol Med. 2008;13:125–35.
56. Donati D, Colangeli M, Colangeli S, Di Bella C, Mercuri M. Allograft-prosthetic composite in the proximal tibia after bone tumor resection. Clin Orthop Relat Res. 2008;466: 459–65.
57. Duthie RB. The formation and operation of a bone bank in Edinburgh. Edinb Med J. 1953;60:316.
58. Eckardt JJ, Eiber FR, Dorey FJ, Mirra JM. The UCLA experience in limb salvage surgery for malignant tumors. Orthopedics. 1985;8:612–21.
59. Eilber F, Giuliano A, Eckhardt J. Adjuvant chemotherapy for osteosarcoma: a randomized prospective trial. J Clin Oncol. 1987;5:21–6.
60. Eilber FR, Mirra JJ, Grant TT, Weisenburger T, Morton DL. Is amputation necessary for sarcomas? A seven-year experience with limb salvage. Ann Surg. 1980;192:431–7.
61. Enneking WF, Campanacci DA. Retrieved human allografts: a clinicopathological study. J Bone Joint Surg Am. 2001;83-A:971–86.
62. Enneking WF, Dunham W, Gebhardt MC, Malawar M, Pritchard DJ. A system for the functional evaluation of reconstructive procedures after surgical treatment of tumors of the musculoskeletal system. Clin Orthop Relat Res. 1993;286:241–6.
63. Enneking WF, Dunham WK. Resection and reconstruction for primary neoplasms involving the innominate bone. J Bone Joint Surg Am. 1978;60-A:731–46.
64. Enneking WF, Kagan A. The implications of "skip" metastases in osteosarcoma. Clin Orthop Relat Res. 1975;111:33–41.
65. Enneking WF, Mindell ER. Observations on massive retrieved human allografts. J Bone Joint Surg Am. 1991;73-A:1123–42.
66. Enneking WF, Spanier SS, Goodman MA. A system for the surgical staging of musculoskeletal sarcoma. Clin Orthop Relat Res. 1980;153:106–20.
67. Evans RG, Nesbit ME, Gehan EA, Garnsey LA, Burgert Jr O, Vietti TJ, et al. Multimodal therapy for the management of localized Ewing's sarcoma of pelvic and sacral bones: a report from the second intergroup study. J Clin Oncol. 1991;9:1173–80.
68. Fletcher BD, Hanna SL, Fairclough DL, Gronemeyer SA. Pediatric musculoskeletal tumors: use of dynamic, contrast-enhanced MR imaging to monitor response to chemotherapy. Radiology. 1992;184:243–8.
69. Friedman MA, Carter SK. The therapy of osteogenic sarcoma: current status and thoughts for the future. J Surg Oncol. 1972;25:489–95.

70. Frouge C, Vanel D, Coffre C, Couanet D, Contesso G, Sarrazin D. The role of magnetic resonance imaging in the evaluation of Ewing sarcoma. A report of 27 cases. Skeletal Radiol. 1988;17:387–92.
71. Fuchs N, Bielack S, Epler D, Bieling P, Delling G, Körholz D, et al. Long-term results of the co-operative German- Austrian-Swiss osteosarcoma study group's protocol COSS-86 of intensive multidrug chemotherapy and surgery for osteosarcoma of the limbs. Ann Oncol. 1998;9:893–9.
72. Gallie WE. The use of boiled bone in operative surgery. Am J Orthop Surg. 1918;16:373.
73. Gao S, Zheng Y, Cai Q, Yao W, Wang J. Preliminary clinical research on epiphyseal distraction in osteosarcoma in children. World J Surg Oncol. 2014;12:251–8.
74. Gebhardt MC, Flugstad DI, Springfield DS, Mankin HJ. The use of bone allografts for limb salvage in high-grade extremity osteosarcoma. Clin Orthop Relat Res. 1991;270:181–96.
75. Getty PJ, Peabody TD. Complications and functional outcomes of reconstruction with an osteoarticular allograft after intra-articular resection of the proximal aspect of the humerus. J Bone Joint Surg Am. 1999;81-A:1138–46.
76. Gilbert HA, Kagan RA, Winkley J. Soft tissue sarcomas of the extremities: their natural history, treatment and radiation sensivity. J Surg Oncol. 1975;7:303–17.
77. Girard C. Desarticulation de l'os Iliaque pour Sarcome. Rev de Chir. 1895;15:952.
78. Girard C. Sur la Desarticulation Interilio-abdominale. Rev de Chir. 1898;18:1141.
79. Gkavardina A, Tsagozis P. The use of megaprostheses for reconstruction of large skeletal defects in the extremities: a critical review. Open Orthop J. 2014;8:384–9.
80. Golfieri R, Baddeley H, Pringle JS, Leung AW, Greco A, Souhami R. MRI in primary bone tumors: therapeutic implications. Eur J Radiol. 1991;12:201–7.
81. Gordon-Taylor G, Wiles PW. Interinnomino- abdominal (Hindquarter) amputation. Br J Surg. 1935;22:671.
82. Gosheger G, Gebert C, Ahrens H, Streitbuerger A, Winkelmann W, Hardes J. Endoprosthetic reconstruction in 250 patients with sarcoma. Clin Orthop Relat Res. 2006;450:164–71.
83. Gottsauner F, Kotz R, Knahr K, Kristen H, Ritschl P, Salzer M. Rotatioplasty for limb salvage in the treatment of malignant tumors in the knee. J Bone Joint Surg Am. 1991;73-A:1365–75.
84. Greenberg DB, Goorin A, Gebhardt MC, Gupta L, Stier N, Harmon D, et al. Quality of life in osteosarcoma survivors. Oncology (Huntingt). 1994;8:19–25.
85. Grimer RJ, Carter SR, Tillman RM, Sneath RS, Walker PS, Unwin PS, Shewell PC. Endoprosthetic replacement of the proximal tibia. J Bone Joint Surg (Br). 1999;81-B:488–94.
86. Grimer RJ. Surgical options for children with osteosarcoma. Lancet Oncol. 2005;6:85–92.
87. Haskell CM, Sullivan A. Comparative survival in tissue culture of normal and neoplastic human cells exposed to adriamycin. Cancer Res. 1974;34:2991–4.
88. Hayes FA, Thompson EI, Meyer WH, Kun L, Parham D, Rao B, et al. Therapy for localized Ewing's sarcoma of bone. J Clin Oncol. 1989;7:208–13.
89. Hillmann A, Hoffmann C, Gosheger G, Krakau H, Winkelmann W. Malignant tumor of the distal part of the femur or the proximal part of the tibia: endoprosthetic replacement or rotationplasty. Functional outcome and quality-of-life measurements. J Bone Joint Surg Am. 1999;81-A:462–8.
90. Holscher HC, Bloem JL, Nooy MA, Taminiau AH, Eulderink F, Hermans J. The value of MR imaging in monitoring the effect of chemotherapy on bone sarcomas. AJR Am J Roentgenol. 1990;154:763–9.
91. Hoption Cann SA, van Netten JP, van Netten C. Dr William Coley and tumor regression: a place in history or in the future. Postgrad Med J. 2003;79(938):672–80. www.postgradmedj.com.
92. Hornicek Jr FJ, Mnaymneh W, Lackman RD, Exner GU, Malinin TI. Limb salvage with osteoarticular allografts after resection of proximal tibia bone tumors. Clin Orthop Relat Res. 1998;352:179–86.
93. Huvos AG. James Ewing: cancer man. Ann Diagn Pathol. 1998;27:57–71.
94. Huvos AG, Rosen G, Marcove RC. Primary osteogenic sarcoma. Pathologic aspects in 20 patients after treatment with chemotherapy, en bloc resection and prosthetic bone replacement. Arch Pathol Lab Med. 1977;101:14–8.

95. Inclan A. The use of preserved bone graft in orthopaedic surgery. J Bone Joint Surg Am. 1942;24:81.
96. Jaffe N. Adjuvant methotrexat and citrovorumfactor treatment of osteogenic sarcoma. N Engl J Med. 1974;291:994–7.
97. Jaffe N, Carrasco H, Raymond K, Ayala A, Eftekhari F. Can cure in patients with osteosarcoma be achieved exclusively with chemotherapy and abrogation of surgery? Cancer. 2002;95:2202–10.
98. Jaffe N, Watts H, Fellows KE, Vawter G. Local en bloc resection for limb preservation. Cancer Treat Rep. 1978;62:217–23.
99. Jaffe N. Recent advances in the chemotherapy of metastatic osteogenic sarcoma. Cancer. 1972;30:1627–31.
100. Jeon DG, Kawai A, Boland P, Healey JH. Algorithm for the surgical treatment of malignant lesions of the proximal tibia. Clin Orthop Relat Res. 1999;358:15–26.
101. Johnson JT. Reconstruction of the pelvic ring following tumourresection. J Bone Joint Surg Am. 1978;60-A:747–51.
102. Jürgens H, Exner U, Gadner H, Harms D, Michaelis J, Sauer R, et al. Multidisciplinary treatment of primary Ewing's sarcoma of bone. A 6-year experience of a European Cooperative Trial. Cancer. 1988;61:23–32.
103. Kaush W. Über Knochenersatz. Beiträge zur Transplantation toten Knochens. Beitr Klin Chir. 1910;68:670.
104. Kinsella TJ, Miser JS, Waller B, Venzon D, Glatstein E, Weaver-McClure L, et al. Long-term follow-up of Ewing's sarcoma of bone treated with combined modality therapy. Int J Radiat Oncol Biol Phys. 1991;20:389–95.
105. Kotoura Y, Yamamuro T, Kasahara K. Histological studies of the effect of intra-operative radiation therapy. In: Abe M, Takahashi M, editors. Intra-operative radiation therapy. New York: Pergamon Press; 1991. p. 373–5.
106. Kotz R, Engel A. Endoprothesen bei großen Knochenresektionen. Öst Ärzteztg. 1981;36:1–7.
107. Kotz R, Ritschl P, Trachtenbrodt J. A modular femur-tibiareconstruction-system. Orthopedics. 1986;9:1639–52.
108. Kotz R, Salzer M. Rotationplasty for chilhood osteosarcoma of the distal part of the femur. J Bone Joint Surg Am. 1982;64-A:959–69.
109. Kotz R, Windhager R, Dominkus M, Robioneck B, Müller-Daniels H. A self-extending paediatric leg implant. Nature. 2000;406:143–4.
110. Krepler P, Dominkus M, Kotz R. Die endoprothetische Versorgung an den Extremitäten bei Kindern nach Resektion primär maligner Knochentumoren. Orthopade. 2003;32:1013–9.
111. Kropej D, Schiller C, Ritschl P, Salzer-Kuntschik M, Kotz R. The management of IIB osteosarcoma. Experience from 1976 to 1985. Clin Orthop Relat Res. 1985;270:40–4.
112. Lane JM, Rosen G, Boland P, Otis J, Abou-Zahr K. Surgical management of osteogenic sarcoma of the lower limb. Bull NY Acad Med. 1985;61:395–404.
113. Lang P, Vahlensieck M, Matthay KK, Johnston JO, Rosenau W, Gooding CA, et al. Monitoring neovascularity as an indicator to response to chemotherapy in osteogenic and Ewing sarcoma using magnetic resonance angiography. Med Pediatr Oncol. 1996;26:329–33.
114. Le Deley MC, Guinebretière JM, Gentet JC, Pacquement H, Pichon F, Marec-Bérard P, et al. SFOP OS94: a randomised trial comparing preoperative high-dose methotrexate plus doxorubicin to high-dose methotrexate plus etoposide and ifosfamide in osteosarcoma patients. Eur J Cancer. 2007;43:752–61.
115. Lee Jr CM, Alt LP. Hemipelvectomy and hip disarticulation for malignant tumors of the pelvis and lower extremity. Ann Surg. 1953;137:704.
116. Lewis IJ, Nooij MA, Whelan J, Sydes MR, Grimer R, Hogendoorn PC, et al. Improvement in histologic response but not survival in osteosarcoma patients treated with intensified chemotherapy: a randomized phase III trial of the European Osteosarcoma Intergroup. J Natl Cancer Inst. 2007;99:112–28.
117. Lexer E. Die Verwendung der freien Knochenplastik nebst Versuchen über Gelenkversteifung und Gelenktransplantation. Arch Klin Chirurg. 1908;68:940.

118. Linberg BE. Interscapulo-thoracic resection for malignant tumours of the shoulder joint region. J Bone Joint Surg. 1928;26:344–9.
119. Lindberg RD. The role of radiation therapy in the treatment of soft tissue sarcoma in adults. In: Proc 7th National Cancer Congress. Philadelphia: JB Lippincott Co; 1972.
120. Link MP, Goorin AM, Miser AW, Green AA, Pratt CB, Belasco JB, et al. The effect of adjuvant chemotherapy on relapse-free survival in patients with osteosarcoma of the extremity. N Engl J Med. 1986;314:1600–6.
121. Malawer MM, Chou LB. Prosthetic survival and clinical results with use of large-segment replacements in the treatment of high-grade bone sarcomas. J Bone Joint Surg Am. 1995;77-A:1154–65.
122. Mankin HJ, Doppelt SH, Sullivan TR, Tomford WW. Osteoarticular and intercalary allograft transplantation in the management of malignant tumors of bone. Cancer. 1982;50:613.
123. Mankin HJ, Gebhardt MC, Jennings LC, Springfield DS, Tomford WW. Long-term results of allograft replacement in the management of bone tumors. Clin Orthop Relat Res. 1996;324:86–97.
124. Mankin HJ, Gebhardt MC, Tomford WW. The use of frozen cadaveric allografts in the management of patients with bone tumors of the extremities. Orthop Clin North Am. 1987;18: 275–89.
125. Mankin HJ, Lange TA, Spanier SS. The Hazards of biopsy in patients with malignant primary bone and soft tissue tumors. J Bone Joint Surg Am. 1982;64-A:1121–7.
126. Mankin HJ, Springfield DS, Gebhardt MC, Tomford WW. Current status of allografting for bone tumors. Orthopedics. 1992;15:1147–54.
127. Marcove R, Lewis MM, Rosen G, Huvos AG. Total femur and total knee replacement. A preliminary report. Clin Orthop Relat Res. 1977;126:147–52.
128. Marcove RC, Mike V, Hajek JV, Levin AG, Hutter RV. Osteogenic sarcoma under the age of twenty-one. A review of one hundred and forty-five operative cases. J Bone Joint Surg Am. 1970;52-A:411–23.
129. Marcove RC, Stovell PB, Huvos AG, Bullough PG. The use of cryosurgery in the treatment of low and medium grade chondrosarcoma. A preliminary report. Clin Orthop Relat Res. 1977;122:147–56.
130. Marulanda GA, Henderson ER, Johnson DA, Letson GD, Cheong D. Orthopedic surgery options for the treatment of primary osteosarcoma. Cancer Control. 2008;15:13–20.
131. Masrouha KZ, Musallam KM, Samra AB, Tawil A, Haidar R, Chakhachiro Z, et al. Correlation of non-mass-like abnormal MR signal intensity with pathological findings surrounding pediatric osteosarcoma and Ewing's sarcoma. Skeletal Radiol. 2012;41:1453–61.
132. McKenna RJ, Schwinn CD, Soong KY, Higinbotham ML. Sarcomata of the ostegenic series: an analysis of 552 cases. J Bone Joint Surg Am. 1966;48-A:1–26.
133. Meyers PA, Gorlick R, Heller G, Casper E, Lane J, Huvos AG, et al. Intensification of preoperative chemotherapy for osteogenic sarcoma: results of the Memorial Sloan – Kettering (T12) protocol. J Clin Oncol. 1998;16:2452–8.
134. Mittermayer F, Krepler P, Dominkus M, Schwameis E, Sluga M, Heinzl H, et al. Long term follow up of uncemented tumor endoprostheses for the lower extremity. Clin Orthop Relat Res. 2001;388:167–77.
135. Moore A, Bohlmann H. Metal hip joint. A case report. J Bone Joint Surg Am. 1943;25-A: 688–92.
136. Morello E, Vasconi E, Martano M, Peirone B, Buracco P. Pasteurized tumoral autograft and adjuvant chemotherapy for the treatment of canine distal radial osteosarcoma: 13 cases. Vet Surg. 2003;32:539–44.
137. Morton JJ. Interinnomino-abdoimiinal (hindquarter) amputation. Ann Surg. 1942;115:628.
138. Morton DL, Eilber FR, Townsend CM, Grant TT, Mirra J, Weisenburger TH. Limb salvage from a multidisciplinary treatment approach for skeletal and soft tissue sarcomas of the extremity. Ann Surg. 1976;184:268–77.
139. Muscolo DL, Ayerza MA, Aponte-Tinao LA. Massive allograft use in orthopedic oncology. Orthop Clin North Am. 2006;37:65–74.

140. Myers GJ, Abudu AT, Carter SR, Tillman RM, Grimer RJ. The long-term results of endoprosthetic replacement of the proximal tibia for bone tumours. J Bone Joint Surg (Br). 2007;89-B:1632–7.
141. Nagashima T, Yamamuro T, Kotoura Y, Takahashi M, Abe M, Nakashima Y. Histological studies on the effect of intra- operative irradiation for osteosarcoma. J Jpn Orthop Assoc. 1983;57:1681–97.
142. Natarajan MV, Sivaseelam A, Rajkumar G, Hussain SH. Custom megaprosthetic replacement for proximal tibial tumours. Int Orthop. 2003;27:334–7.
143. Nilsonne U, Kreicbergs A, Olsson E, Stark A. Function after pelvic tumour resection involving the acetabular ring. Int Orthop. 1982;6:27–33.
144. Ottolenghi CE. Massive osteo and osteo-articular bone grafts: technique and results of 62 cases. Clin Orthop Relat Res. 1972;87:156–64.
145. Parrish FF. Allograft replacement of all or part of the end of a long bone following excision of a tumor. J Bone Joint Surg Am. 1973;55-A:1–22.
146. Patel SJ, Lynch JW, Johnson T, Carroll RR, Schumacher C, Spanier S. Dose-intense ifosfamide/doxorubicin/cisplatin based chemotherapy for osteosarcoma in adults. Am J Clin Oncol. 2002;25:489–95.
147. Paulussen M, Ahrens S, Burdach S, Craft A, Dockhorn-Dworniczak B, Dunst J, et al. Primary metastatic (stage IV) Ewing tumor: survival analysis of 171 patients from the EICESS studies. Ann Oncol. 1998;9:275–81.
148. Picci P, Bacci G, Campanacci M, Gasparini M, Pilotti S, Cerasoli S, et al. Histologic evaluation of necrosis in osteosarcoma induced by chemotherapy. Regional mapping of viable and nonviable tumor. Cancer. 1985;56:1515–21.
149. Picci P, Sangiorgi L, Rougraff BT, Neff JR, Casadei R, Campanacci M. Relationship of chemotherapy-induced necrosis and surgical margins to local recurrence in osteosarcoma. J Clin Oncol. 1994;12:2699–705.
150. Pinedo HM, Kenis Y. Chemotherapy of advanced soft tissue sarcoma in adults. Cancer Treat Rev. 1977;4:67–86.
151. Pinedo HM, Vendrik CP, Staquet M, Kenis Y, Sylvester R. EORTC protocol for therapy of metastatic soft tissue sarcoma: a randomized trial. Eur J Cancer. 1977;13:756–71.
152. Pratt CB, Rivera G, Shanks E, Kumar AP, Green AA, George S. Combination chemotherapy for osteosarcoma. Cancer Treat Rep. 1978;62:251–8.
153. Price CH, Thuber K, Saizer-Kuntachik M, Salzer M, Willert HG, Immenkamp M, et al. Osteosarcoma in children. J Bone Joint Surg (Br). 1975;57-B:341–5.
154. Ransohoff J. Interilio-abdominal amputation. With report of a case. Ann Surg. 1909;50:925.
155. Ravitch MM. Hemipelvectomy. Surgery. 1949;26:199.
156. Ravitch MM. Radical treatment of massive mixed angiomas (hemolymph angiomas) in infants and children; with report of hemipelvectomy in a 13-day-old infant. Ann Surg. 1951;134:228.
157. Rella W, Kotz R, Arbes H, Leber H. Tumor-specific immunity in sarcoma patients. Oncology. 1977;34:219–23.
158. Rosen G. Disease-free survival in children with Ewing's sarcoma treated with radiation therapy and adjuvant four-drug sequential chemotherapy. Cancer. 1974;33:384–93.
159. Rosen G, Caparros B, Groshen S, Nirenberg A, Cacavio A, Marcove RC, et al. Primary osteosarcoma of the femur: a model for the use of preoperative chemotherapy in high risk malignant tumors. Cancer Invest. 1984;2:181–92.
160. Rosen G, Caparros B, Huvos AG, Kosloff C, Nirenberg A, Cacavio A, et al. Preoperative chemotherapy for osteogenic sarcoma: selection of postoperative adjuvant chemotherapy based on the response of the primary tumor to preoperative chemotherapy. Cancer. 1982;49:1221–30.
161. Rosen G, Marcove RC, Huvos AG. Primary osteogenic sarcoma: eight year experience with adjuvant chemotherapy. J Cancer Res Clin Oncol. 1983;106:55–67.
162. Rosen G, Murphy ML, Huvos AG, Gutierrez M, Marcove RC. Chemotherapy, en bloc resection, and prosthetic bone replacement in the treatment of osteogenic sarcoma. Cancer. 1976; 37:1–11.

163. Rosen G, Tan C, Sanmaneechai A, Beattle Jr EJ, Marcove RC, Murphy ML. The rationale for multiple drug chemotherapy in the treatment of osteogenic sarcoma. Cancer. 1975;35:936–45.
164. Rougraff BT, Simon MA, Kneisl JS, Greenberg DB, Mankin HJ. Limb salvage compared with amputation for osteosarcoma of the distal end of the femur. A long-term oncologic al, functional, and quality-of-life study. J Bone Joint Surg Am. 1994;76-A:649–56.
165. Rubin P, Andrews JR, Swarm R, Gump H. Radiation induced dysplasias of bone. AJR. 1959;82:206–16.
166. Rusell WO, Cohen J, Enzinger F, Hajdu SI, Heise H, Martin RG, et al. A clinical and pathological staging system for soft tissue sarcoma. Cancer. 1977;40:1562–70.
167. Salzer M, Knahr K, Locke H, Stärk N, Matejovsky Z, Plenk Jr H, et al. A bioceramic endoprosthesis for the replacement of the proximal humerus. Arch Orthop Trauma Surg. 1979;93:169–84.
168. Salzer M, Salzer-Kuntschik M. Das Wiener Knochengeschwulstregister. Wien Klin Wochenschr. 1968;80:401–2.
169. San Julian Aranguren M, Leyes M, Mora G, Cañadell J. Consolidation of massive bone allografts in limb-preserving operations for bone tumours. Int Orthop. 1995;19:377–82.
170. San Julian M, Dolz R, Garcia-Barrecheguren E, Noain E, Sierrasesumaga L, Cañadell J. Limb salvage in bone sarcomas in patients younger tan age 10. A 20 years of experience. J Pediatr Orthop. 2003;23:753–62.
171. San-Julian M, Aquerreta JD, Benito A, Cañadell J. Indications for epiphyseal preservation in metaphyseal malignant bone tumors of children: relationship between image methods and histological findings. J Pediatr Orthop. 1999;19:543–8.
172. San-Julian M, Cañadell J. Fractures of allografts used in limb preserving operations. Int Orthop. 1998;22:32–6.
173. Sanchís Olmos V. El banco de huesos del Hospital Provincial de Madrid. Acta Ortop Traum Ibérica. 1953;1:3–12.
174. Sauerbruch F. Die Extirpation des Femurs mit Umkippplastik des Unterschenkels. Dtsch Z Chir. 1922;169:1–2.
175. Savariaud M. Un cas de desarticulation interilio abdominale. Procede a lambeau interne. Rev de Chir. 1902;26:345.
176. Scales JT, Sneath RS, Wright KW. Design and clinical use of extending prostheses. In: Enneking WF, editor. Limb salvage in musculoskeletal oncology. New York/Edinburgh/London/Melbourne: Churchill Livingstone; 1987. p. 52–61.
177. Schrager J, Patzer RE, Mink PJ, Ward KC, Goodman M. Survival outcomes of pediatric osteosarcoma and Ewing's sarcoma: a comparison of surgery type within the SEER database, 1988–2007. J Registry Manag. 2011;38:153–61.
178. Schwartz AJ, Kabo JM, Eilber FC, Eilber FR, Eckardt JJ. Cemented distal femoral endoprostheses for musculoskeletal tumor: improved survival of modular versus custom implants. Clin Orthop Relat Res. 2010;468:2198–210.
179. Shehadeh A, Noveau J, Malawer M, Henshaw R. Late complications and survival of endoprosthetic reconstruction after resection of bone tumors. Clin Orthop Relat Res. 2010;34:871–6.
180. Shiu MH, Castrol EB, Hadju SI, Fortner JG. Surgical treatment of 297 soft tissue sarcomas of the lower extremity. Ann Surg. 1975;182:597–602.
181. Sim FH, Beauchamp CP, Chao EY. Reconstruction of musculoskeletal defects about the knee for tumor. Clin Orthop Relat Res. 1987;221:188–201.
182. Sim FH, Chao EY. Hip salvage by proximal femoral replacement. J Bone Joint Surg (Br). 1981;63-B:1228–39.
183. Sim FH, Frassica FJ. Use of allografts following resection of tumors of the musculoskeletal system. Instr Course Lect. 1993;42:405–13.
184. Simon MA, Hecht JD. Invasion of joints by primary sarcoma in adults. Cancer. 1980;50:1649–55.
185. Springfield DS, Schmidt R, Graham-Pole J, Marcus Jr RB, Spanier SS, Enneking WF. Surgical treatment for osteosarcoma. J Bone Joint Surg Am. 1988;70-A:1124–30.

186. Steel HH. Partial or complete resection of the hemi-pelvis: an alternative to hindquarter amputation for peri-acetabular chondrosarcoma of the pelvis. J Bone Joint Surg Am. 1978;60-A:719–30.
187. Stein JJ. Osteogenic sarcoma (osteosarcoma): results of therapy. Am J Roentgenol. 1975;123: 607–13.
188. Steinman RM, Hemmi H. Dendritic cells: translating innate to adaptive immunity. Curr Top Mocrobiol Immunol. 2006;311:17–58.
189. Suit HD, Rusell WO. Radiation therapy of soft tissue sarcomas. Cancer. 1975;36:759–64.
190. Suit HD, Russell WO, Martin RG. Sarcoma of soft tissue: clinical and histopathological parameters and response to treatment. Cancer. 1975;35:1478–83.
191. Sung HW, Wang HM, Kuo DP, Hsu WP, Tsai YB. EAR method: an alternative method of bone grafting following bone tumor resection (a preliminary report). Semin Surg Oncol. 1986;2:90–8.
192. Sutow WW, Gehan EA, Dyment PG, Vietti T, Miale T. Multidrug adjuvant chemotherapy for osteosarcoma: interim report of the Southwest Oncology Group Studies. Cancer Treat Rep. 1978;62:265–9.
193. Sweetham R, Knowelden J, Seddon H. Bone sarcoma: treatment by irradiation, amputation, or a combination of the two. BMJ. 1971;2:363–7.
194. Sweetman R. Amputation in osteosarcoma. J Bone Joint Surg (Br). 1973;55B:189–92.
195. Szendröi M. Advances in orthopaedic oncology. Int Orthop. 2002;26:195–6.
196. Traina F, Errani C, Toscano A, Pungetti C, Fabbri D, Mazzotti A, et al. Current concepts in the biopsy of musculoskeletal tumors: AAOS exhibit selection. J Bone Joint Surg Am. 2015;97-A:7.
197. Trifaud A, Meary R. Prognostic et traitement des sarcomes osteogeniques. Paris: Masson; 1972.
198. Tsuboyama T, Toguchida J, Kotoura Y, Kasahara K, Hiraoka M, Nakamura T. Intra-operative radiation therapy for osteosarcoma in the extremities. Int Orthop. 2000;24:202–7.
199. Tsuchiya H, Tomita K. Prognosis of osteosarcoma treated by limb-salvage surgery: the ten-year intergroup study in Japan. Jpn J Clin Oncol. 1992;22:347–53.
200. Unwin PS, Cannon SR, Grimer RJ, Kemp HB, Sneath RS, Walker PS. Aseptic loosening in cemented custom-made prosthetic replacements for bone tumours of the lower limb. J Bone Joint Surg (Br). 1996;78-B:5–13.
201. Uyttendaele D, de Schryver A, Classens H, Roels H, Berkvens P, Mondelaers W. Limb conservation in primary bone tumours by resection extracorporeal irradiation and re-implantation. J Bone Joint Surg (Br). 1988;70-B:348–53.
202. van der Woude HJ, Bloem JL, Verstraete KL, Taminiau AH, Nooy MA, Hogendoorn PC. Osteosarcoma and Ewing's sarcoma after neoadjuvant chemotherapy: value of dynamic MR imaging in detecting viable tumor before surgery. AJR Am J Roentgenol. 1995;165:593–8.
203. Van Nes CP. Rotationplasty for congenital defects of the femur. Making use of the ankle of the shortened limb to control the knee joint of a prosthesis. J Bone Joint Surg (Br). 1950;32-B:12–6.
204. Volkov M. Allotransplantation of joints. J Bone Joint Surg (Br). 1970;52-B:49.
205. Wilkins RM. Complications of allograft reconstructions. In: Simon MA, Springfield D, editors. Surgery for bone and soft-tissue tumors. Philadelphia: Lippincott-Raven Pub; 1998. p. 487–96.
206. Wilson PD. Experiences with a bone bank. Ann Surg. 1947;126:932.
207. Windhager R, Karner J, Kutschera HP, Polterauer P, Salzer-Kuntschik M, Kotz R. Limb salvage in periacetabular sarcomas. Clin Orthop Relat Res. 1996;331:265–76.
208. Windhager R, Millesi H, Kotz R. Resection-replantation for primary malignant tumors of the arm. An alternative to fore-quarter amputation. J Bone Joint Surg (Br). 1995;77-B:176–84.
209. Winkelmann WW. Type-B-a-IIIa hip rotationplasty: an alternative operation for the treatment of malignant tumors of the femur in early childhood. J Bone Joint Surg Am. 2000;82-A:814–28.
210. Winkler K, Beron G, Kotz R, Salzer-Kuntschik M, Beck J, Beck W, et al. Neoadjuvant chemotherapy for osteogenic sarcoma. Results of a cooperative German/Austrian study. J Clin Oncol. 1984;2:617–24.

211. Wu CC, Henshaw RM, Pritsch T, Squires MH, Malawer MM. Implant design and resection length affect cemented endoprosthesis survival in proximal tibial reconstruction. J Arthroplasty. 2008;23:886–93.
212. Wunder JS, Leitch K, Griffin AM, Davis AM, Bell RS. Comparison of two methods of reconstruction for primary malignant tumors at the knee: a sequential cohort study. J Surg Oncol. 2001;77:89–99.
213. Wunder JS, Paulian G, Huvos AG, Heller G, Meyers PA, Healey JH. The histological response to chemotherapy as a predictor of the oncological outcome of operative treatment of Ewing sarcoma. J Bone Joint Surg Am. 1998;80-A:1020–33.
214. Zatsepin ST. Conservative operation for pelvic bone tumours. Int Orthop. 1981;4:259–68.
215. Zeltzer L, Kellerman J, Ellenberg L, Dash J, Rigler D. Psychologic effects of illness in adolescence. II. Impact of illness in adolescents. Crucial issues and coping styles. J Pediatr. 1980;97:132–8.
216. Zwart HJ, Taminiau AH, Schimmel JW, van Horn JR. Kotz modular femur and tibia replacement. 28 tumor cases followed for 3 (1–8) years. Acta Orthop Scand. 1994;65:315–8.

Chapter 2
Non-surgical Treatment of Pediatric Bone Sarcomas

Luis Sierrasesúmaga, Isabel Martin, and Moira Garraus

Abstract The functional results of surgery are important, but only when survival of a patient is achieved. The key to success in the overall treatment of malignant bone tumors in children lies in multi-disciplinarity. A good response to chemotherapy together with function-preserving surgery of quality (that assures local control of the disease) are both fundamental to treatment success.

Keywords Chemotherapy • Bone sarcomas • Radiotherapy • Local Control • Relapse • Osteosarcoma • Ewing's Sarcoma • Limb Salvage

2.1 Introduction

Pediatric bone sarcomas are malignant tumors of the bone. The optimum treatment of bone tumors affecting children and adolescents requires a multidisciplinary approach combining surgery, radiotherapy and chemotherapy. Treatment success is based on early diagnosis and on adequate experience of the medical team; for this reason it is advisable that these cases be treated in centers highly specialized in the management of this pathology [1, 2].

Not all bone tumors are malignant. Benign bone tumors are more common than malignant ones [3]. There are no epidemiology data specifically comparing pseudotumoral and benign bone lesions. Benign conditions are 100 times more frequent than malignant primary bone tumors. Simple bone cyst and Langerhans cells

L. Sierrasesúmaga, MD, PhD (✉)
Department of Pediatrics, University Clinic of Navarra
Avda. Pio XII s/n 31080, Pamplona, Navarra E31080, Spain
e-mail: lsierra@unav.es

I. Martin, MD, PhD
Centro de salud de La Rochapea, Pamplona, Spain

M. Garraus, MD, PhD
Department of Pediatrics, Hospital San Joan de Deu, Barcelona, Spain

M. San-Julian (ed.), *Cañadell's Pediatric Bone Sarcomas: Epiphysiolysis before Excision*, DOI 10.1007/978-3-319-24220-0_2

histiocytosis represent more than 50 % of all pseudotumoral lesions; typically, they affect children and teenagers with a median age of 12 years. With respect to benign lesions, the most frequent are the benign chondroblastic lesions (osteochondromas and chondromas) and osteoid osteoma. Aneurysmal bone cyst is also considered a benign entity.

Malignant bone tumors, with average rates in Europe of the order of 6–7 cases per million, generally represent between 5 and 7 % of childhood cancers. The two most frequent types are osteosarcomas and Ewing's tumors. The former constitute a little more than half of bone tumors, the Ewing's tumors over 40 %. Chondrosarcomas represent about 2 % (rates of the order of 0.1 cases per million). Bone tumors are very infrequent in babies and infants. Incidence increases with age, peaking in the age range of 10–14 years, in which a little over 10 % of all such tumors occur. Osteosarcomas are rare before 5 years of age. Until that age, Ewing's tumors are slightly more frequent than osteosarcomas. The incidence of both types becomes practically equal in the 5–9 year-old group and, in the 10–14 year-old group the incidence of osteosarcoma (OS) overtakes that of the Ewing's tumors. Ewing's sarcomas (ES) are slightly more predominant in males [4].

2.2 Treatment of Osteosarcoma (OS)

The bad prognosis initially associated with OS treated exclusively with local therapy (radical surgery) took a turn for the better when systemic chemotherapy was introduced into the treatment schemes in the 1980s. The majority of patients with localized disease develop metastasis within 1 year if they only receive local treatment. However, at the time of diagnosis, the best available methods only detect metastatic disease in 10–20 % of cases [5]. This means that micro metastases exist at the moment of diagnosis in the majority of patients [6]. Currently, treatments based on chemotherapy in conjunction with surgery achieve a 5-year event-free survival rate of 60–70 % in extremity localized, non-metastatic disease. Two major problems are the poor prognosis after metastatic relapse or recurrence, and the poor prognosis for patients with unresectable axial tumors [7].

2.2.1 Surgery

The objective of surgery is to achieve en-bloc resection of the tumor and preserve as much function as possible. Complete surgical resection, if feasible, remains essential for cure. Local control can only be achieved with complete resection margins [8]. In accordance with the definitions of Enneking, complete resection implies the total extirpation of the tumoral tissue (including the biopsy scar) surrounded by an envelope of normal healthy tissue [9]. In the case of a localized OS, as opposed to other sarcomas, achieving surgical remission is important for the overall cure, and so the fundamental objective is to establish adequate surgical margins at the time of local control surgery. In the past, there was controversy over the suitability of conservative surgery as opposed to amputation; currently, with modern treatments for conservation of the extremity, local relapse occurs in 4–10 % of patients, and there do not seem to be clear differences in this respect between ablation surgery and limb salvage surgery [8]. One study found local recurrence rates of 2–3 % after amputation and 5–7 % after conservative surgery, with no significant differences in survival [10]. Amputation is currently reserved for those cases in which it not considered possible to resect the primary tumor; in the great majority of cases it is possible to use surgical techniques that conserve the extremity [11, 12]. During the last few years, the role of conservation surgery has increased markedly. As a result of refinements in neoadjuvant chemotherapy, biomechanical engineering and imaging studies, approximately 80–90 % of patients with OS are now candidates for conservation surgery [13]. Local recurrence has been attributed to insufficient surgical margins, with only a wide margin being considered appropriate [14], although no general agreement exists on what constitutes an adequate margin thickness. Also, surgical margin width in bone has been found not to correlate with the local recurrence rate [15].

At the time of OS diagnosis, about 10–20 % of patients present macroscopic evidence of metastatic disease, most commonly (90 %) in the lungs, but metastases can also develop in bone (8–10 %) and rarely in lymph nodes [13]. The treatment of pulmonary metastases is surgical resection (thoracotomy with metastasectomy) plus effective adjuvant chemotherapy [16].

2.2.2 Radiotherapy

OS is considered a radioresistant tumor [17]. However, radiotherapy can be an adjuvant option as local treatment of unresectable tumors, or as palliation of symptomatic metastases. Conventional external beam radiotherapy with systemic chemotherapy treatment may provide a successful multimodal approach to local control and symptom relief [18]. Proton therapy to deliver high radiotherapy doses has been successfully used as local treatment for some patients with unresectable or incompletely resected OS [19].

2.2.3 Chemotherapy

Before the introduction of adjuvant chemotherapy, more than 80 % of osteosarcoma patients developed metastatic disease. The first studies using individual agents began in the 1960s and 1970s and established, on a non-randomized basis, the role of chemotherapy in the management of osteosarcoma. Prior to the 1960s, OS was considered a chemo resistant tumor. The agents initially investigated yielded inconsistent results. They included l-phenylalanine mustard (with a response rate of 16 %), mitomycin C (response, 24 %), cyclophosphamide (response, 15 %), vincristine, 5-fluorouracil and nitrogen mustard [20]. A regimen comprising mitomycin C, phenylalanine mustard, and vincristine proved fruitless [20]. Responses to individual chemotherapeutic agents, such as, high doses of methotrexate or doxorubicin, were described in 20–40 % of patients with metastatic disease [21].

However, the demonstration of the importance of systemic treatment in the management of osteosarcoma was not established definitively until the publication of the results of a multi-institutional study, which randomized patients with exclusively surgical treatment versus surgery combined with chemotherapy [22].

Current chemotherapy protocols include combinations of the following agents: high dose methotrexate, doxorubicin, cyclophosphamide, cisplatin, ifosfamide, etoposide, and carboplatin, which cure 50–75 % of patients with localized disease. Regimens containing three active chemotherapy agents have been shown to be superior to regimens containing two active agents; regimens with four active agents were not superior to regimens with three active agents; the meta-analysis suggested that three drug regimens that did not include high dose methotrexate were inferior to three drug regimens that did include high dose methotrexate [23–32]. Chemotherapeutic agents such as bleomycin, cyclophosphamide, and dactinomycin (actinomycin D) have been largely abandoned, as they have not proved to be as effective as the other aforementioned drugs [33].

Preoperative, or *neoadjuvant,* chemotherapy is generally administered for a period of about 8–10 weeks prior to surgery. Following surgical resection and a brief break to allow for wound healing, postoperative adjuvant chemotherapy is continued for a period of another 12–29 weeks [34]. The preoperative chemotherapeutic treatment allows time to plan limb salvage surgery and reconstructive procedures and to study the histological effect of preoperative chemotherapy on the primary tumor so that adjustment of postoperative chemotherapy can be considered [35].

2.2.4 Lessons from the T-10 Protocols

For over two decades, the treatment of OS has followed the basic principles dictated by the T-10 protocol [35]. The T-10 protocol and its variants consist in a chemotherapy regimen with high doses of methotrexate, doxorubicin, cisplatin and a combination of bleomycin, cyclophosphamide and dactinomycin. With the T-10 protocol, the disease-free survival (DFS) at 5 years, as described by its authors, approximates to 70 % [35]. In a study undertaken by the European Osteosarcoma Intergroup (EOI), patients were randomized to receive the T-10 protocol or a simpler protocol, with six cycles of a combination of cisplatin and doxorubicin. The final DFS results were equal in the two branches, which suggests that a simple regimen, with cisplatin and doxorubicin, can cure more than half non-metastatic osteosarcoma patients [36].

One of the greatest contributions of T-10 and its predecessor, T-7, has been the finding that the histological response to the neoadjuvant chemotherapy is the most important prognostic factor in patients with localized disease [37, 38].

Intensification of post-operative or pre-operative therapy with doxorubicin, cisplatin and ifosfamide (IFX) was not found to improve upon T-10 results [38–40]. In the overall setting of intensive multidrug treatment (with high-dose methotrexate [HDMTX], doxorubicin, cisplatin, and ifosfamide), there was no detectable correlation between higher dose intensities and better outcomes [41]. This conclusion is supported by the results of studies by the European Osteosarcoma Intergroup (EOI), the Italian Sarcoma Group (ISG) and the Scandinavian Sarcoma Group (SSG) [7].

A delay of more than 21–24 days in the resumption of chemotherapy after surgery – especially for patients with lower degrees of necrosis – was associated with an increased risk of recurrence and death [37, 42].

2.2.5 *Ifosfamide or the Ifosfamide/Etoposide Combination in the Treatment of OS*

Ifosfamide (IFX) has been incorporated in osteosarcoma treatment regimens. As a consequence of the first studies, which indicated that IFX as sole agent achieved response rates of 10–60 % in patients with refractory disease, some researchers began to use the drug in the rescue of patients with a poor histological response [43]. Originally, IFX doses of 5–8 g/m^2 were used although higher doses (12–18 g/m^2) may be more effective [44]. A study by the Pediatric Oncology Group (POG) in patients with previously untreated metastatic disease demonstrated responses in 27 % of cases; the dose used was 12 g/m^2 [45]. More recently, IFX has been incorporated as a frontline therapy in the treatment of OS under many regimens [33]. However, the final impact of this incorporation is still not clear [45].

The finding that administration of an alkylating agent with etoposide has a synergistic anti-tumoral effect has led to the combined administration of IFX and etoposide in fractionated form over a period of 3–5 days. In patients with refractory OS and who had previously received IFX, the IFX-etoposide combination achieved response rates of 15–48 % [46]. Recently, for patients with metastatic OS, researchers at the POG incorporated the IFX-etoposide combination in the basic treatment with cisplatin, doxorubicin and high dose methotrexate and achieved responses in 62 % of patients; the DFS at 2 years was 45 % [44]. In patients with metastatic OS, the combination of IFX with etoposide seems to be more effective than that of IFX alone. These results suggest that future studies should investigate this combination in the treatment of patients with localized disease. In particular, the use of the IFX-etoposide combination is being used more frequently for the rescue of patients with a poor histological response; however, there is no evidence that this modification to the treatment improves survival rates. A joint European-American (EURAMOS-1) study found that adding ifosfamide and etoposide to MAP (high-dose methotrexate, cisplatin, and doxorubicin) was associated with additional morbidity and had no effect on survival outcome [47]. Evidence from EURAMOS-1 does not support adaptation of postoperative chemotherapy based on histological response [47].

2.2.6 The Role of Methotrexate in the Treatment of OS

Methotrexate was one of the first drugs demonstrated to be active in OS [6] and has occupied a primordial role in the treatment of OS since then. A meta-analysis [32] of protocols for the treatment of OS concluded that three drug regimens that did not include high dose methotrexate were inferior to three drug regimens that did. Furthermore, certain evidence suggests that the pharmokinetics of methotrexate can influence the final result, although any such influence is inferior and less clear in the context of more-intensive protocols [48, 49]. In any case, the action of methotrexate seems to require that it be administered in high doses (normally 12 g/m^2), and administration of lower doses apparently has less impact [50].

The role of HDMTX has not yet been fully clarified [31]. The first EOI study randomized patients to receive six cycles of cisplatin and doxorubicin or four courses of the same combination each preceded by a cycle of HDMTX [36]. In this study, cisplatin-doxorubicin without HDMTX gave better results: DFS at 5 years was 57 % without HDMTX versus 41 % with. A possible reading of these results is that high doses of methotrexate may not be necessary if other agents are intensified. This interpretation may principally be valid when treatment protocols are followed in countries with fewer resources: monitorization of levels is not possible. In Latin America excellent results have been obtained using protocols without methotrexate, protocols that intensify cisplatin, doxorubicin, IFX and etoposide [51]. Daw et al. [31] conducted a multi-institutional trial (OS99) that evaluated the efficacy of carboplatin, ifosfamide, and doxorubicin without HDMTX in patients with newly diagnosed, localized, resectable OS. The regimen used was found to produce outcomes comparable to the outcomes of regimens containing cisplatin or HDMTX. Carboplatin, ifosfamide, and doxorubicin given without HDMTX resulted in 5-year event-free survival (EFS) estimates of 66.7 % and survival estimates of 78.9 %.

2.2.7 Cisplatin and Carboplatin

Cisplatin is one of the most effective agents against osteosarcoma. However, the toxicity of this agent is significant; it can cause loss of hearing and renal failure, both of which can be permanent in some cases. Toxicity can be reduced by using prolonged infusions. The substitution of carboplatin for cisplatin has been recently evaluated at the St. Jude Children's Research Hospital. In the context of an intense regimen with high doses of methotrexate, IFX and doxorubicin, the use of carboplatin resulted in a DFS at 3 years of 72 %, results comparable to treatments using cisplatin, but with much lower toxicity [45]. However, the incorporation of carboplatin in treatment protocols requires further careful evaluation because other recent studies have demonstrated low anti-tumoral effect when it is used alone in patients with metastatic disease [52]. Additionally, even in the context of a multiple agent regimen, carboplatin is inferior to cisplatin for patients with non-resectable or metastatic osteosarcoma [53].

2.2.8 Pre-/Post-operative Chemotherapy and Intra-arterial Chemotherapy

One of the greatest findings to come out of the T-10 protocol was that the grade of histological response to pre-operative chemotherapy is the most important prognostic factor in patients with localized disease [37]. To date this understanding still holds true, with patients who achieve a good histological response (usually defined as >90 % necrosis) having a better prognosis than those who do not [54, 55]. Studies have consistently demonstrated 5-year EFS rates of 35–45 % for poor responders and 70–80 % for good responders [56]. This observation has determined most current treatments; however, some findings suggest that although intensified chemotherapeutic regimens increased tumor necrosis, the overall survival remained unchanged [57]. Intensification of pre-operative chemotherapy with cisplatin, doxorubicin and IFX gives rise to a modest increase in the proportion of good responders, but the final impact is minimal. Modification of post-operative therapy by intensifying the use of cisplatin, doxorubicin or, more recently, with the incorporation of new agents such as IFX and etoposide have not resulted in significant improvement in the prognosis for patients with poor histological response [25, 40]. Exposure of tumoral cells to sub-optimal cytotoxic levels during pre-operative treatment can give rise to the development of chemo-resistance and increase the propensity to metastatic dissemination. Modification of postoperative therapy cannot reverse such adverse effects. Following this line of reasoning, the achievement of a fast, early response should be the principal objective. Alternatives to intensification of adjuvant chemotherapy could focus, therefore, on improving the pre-operative treatment.

In the 1980s, Jaffe et al. [58] demonstrated that with intra-arterial administration it was possible to achieve high concentrations of cisplatin in a tumor without compromising systemic exposure. Following this, various groups included intra-arterial administration of cisplatin in their treatment of osteosarcoma. Despite the relevance of this development, only two teams endeavored to investigate the matter in a randomized manner. One of these teams, researchers at the Instituto Ortopédico Rizzoli, randomized patients to receive cisplatin intra-arterially or intravenously under the IOR/OS-3 and IOR/OS-5 protocols. Under both protocols, the pre- and post- operative chemotherapy included doxorubicin and high doses of methotrexate, with the addition of IFX in the second protocol. Under both protocols, the proportion of good responders was greater in the group of patients treated with intra-arterial cisplatin, but the final results were similar in both groups [59]. Using a similar design, the other team, a German study, COSS-86, also failed to demonstrate any advantage to intra-arterial administration [60]. In a recent study, however, Wilkins et al. have described excellent results with this technique [61].

2.3 Treatment of Patients with Metastatic Disease

2.3.1 Metastatic Disease at Diagnosis

At the time of OS diagnosis, about 10–20 % of patients present with macroscopic evidence of metastatic disease, most commonly (90 %) in the lungs, but metastases can also develop in bone (8–10 %) and rarely in lymph nodes [62, 63]. However, the remaining 80–90 % of patients are assumed to have micrometastatic disease, which is subclinical or undetectable using current diagnostic equipment. In view of the poor prognosis, treatment of OS patients with observed metastatic disease must include an aggressive, multi-disciplinary approach with intensive pre-operative and post-operative chemotherapy and resection of both the primary tumor and metastases [62, 63]. Using this approach, contemporary protocols that incorporate IFX or the combination of IFX with etoposide, as well as methotrexate, doxorubicin and cisplatin, have been described to attain rates of DFS at 2 or 5 years of 25–45 % [62–64]; a longer follow-up, however, is necessary.

The addition of either muramyl tripeptide or ifosfamide to a standard chemotherapy regimen that included cisplatin, high dose methotrexate, and doxorubicin was evaluated using a factorial design in patients with metastatic osteosarcoma [65]. The appropriate role of muramyl tripeptide in the treatment of osteosarcoma remains under discussion.

Some authors have investigated the use of high-dose chemotherapy and autologous rescue of hematopoietic cells. Whilst this approach is reasonable and practicable, it does not seem to confer any advantage over the conventional treatment [66, 67].

Complete resection of pulmonary metastatic disease can be achieved in a high percentage of patients with residual lung nodules after preoperative chemotherapy. Multiple metastatic nodules imply a worse prognosis than do just one or two nodules, and bilateral lung involvement is worse than unilateral. Patients with peripheral lung lesions may have a better prognosis than patients with central lesions. Patients with fewer than three nodules confined to one lung have been found to have 5-year EFS of approximately 40–50 % [68].

After the lung, the second most common site of metastasis is another bone. The prognosis is poor for patients with metastasis to other bones distant from the primary tumor or with transarticular skip lesions [69, 70].

Multifocal OS is a different entity, and patients have an extremely poor prognosis. No patient with synchronous multifocal OS has ever been reported to be cured, but systemic chemotherapy and aggressive surgical resection may achieve significant prolongation of life [71].

2.3.2 Recurrent OS

Approximately 50 % of relapses occur within 18 months of therapy termination, and only 5 % of recurrences develop after five or more years [72]. The incidence of recurrence by site has been estimated as follows: lung (65–80 %), bone (8–10 %), local (4–7 %), and combined relapse (10–15 %) [72]. Other localizations of metastases are rare but may occur as late as 4 years after diagnosis [73].

For patients with OS in relapse, a very aggressive surgical approach is recommended. The survival rate at 4 years after relapse, for patients in whom it is possible to obtain a complete new remission, is approximately 30–40 %; it is 0 % for patients in whom the disease cannot be resected [74]. The role of systemic chemotherapy for the treatment of patients with recurrent osteosarcoma is not well defined. The choice of systemic treatment depends on the previous primary treatment. Ifosfamide (in combination with etoposide) has proved active in as many as one third of recurrent OS patients who had not previously received ifosfamide [75]. Cyclophosphamide and etoposide are active in recurrent OS, as is the combination of gemcitabine and docetaxel [76, 77]. Grignani et al. [78] reported rare objective responses and disease stabilization with sorafenib in patients with recurrent OS.

The prognostic factors for survival after relapse include the presence of isolated pulmonary metastasis: patients with metastases limited to the lungs have a better outcome than do patients with metastases to other sites or to the lungs combined with other sites [79]; late relapse (>24 months); and a low number of pulmonary lesions [16]. Bielack et al. [80] reported survival estimates with second and subsequent OS recurrences. Five-year overall survival (OAS) and EFS rates were 16 % and 9 % for second, 14 % and 0 % for third, 13 % and 6 % for fourth, and 18 % and 0 % for fifth recurrences, respectively [80]. The median interval from first to second recurrence was 9 months, and the median interval between subsequent recurrences was approximately 6 months [80].

2.3.3 Future Treatments

The survival rates for patients with metastatic disease at the time of diagnosis and for those in relapse are very low: less than 30 % survive [80]. For this reason it is necessary to develop new strategies, for example, strategies based on new drugs or new combinations of existing drugs, to treat patients with poor prognosis. The fractionated administration of cyclophosphamide with the inhibitor of topoisomerase, topotecan, seems to be a promising combination for the treatment of many pediatric neoplasias. However, in relapsed osteosarcoma patients, the rate of response was only 11 %, a response far lower than that observed in other neoplasias [81]. Sequential administration of gemcitabine and docetaxel has been demonstrated to be quite effective in the treatment of sarcomas in relapse [77]. In a study of a group of 35 adult patients with various relapsed sarcomas, the response rate was 43 %; the study included four patients with refractory osteosarcoma, of which two gave partial responses and two attained stable disease states [82].

Another agent that proved to have good activity *in vitro* against osteosarcoma is ecteinascidin-743 (ET-743). However, in spite of the promising results of preclinical studies, a phase II study in patients with recurrent osteosarcoma did not demonstrate any activity [83].

The majority of patients who relapse do so with lung metastases. In fact, most patients are considered to have micro metastatic lung disease at the moment of diagnosis. The possibility of controlling this microscopic lung disease on finalizing treatment for the primary tumor could give rise to a substantial improvement in survival. In an animal model, the administration of muramyl tripeptide encapsulated in liposomes (L-MTP-PE) activated pulmonary macrophages and brought about the eradication of lung micro metastases [84]. The Children's Oncology Group (COG) performed a prospective randomized trial in newly diagnosed children and young adults with localized OS. All patients received cisplatin, doxorubicin, and high dose methotrexate. One half of the patients were randomly assigned to receive ifosfamide. In a second randomization, one half of the patients were assigned to receive L-MTP-PE beginning after definitive surgical resection. The addition of ifosfamide did not improve outcome. The group that received L-MTP-PE had a longer EFS, but the improvement did not meet the conventional standard for statistical significance ($P=0.08$). The group did, however, show a significant improvement in OS (78 % vs. 70 %; $P=0.03$) [85]. The appropriate role of L-MTP-PE in the treatment of osteosarcoma remains under discussion.

It is possible that one might effect an activation of alveolar macrophages with nebulized GM-CSF. In a phase I study carried out in patients with lung metastasis of various refractory neoplasias, nebulized GM-CSF was successfully administered with minimal toxicity. The dose tolerated was 250 mcg/dose, twice a day for seven consecutive days every other week. Only two patients with OS were treated in the study, and in one of them the disease was stabilized for over 11 months [86].

Another interesting approach, which has been developed in an animal model, is gene transfer of IL-12 by nebularization using a non-viral vector, such as the cationic DNA transporter polyethylenimine (PEI). Therapy with IL-12 is based on the known anti-tumoral activity of this cytokine. However, the clinical use of IL-12 in a systemic way is limited by its toxicity. Using the technology of PEI-based IL-12 transfer in immunosuppressed mice with OS lung metastasis, researchers demonstrated an increase in the expression of IL-12 in lung tissue, accompanied by an increase in tissue levels of IL-12. It is important to note that an increased expression of IL-12 in the liver was not observed, which suggests that the systemic effects were minimal. In this animal model, the aerosol therapy brought about a significant decrease in the number of metastatic nodules. Also, it has been demonstrated that IL-12 increases, *in vitro*, the sensitivity of osteosarcoma to alkylating agents. This occurs through a mechanism involving activation of the Fas pathway. The implication is that IL-12, by aerosol, could have a synergistic effect with IFX. The same PEI transfer technique has been used for transfection of p53, which demonstrated anti-tumoral activity [87].

Aerosolization technology has extended to the administration of chemotherapeutic agents directly to the lungs. For example, 9-nitrocamptothecin was nebulized into either mice with subcutaneous xenoinserts of a variety of neoplasias or mice with osteosarcoma lung lesions. There was good anti-tumoral effect on both the subcutaneous and the lung tumors, which suggests that there is not only a local effect but also a systemic one. Based on these preliminary studies, a phase I study in patients with lung metastasis from refractory neoplasias has recently been completed; phase II studies are being developed [88].

The degree of necrosis observed in the primary tumor after an initial period of chemotherapy correlates with subsequent EFS and OS. An international consortium (EURAMUS) was formed to conduct a large prospective randomized trial. All patients received initial therapy with cisplatin, doxorubicin, and high dose methotrexate. Patients with more than 90 % necrosis were randomly assigned to continue the same chemotherapy after surgery or to receive the same chemotherapy with the addition of interferon. The addition of interferon did not improve the probability of EFS [89]. Patients with less than 90 % necrosis were randomly assigned to continue the same chemotherapy or to receive the same chemotherapy with the addition of high dose ifosfamide and etoposide.

Reports on the use of high dose samarium-153-EDTMP radioisotope therapy as a method to provide palliation for patients with bone metastases indicate feasibility, but so far the role of this treatment modality is not well defined [90]. In addition, high doses of samarium-153-EDTMP are being used increasingly as a therapeutic agent.

2.4 Treatment of Ewing's Sarcoma (ES)

In his initial description of ES as a diffuse endothelioma of the bone, James Ewing pointed out, among other characteristics of this tumor, that it has an elevated susceptibility to radiation therapy [91]. Over the following 50 years, radiotherapy continued to be the predominant way of treating ES, although 80 % of patients died after local relapse or metastatic disease during the 2 years after diagnosis.

The current therapeutic approach, which gives cause for much greater optimism in terms of cure rates, seeks to cure the patient while preserving the functionality of the affected body part and to minimize late secondary effects.

The approach comprehends a multi-disciplinary focus based on the following concepts:

1. ES has a systemic character at the time of diagnosis. The therapeutic approach requires adequate local control of the macroscopic disease, together with systemic control of micrometastasis.
2. Local control of the macroscopic disease must be multi-disciplinary: combining, according to necessity, surgery, radiotherapy and chemotherapy. The response to neoadjuvant chemotherapy and the surgical possibilities determine the doses and

fields of radiotherapy. Local control measures must not compromise systemic control.
3. Systemic control of micrometastasis must be carried out through the administration of a protocol of intensive cyclic polychemotherapy comprising agents of the greatest anti-tumoral activity available.
4. Treatment must be adapted to the characteristics of each patient, taking into account the primary localization, the size of the lesion, the staging and therapeutic possibilities according to age. This tailoring is necessary to obtain the maximum therapeutic benefit with the best possible functional result.

2.4.1 Chemotherapy for ES

Current protocols of chemotherapy for ES include vincristine, doxorubicin, ifosfamide/cyclophosphamide, and etoposide [92–94]. The mode of administration and dose intensity of chemotherapy within courses differs markedly between protocols. A European Intergroup Cooperative Ewing Sarcoma Study (EICESS) trial suggested that 1.2 g of cyclophosphamide produced a similar event free survival (EFS) as 6 g of ifosfamide in patients with lower risk disease. The same study also identified a trend toward better EFS for patients with localized ES, and a tendency for patients with higher-risk disease to receive a treatment that included etoposide [95]. Protocols in the USA generally alternate courses of vincristine, cyclophosphamide, and doxorubicin with courses of ifosfamide/etoposide [96], while European protocols generally combine vincristine, doxorubicin, and an alkylating agent with or without etoposide in a single treatment cycle [97].

Standard chemotherapy in current protocols includes vincristine, doxorubicin, and cyclophosphamide, also known as the VAdriaC or VDC regimen, alternating with ifosfamide and etoposide (IE) [98]. The combination of IE has shown activity in Ewing sarcoma, and a large randomized clinical trial and a nonrandomized trial demonstrated that outcome was improved when IE was alternated with VAdriaC [92–94]. Dactinomycin is no longer used in the United States but continues to be used in EuroEwing studies. In a meta-analysis of studies that had been undertaken before the standard use of ifosfamide and etoposide, increased dose intensity of doxorubicin during the initial months of therapy was associated with an improved outcome [99]. A 4-year EFS of 82 % has been reported for high dose VAdriaC and IE [100]. However, in an intergroup trial of the Pediatric Oncology Group and the Children's Cancer Group, which compared a dose-intensified chemotherapy regimen of vincristine, doxorubicin, cyclophosphamide, ifosfamide, and etoposide (VDC/IE) with standard doses of the same regimen, no differences in outcome were observed [101]. In a COG trial, patients were randomly assigned to receive chemotherapy (VAdriaC alternating with IE) given every 2 weeks (interval compression) versus every 3 weeks (standard). Patients treated every 2 weeks had an improved 5-year EFS relative to those treated every 3 weeks (73 % vs. 65 %, $P = .048$). There was no increase in toxicity observed with the every-2-week schedule [97]. The duration of primary chemotherapy ranges from 6 months to approximately 1 year.

For patients with a high risk of relapse with conventional treatments, certain researchers have utilized high-dose chemotherapy with hematopoietic stem cell transplant (HSCT) as consolidation treatment, in an effort to improve outcome [102–113]. A retrospective review using international bone marrow transplant registries compared, for patients with Ewing sarcoma at high risk for relapse, reduced intensity conditioning with high intensity conditioning followed by allogeneic stem cell transplant; outcomes were not found to differ [114]. Multiple small studies that report benefits achieved with HSCT have been published. However, these results are difficult to interpret because only patients who have a good initial response to standard chemotherapy are considered for HSCT [110].

2.4.2 *Treatment Response Factors to Preoperative Therapy*

Multiple studies have shown that patients with minimal or no residual viable tumor after presurgical chemotherapy have significantly better event free survival than patients with larger amounts of remaining viable tumor [115, 116]. For patients who receive preinduction and postinduction chemotherapy positron emission tomography (PET) scans, decreased FDG uptake after chemotherapy correlated with good histologic response and better outcome [117]. Patients with poor response to presurgical chemotherapy have a higher risk of local recurrence [118].

2.4.3 *Local Control of Disease*

Analysis of local control in ES is complicated because of the difficulties involved in the interpretation of the radiological studies typically used in follow-up, after administration of combined treatments. On many occasions, after surgery, radiotherapy and chemotherapy, the imaging signal obtained is not that of normal bone and is difficult to interpret. Persistence of residual material corresponding to fibrosis, necrosis or both is frequent. In this respect, studies with magnetic resonance after administration of gadolinium are more reliable than other imaging techniques.

The analysis of results in terms of local control referred to in the various reported series, which are generally lacking in biopsy/necropsy studies, can under- or overestimate the degree of control. Fernández et al. [119] registered a rate of clinical local relapse of 37.5 %, which after necroscopic studies increased to 47.5 %. In other studies, even larger differences have been detected: for example, a rate of local relapse being 65 % while clinical diagnoses suggested a rate of scarcely 25 % [120].

It is important to note that local control, while an indispensable condition for obtaining a full cure, can, however, accompany a prognosis of death. In the pre-chemotherapy era, rates of local control of 60–70 % were reported for series in which the rates of survival were below 20 % [121].

2.4.4 *Therapeutic Strategy to Obtain Local Control*

2.4.4.1 Radiotherapy

While surgery is effective and appropriate for patients who can undergo complete resection with acceptable morbidity, children who have unresectable tumors or who would suffer loss of function are treated with radiation therapy alone. Those who undergo gross resections with microscopic residual disease may benefit from adjuvant radiation therapy. Randomized trials that directly compare both modalities (i.e. resection with or without radiation therapy) do not exist, and so the relative roles of gross resection and radiotherapy remain controversial. Research addressing this issue are retrospective and nonrandomized, limiting their value. Krasin et al. [122] reported on a series of patients with localized ES who received both surgery and radiation. Local failure for patients with positive and negative margins was 17 % and 5 %, respectively, and overall survival (OS) was 71 % and 94 %, respectively. However, in a large retrospective study, 45 Gy adjuvant radiation therapy for patients with inadequate margins did not appear to improve either local control or disease free survival [123]. It is not known whether higher doses of radiation therapy could improve outcome. Adjuvant radiation therapy should be considered for patients with residual microscopic disease, inadequate margins, or viable tumor in the resected specimen and close margins. When preoperative assessment has suggested a high probability that surgical margins will be close or positive, preoperative radiation therapy has been used to shrink the tumor, thereby enabling surgical resection with clear margins [124].

Data for patients with pelvic primary ES from a North American intergroup trial showed no difference in local control or survival based on local control modality: surgery alone, radiation therapy alone, or radiation plus surgery [125]. For young children with ES, surgery may be a less morbid therapy than radiation therapy because radiation causes retardation of bone growth. Another potential advantage of surgical resection of the primary tumor is the information it can provide concerning the amount of necrosis in the resected tumor. Patients with residual viable tumor in the resected specimen have a worse outcome than those with complete necrosis. In a French Ewing study (EW88), EFS for patients with less than 5 % viable tumor, 5 % to 30 % viable tumor, and more than 30 % viable tumor was 75 %, 48 %, and 20 %, respectively [116].

ES shows great sensitivity to radiation [126]. The local control obtainable with irradiation is directly proportional to the dose administered and to the volume of tissue included in the field. The percentage of patients for whom radiotherapy alone achieves local control is between 50 and 80 %. With doses above 40 Gy, high percentages of local control are obtained. With lower doses, even when rapid clinical improvement and disappearance of macroscopic lesions are observed, the incidence of local relapse is very high [122].

For patients with residual disease after an attempt at surgical resection, the Intergroup Ewing Sarcoma Study recommends 45 Gy to the original disease site plus a 10.8 Gy boost for patients with gross residual disease and 45 Gy plus a 5.4 Gy boost for patients with microscopic residual disease. Radiation therapy is not recommended for those who have no evidence of microscopic residual disease following surgical resection. Radiation therapy is associated with the development of secondary malignant neoplasms. A retrospective study noted that the incidence of a secondary malignancy was 20 % for patients who had received 60 Gy or more and 5 % for those who received 48–60 Gy; none of those who received less than 48 Gy developed a second malignancy [127].

Hyperfractionated radiation therapy has not been associated with improved local control or decreased morbidity. A comparison of proton beam radiation therapy and intensity modulated radiation therapy (IMRT) has shown that proton beam radiation therapy can spare more normal tissue adjacent to the primary Ewing sarcoma than IMRT [128]. The study's follow-up was relatively short, and there are no data available to indicate whether the reduction in dose to adjacent tissue will result in improved functional outcome or reduce the risk of secondary malignancy.

2.4.4.2 Chemotherapy Plus Radiotherapy

The addition of chemotherapy protocols to local irradiation have not only meant an advance in the control of systemic disease but have also increased the rates of local disease control. Numerous authors have demonstrated the beneficial effect of this therapeutic association, in comparison with historical series. Consequently, over the last 20 years, this therapeutic approach: the combination of high-dose irradiation with systemic chemotherapy has been considered as optimum in the treatment of ES [129].

The rate of local control that can be expected with combination of chemotherapy plus radiotherapy is between 75 and 90 % [129–132].

2.4.4.3 Chemotherapy Plus Surgery

With the combination of neoadjuvant chemotherapy plus surgery, local control rates similar to those obtained with radiotherapy (alone) have been reported [133]. However, it is difficult to compare the two approaches because no randomized comparative study has ever been undertaken. The data of CESS-86 are the closest approximation to a comparative study; differences between both groups were not found (DFS at 5 years was 67 % with chemotherapy versus 65 % with radiotherapy) [134]. Scrutiny of published comparative works indicates a clear selection of patients. The tendency has been to use surgery (with chemotherapy) for peripheral tumors or for localized tumors of reduced dimensions, which have a better prognosis than central tumors of greater volume [115]. In general there seems to be agreement in the idea of avoiding radiation in patients whose young age leads one to predict serious sequelae.

2.4.4.4 Chemotherapy ± Surgery ± Radiotherapy

Patients who, after induction chemotherapy, demonstrate a high percentage (>30 %) of tumor-cell viability in the surgical piece have a bad prognosis. The presence of more than 5 % viable tumor is related to low DFS. In one study, when <5 % of the resected tumor was viable, the DFS was 75 %; when >5 % was viable, the DFS was 48 % [135]. Similarly, the presence of residual disease in surgical margins or the impossibility of carrying out a complete block resection is associated with a high probability of local relapse [136].

The majority of authors agree on the use of radiotherapy in the following types of patients [136]:

1. Patients for whom there is no surgical option, either initially or after the administration of neoadjuvant chemotherapy.
2. Patients with a bad response to neoadjuvant chemotherapy.
3. Patients with refractory disease in general.
4. Patients in whom there remains residual disease, whether macroscopic or microscopic, in the tumoral bed after surgery.

The rates of local control of disease in patients treated with radiotherapy and chemotherapy are lower for pelvic and proximal locations in comparison to distal locations and for tumors of large initial volume. Various groups have proposed carrying out surgical resection of the zones previously affected by tumor in high-risk patients treated with radiation and chemotherapy. The data obtained in the corresponding series demonstrate a clear advantage in terms of DFS for patients receiving such resection [137].

2.4.5 *Systemic Control of Disease*

In the pre-chemotherapy era, survival at 5 years for patients with ES treated with surgery and radiotherapy was less than 10 % of cases [138]. As with other childhood solid tumors, phase II studies with sole agents began in the 1960s. All the agents with known activity against solid tumors have been tested, and many of them, as sole agents, demonstrated activity against ES. Out of all of them, cyclophosfamide, IFX, melphalan in high doses and Adriamycin have demonstrated special activity. Other agents such as dactinomycin, BCNU, 5-FU, daunomycin, mitramycin, cisplatin and derivatives of the epipodophyllotoxins have shown different degrees of activity. A combination with surprisingly marked activity, even in patients who are resistant to other drugs, is IFX with etoposide [92].

2.4.6 The Role of Chemotherapy in Localized Disease

With the anti-tumoral activity of chemotherapy against macroscopic disease proven, in 1964 two of the first studies with complementary chemotherapy were initiated in the St. Jude Children's Research Hospital [139] and in the National Cancer Institute [120]. Patients were treated with VAC (vincristine, actinomycin D, cyclophosfamide) with or without Adriamycin (Adr), at doses which we today consider subtherapeutical. Survival was 33 %. In 1973 the first cooperative multi-center study, denominated IESS-I, began. The study concluded that the addition of Adr to the VAC protocol is effective and better than prophylactic irradiation of the lungs: with the VAC + Adr combination, DFS at 5 years was 60 % [129].

IESS-I lead on to a second study, the IESS-II, which evaluated the role of intensification of Adr. An increase of 150 % of the previously used dose improved the DFS at 5 years: 73 % with intensification versus 56 % without [140]. Studies by other groups with VAC + Adr with and without intensification achieved very similar results to those obtained in IESS-II [141]. The importance of administering Adr, with VAC, in the highest tolerable doses during the initial stages of treatment is well established. The development of IFX and the data obtained from phase II studies lead to the idea of substituting cyclophosfamide with IFX. None of the three big studies carried out to evaluate this was able to demonstrate any clear benefit of the substitution. In the control of ES, cyclophosphamide is as effective as IFX in VAC + Adr combinations [142, 143].

In view of good results obtained with IFX + VP-16, IESS-III studied the possible benefit of adding this combination to VAC + Adr. A significant increase in the DFS at 5 years was obtained (68 % versus 54 %) [100].

Currently, for non-metastatic ES chemotherapy treatment, we consider protocols that combine VAC + Adr (in high doses) with IFX + VP-16 as being standard. In a recent study, a combination of this protocol with surgery and radiotherapy achieved a DFS at 4 years of 82 % [100].

The COG (Children Oncology Group) has proposed carrying out a randomized study to compare the administration of VAC + Adr plus IFX + VP-16 using filgastrim as support, with shorter periods between cycles (14 days versus 21 days), in order to evaluate whether such intensification of doses has an effect on survival. The proposed study is based on the experience of a pilot study by Womer et al. [144], who with this approach obtained a rate of DFS at 30 months of 73 %.

2.4.7 Control of Metastatic Disease

The prognosis for patients with metastatic disease is poor. In the majority of series, survival at 3 years is less than 30 % [145, 146]. Current therapies for patients who present with metastatic disease achieve 5-year EFS of approximately 28 % and overall survival (OS) of approximately 30 % [145, 146]. For patients with lung/

pleural metastases only, 5-year EFS is approximately 40 % when treatment includes bilateral lung irradiation [147]. In contrast, patients with bone/bone marrow metastases have a 5-year EFS of approximately 25 %, and patients with combined lung and bone/bone marrow metastases have a 5 year EFS of approximately 14 % [148]. Factors such as age being over 14 years, a primary tumor volume of more than 200 mL, more than one bone metastatic site, bone marrow metastases, and additional lung metastases all independently predict a poor outcome in patients presenting with metastatic disease [149].

The best results with patients with metastatic disease were obtained in a study in the SJCRH by Hayes et al. [141], applying an induction regimen with sequential cyclophosphamide and Adriamycin. The authors report DFS at 47 months of follow-up of 55 %. Other authors have not been able to reproduce these results [150]. The IESS found no benefit for patients with metastatic disease in the addition of ifosfamide and etoposide to a standard regimen of vincristine, doxorubicin, cyclophosphamide, and actinomycinD [151]. In another Intergroup study, increasing the dose intensities of cyclophosphamide, ifosfamide, and doxorubicin did not improve outcome relative to regimens utilizing standard dose intensities. This regimen increased toxicity and risk of second malignancy without improving EFS or OS [145].

Patients with metastasis exclusively to the lung or pleura or both have a better prognosis than patients with metastasis to other sites: cure rates reach 30 %. These patients must be treated with lung irradiation [152].

For patients with metastasis to bone or bone marrow, the cure rate is 20–25 %. The probabilities of cure for patients with combined forms of metastasis to bone or bone marrow and lung are less than 15 % [153].

The approach to radiotherapy in the treatment of metastatic disease is based on applying the known criteria for localized disease to each of the affected zones. In this way there is an attempt to obtain adequate local control on an area-by-area basis. In most cases it is possible to obtain this control with acceptable morbidity [154]. Metastatic sites of disease in bone and soft tissues should receive fractionated radiation therapy doses totaling between 45 and 56 Gy [154].

The problem with carrying out high-dose irradiation of several fields is the limitation this puts on the joint administration of chemotherapy: radiotherapy can be highly toxic to bone marrow. In patients with lung metastasis, it is necessary to irradiate both pulmonary fields irrespective of whether the nodules disappear as a result of chemotherapy. The doses recommended are between 12 and 15 Gy and must be adjusted according to the existing pulmonary function [154].

Intensive therapies, many of which incorporate high dose chemotherapy with or without total body irradiation in conjunction with stem cell support, have not shown improvement in EFS rates for patients with bone and/or bone marrow metastases [114]. The impact of high dose chemotherapy with peripheral blood stem cell support for patients with lung metastases is unknown and is being studied in the EURO-EWING INTERGROUP-EE99 trial [155].

Melphalan, at non-myeloablative doses, has proved to be an active agent in an upfront window (i.e. first-line treatment) study of patients with metastatic disease at diagnosis; However, the cure rate remained extremely low [156].

2.4.8 Relapse or Progression of Disease

Despite the extensive therapeutic efforts carried out in the treatment of ES, between 30 and 40 % of patients relapse. The prognosis for patients who present relapse or disease progression before having attained complete remission is very poor. This prognosis is especially bad if progression occurs during chemotherapy treatment [157].

Patients with late relapse, that is, relapse at least 24 months after diagnosis, have a better prognosis than those with early relapse (34.9 % ± 8.5 % versus 5 % ± 2.8 %) [149].

Multiple relapses, local and systemic, are associated with lower rates of survival at 5 years (12.5 % ± 8.3 %) than local relapse alone (21.7 % ± 7.8 %) or relapse at a distance alone (17.6 % ± 6.1 %) [158].

For patients with local relapse, radical rescue surgery is the treatment that offers the highest probability of survival at 5 years (31.4 % ± 11.6 %); alternative treatments are less effective (9.1 % ± 6.1 %). Lung irradiation significantly improves survival of patients with progression exclusively in this area (DFS at 5 years of 30.3 % ± 12.5 % versus 16.7 % ± 10.8 %). Isolated pulmonary recurrence has been found not to be an important prognostic factor [159].

The approach to treatment aimed at the reinduction of remission is variable and depends on the situation of the patient, on the localization of the relapse, and on treatment previously received. In patients who have not received it previously, the combination of IFX with etoposide is active: response rates of 80 %, the majority partial and 12 % complete, have been described [151]. In addition, there are reports of responses to the combination of cyclophosfamide with topotecan, with combined rates of complete and partial remission of 35 % [160]. The combination of gemcitabine and docetaxel has achieved objective responses in relapsed Ewing sarcoma [161, 162]. High dose ifosfamide (3 g/m^2/day for 5 days = 15 g/m^2) has shown activity in patients with relapse after therapy that included standard ifosfamide (1.8 g/m^2/day for 5 days) [163]. Combinations of irinotecan and temozolomide with or without vincristine are active in recurrent Ewing sarcoma and can be considered for patients in relapse [164–166].

Aggressive attempts to control disease progression, including myeloablative regimens, have been used, but there is no evidence at this time to conclude that myeloablative therapy is superior to standard chemotherapy. Treatments with high-dose chemotherapy and rescue with hematopoietic stem cells have been applied by multiple workgroups. The results are better if the procedure is carried out with the patient in complete remission, or at least in a phase in which the disease is contained [106, 167, 168].

2.4.9 New Biological Approaches

In a search for new treatments, Mitsiades et al. [169], after demonstrating that TRAIL (TNF-related apoptosis-inducing ligand) bound with the DR4 and DR5 cellular death receptors, found an elevated expression of DR4/DR5 in samples of ES and high sensitivity to TRAIL in cell cultures. Given the low toxicity of TRAIL, these authors suggested its use as an anti-tumoral agent.

Zhou et al. [170] maintain the theory that over-expression of the HER2/neu oncogene is associated with tumorigenicity and resistance to drugs in many human tumors. In three cell lines of human ES it has been demonstrated that the over-expression of the HER2/neu gene can be reduced by transduction, using an adeno-viral vector, with the gene E1A. In this way it is possible to increase the activity of cytostatic agents and reinforce expression of topoisomerase II-alpha. Apoptosis is increased in the tumoral cell lines, and there is improved sensitivity to etoposide and Adriamycin.

The receptor for stem-cell factor/KIT could represent a new target for ES treatments of the biological type. Of Ewing's tumors, 44.5 % express KIT. Treatments with the tyrosine kinase inhibitor of KIT, imatinib, induce a slowing down in the phosphorylation of KIT and a dose-response inhibition of cellular proliferation. Imatinib administered alone does not induce an important increase of cellular apoptosis, but it has been demonstrated that it increases the toxic action of cytostatic agents such as vincristine and Adriamycin. Through this mechanism, imatinib could play an important role in the treatment of ES [171].

Monoclonal antibodies against the insulin-like growth factor 1 receptor (IGF1R) are reported to produce objective responses in metastatic recurrent Ewing sarcoma in roughly 10 % of cases [172–175]. A phase I trial of IGF1R antibodies combined with the mTOR inhibitor temsirolimus achieved two complete responses and three minor responses in 17 patients with metastatic recurrent Ewing sarcoma [176].

References

1. Guidelines for the pediatric cancer center and role of such centers in diagnosis and treatment. A. A. P. Section Statement Section on Hematology/Oncology. Pediatrics. 1997;99(1):139–41.
2. Bielack SS, Machatschek JN, Flege S, Jürgens H. Delaying surgery with chemotherapy for osteosarcoma of the extremities. Expert Opin Pharmacother. 2004;5:1243–56.
3. Whelan J, McTiernan A, Cooper N, Wong YK, Francis M, Vernon S, Strauss J. Incidence and survival of malignant bone sarcomas in England 1979–2007. Int J Cancer. 2012;131:E504–17.
4. Peris-Bonet R, Giner Ripoll B, García Cano A. Registro Nacional de Tumores Infantiles (RNTISEOP). Estadísticas Básicas 4. 1980–2001. Supervivencia 1980–1997. Valencia: Universitat de Valencia; 2003 (CD-ROM).
5. Jeffree GM, Price CH, Sissons HA. The metastatic patterns of osteosarcoma. Br J Cancer. 1975;32:87–107.
6. Jaffe N, Frei E, Traggis D, Bishop Y. Adjuvant methotrexate and citrovorum-factor treatment of osteogenic sarcoma. N Engl J Med. 1974;291:994–7.
7. Luetke A, Meyers P, Lewis I, Jürgen's H. Osteosarcoma treatment – where do we stand? A state of the art review. Cancer Treat Rev. 2014;40:523–32.
8. Reddy K, Wafa H, Gaston C, Grimer R, et al. Does amputation offer any survival benefit over limb salvage in osteosarcoma patients with poor chemonecrosis and close margins? Bone Joint J. 2015;97-B:115–20.
9. Enneking WF, Spanier SS, Goodman MA. A system for the surgical staging of musculoskeletal sarcoma. Clin Orthop. 1980;153:106–20.

10. Bacci G, Ferrari S, Longhi A, et al. Pattern of relapse in patients with osteosarcoma of the extremities treated with neoadjuvant chemotherapy. Eur J Cancer. 2001;37:32–8.
11. Bielack SS, Kempf-Bielack B, Delling G, et al. Prognostic factors in high-grade osteosarcoma of the extremities or trunk: an analysis of 1,702 patients treated on neoadjuvant Cooperative Osteosarcoma Study Group Protocols. J Clin Oncol. 2002;20:776–90.
12. Jaffe N. Osteosarcoma: review of the past, impact on the future. The American experience. Cancer Treat Res. 2009;152:239–62.
13. Bielack S, Jürgens H, Jundt G, et al. Osteosarcoma: the COSS experience. Cancer Treat Res. 2009;152:289–308.
14. Grimer RJ, Taminiau AM, Cannon SR, Surgical Subcommitte of the European Osteosarcoma Intergroup. Surgical outcomes in osteosarcoma. J Bone Joint Surg Br. 2002;84:395–400.
15. Andreou D, Bielack SS, Carrle D, et al. The influence of tumor and treatment related factors on the development of local recurrence in osteosarcoma after adequate surgery. An analysis of 1355 patients treated on neoadjuvant Cooperative Osteosarcoma Study Group protocols. Ann Oncol. 2011;22:1228–35.
16. Bacci G, Rocca M, Salone M, et al. High grade osteosarcoma of the extremities with lung metastases at presentation: treatment with neoadjuvant chemotherapy and simultaneous resection of primary and metastatic lesions. J Surg Oncol. 2008;98:415–20.
17. DeLaney TF, Park L, Goldberg SI, et al. Radiotherapy for local control of osteosarcoma. Int J Radiat Oncol Biol Phys. 2005;61:492–8.
18. Mahajan A, Woo SY, Kornguth DG, et al. Multimodality treatment of osteosarcoma: radiation in a high-risk cohort. Pediatr Blood Cancer. 2008;50:976–82.
19. Ciernik IF, Niemierko A, Harmon DC, et al. Proton-based radiotherapy for unresectable or incompletely resected osteosarcoma. Cancer. 2011;117:4522–30.
20. Sutow WW, Vietti TJ, Fernbach DJ, et al. Evaluation of chemotherapy in children with metastatic Ewing's sarcoma and osteogenic sarcoma. Cancer Chemother Rep. 1971;55:67–81.
21. Cortes EP, Holland JF, Wang JJ, et al. Amputation and Adriamycin in primary osteosarcoma. N Engl J Med. 1974;291:998–1000.
22. Link MP, Goorin AM, Miser AW, et al. The effect of adjuvant chemotherapy on relapse-free survival in patients with osteosarcoma of the extremity. N Engl J Med. 1986;314:1600–6.
23. Cassano WF, Graham-Pole J, Dickson N. Etoposide, cyclophosphamide, cisplatin, and doxorubicin as neoadjuvant chemotherapy for osteosarcoma. Cancer. 1991;68:1899–902.
24. Bacci G, Picci P, Avella M, et al. Effect of intraarterial versus intravenous cisplatin in addition to systemic Adriamycin and highdose methotrexate on histologic tumor response of osteosarcoma of the extremities. J Chemother. 1992;4:189–95.
25. Provisor AJ, Ettinger LJ, Nachman JB, et al. Treatment of nonmetastatic osteosarcoma of the extremity with preoperative and postoperative chemotherapy: a report from the Children's Cancer Group. J Clin Oncol. 1997;15:76–84.
26. Fuchs N, Bielack SS, Epler D, et al. Long term results of the cooperative German-Austrian-Swiss osteosarcoma study group's protocol COSS86 of intensive multidrug chemotherapy and surgery for osteosarcoma of the limbs. Ann Oncol. 1998;9:893–9.
27. Voûte PA, Souhami RL, Nooij M, et al. A phase II study of cisplatin, ifosfamide and doxorubicin in operable primary, axial skeletal and metastatic osteosarcoma. European Osteosarcoma Intergroup (EOI). Ann Oncol. 1999;10:1211–8.
28. Zalupski MM, Rankin C, Ryan JR, et al. Adjuvant therapy of osteosarcoma. A Phase II trial: Southwest Oncology Group study 9139. Cancer. 2004;100:818–25.
29. Meyers PA, Schwartz CL, Krailo M, et al. Osteosarcoma: a randomized, prospective trial of the addition of ifosfamide and/or muramyl tripeptide to cisplatin, doxorubicin, and highdose methotrexate. J Clin Oncol. 2005;23:2004–11.
30. Ferrari S, Smeland S, Mercuri M, et al. Neoadjuvant chemotherapy with highdose Ifosfamide, highdose methotrexate, cisplatin, and doxorubicin for patients with localized osteosarcoma of the extremity: a joint study by the Italian and Scandinavian Sarcoma Groups. J Clin Oncol. 2005;23:8845–52.

31. Daw NC, Neel MD, Rao BN, et al. Frontline treatment of localized osteosarcoma without methotrexate: results of the St. Jude Children's Research Hospital OS99 trial. Cancer. 2011;117:2770–8.
32. Anninga JK, Gelderblom H, Fiocco M, et al. Chemotherapeutic adjuvant treatment for osteosarcoma: where do we stand? Eur J Cancer. 2011;47:2431–45.
33. Hattinger CM, Pasello M, Ferrari S, Picci P, Serra M. Emerging drugs for highgrade osteosarcoma. Expert Opin Emerg Drugs. 2010;15:615–34.
34. Carrle D, Bielack SS. Current strategies of chemotherapy in osteosarcoma. Int Orthop. 2006;30:445–51.
35. Rosen G, Caparros B, Huvos AG, et al. Preoperative chemotherapy for osteogenic sarcoma: selection of postoperative adjuvant chemotherapy based on the response of the primary tumour to preoperative chemotherapy. Cancer. 1982;49:1221–30.
36. Bramwell VHC, Burgers M, Senath R, et al. A comparison of two short intensive adjuvant chemotherapy regimens in operable osteosarcoma of limbs in children and young adults: the first study of the European Osteosarcoma Intergroup. J Clin Oncol. 1992;10:1579–91.
37. Meyers PA, Heller G, Healey J, et al. Chemotherapy for non-metastatic osteogenic sarcoma: the Memorial Sloan-Kettering Experience. J Clin Oncol. 1992;10:5–15.
38. Winkler K, Beron G, Delling G, et al. Neoadjuvant chemotherapy of osteosarcoma: results of a randomized cooperative trial (COSS-82) with salvage chemotherapy based on histological tumour response. J Clin Oncol. 1988;6:329–37.
39. Janeway KA, Barkauskas DA, Krailo MD, et al. Outcome for adolescent and young adult patients with osteosarcoma: a report from the Children's Oncology Group. Cancer. 2012;118:4597–605.
40. Ferrari S, Bacci G, Picci P, et al. Long-term follow-up and post-relapse survival in patients with non-metastatic osteosarcoma of the extremity treated with neoadjuvant chemotherapy. Ann Oncol. 1997;8:765–71.
41. Eselgrim M, Grunert H, Kühne T, et al. Dose intensity of chemotherapy for osteosarcoma and outcome in the Cooperative Osteosarcoma Study Group (COSS) trials. Pediatr Blood Cancer. 2006;47:42–50.
42. Imran H, Enders F, Krailo M, et al. Effect of time to resumption of chemotherapy after definitive surgery on prognosis for non-metastatic osteosarcoma. J Bone Joint Surg Am. 2009;91:604–12.
43. Harris MB, Cantor AB, Goorin AM, et al. Treatment of osteosarcoma with ifosfamide: comparison of response in pediatric patients with recurrent disease versus patients previously untreated: a Pediatric Oncology Group study. Med Pediatr Oncol. 1995;24:87–92.
44. Goorin AM, Harris MB, Bernstein M, et al. Phase II/III trial of etoposide and high-dose ifosfamide in newly diagnosed metastatic osteosarcoma: a Pediatric Oncology Group trial. J Clin Oncol. 2002;20:426–33.
45. Meyer WH, Pratt CB, Poquette CA, et al. Carboplatin/ifosfamide window therapy for osteosarcoma: results of the St Jude Children's Research Hospital OS-91 trial. J Clin Oncol. 2001;19:171–82.
46. Gentet J-C, Brunat-Mentigny M, Demaille MC, et al. Ifosfamide and etoposide in childhood osteosarcoma. A phase II study of the French Society of Paediatric Oncology. Eur J Cancer. 1997;33:232–7.
47. Whelan JS, Bielack SS, Marina N, et al. EURAMOS-1, an international randomised study for osteosarcoma: results from pre-randomisation treatment. Ann Oncol. 2015;26:407–14.
48. Graf N, Winkler K, Betlemovic M, Fuchs N, Bode U. Methotrexate pharmacokinetics and prognosis in osteosarcoma. J Clin Oncol. 1994;12:1443–51.
49. Crews KR, Liu T, Rodríguez-Galindo C, et al. High-dose methotrexate pharmacokinetics and outcome of children and young adults with osteosarcoma. Cancer. 2004;100:1723–33.
50. Bacci G, Picci P, Ruggieri P, et al. Primary chemotherapy and delayed surgery (neoadjuvant chemotherapy) for osteosarcoma of the extremities. Cancer. 1990;65:2539–53.
51. Petrilli AS, Oliveira DT, Ginani VC, et al. Use of amifostine in the therapy of osteosarcoma in children and adolescents. J Pediatr Hematol Oncol. 2002;24:188–91.

52. Ferguson WS, Harris MB, Goorin AM, et al. Presurgical window of carboplatin and surgery and multidrug chemotherapy for the treatment of newly diagnosed metastatic or unresectable osteosarcoma: Pediatric Oncology Group trial. J Pediatr Hematol Oncol. 2001;23: 340–8.
53. Daw NC, Rodríguez-Galindo C, Billups CA, et al. Metastatic osteosarcoma: results of two consecutive therapeutic trials at St. Jude Children's Research Hospital. Proc Ann Meet Am Soc Clin Oncol. 2002:1556 (Abstr).
54. Jawad MU, Cheung MC, Clarke J, Koniaris LG, Scully SP. Osteosarcoma: improvement in survival limited to high-grade patients only. J Cancer Res Clin Oncol. 2011;137:597–607.
55. Pakos EE, Nearchou AD, Grimer RJ, et al. Prognostic factors and outcomes for osteosarcoma: an international collaboration. Eur J Cancer. 2009;45:2367–75.
56. Whelan J, Seddon B, Perisoglou M. Management of osteosarcoma. Curr Treat Options Oncol. 2006;7:444–55.
57. Meyers PA, Gorlick R, Heller G, et al. Intensification of preoperative chemotherapy for osteogenic sarcoma: results of the Memorial Sloan-Kettering (T12) protocol. J Clin Oncol. 1998;16:2452–8.
58. Jaffe N, Knapp J, Chuang VP, et al. Osteosarcoma: intra-arterial treatment of the primary tumour with cis-diammine-dichloroplatinum II (CDP). Cancer. 1983;51:402–7.
59. Bacci G, Ferrari S, Tienghi A, et al. A comparison of methods of loco-regional chemotherapy combined with systemic chemotherapy as neo-adjuvant treatment of osteosarcoma of the extremity. Eur J Surg Oncol. 2001;27:98–104.
60. Winkler K, Bielak S, Delling G, et al. Effect of intraarterial versus intravenous cisplatin in addition to systemic doxorubicin, high-dose methotrexate, and ifosfamide on histologic tumor response in osteosarcoma (study COSS-86). Cancer. 1990;66:1703–10.
61. Wilkins RM, Cullen JW, Odom L, et al. Superior survival in treatment of primary nonmetastatic pediatric osteosarcoma of the extremity. Ann Surg Oncol. 2003;10:498–507.
62. Kager L, Zoubek A, Pötschger U, et al. Primary metastatic osteosarcoma: presentation and outcome of patients treated on neoadjuvant Cooperative Osteosarcoma Study Group protocols. J Clin Oncol. 2003;21:2011–8.
63. Bacci G, Briccoli A, Rocca M, et al. Neoadjuvant chemotherapy for osteosarcoma of the extremities with metastases at presentation: recent experience at the Rizzoli Institute in 57 patients treated with cisplatin, doxorubicin, and a high dose of methotrexate and ifosfamide. Ann Oncol. 2003;14:1126–34.
64. Bacci G, Briccoli A, Ferrari S, et al. Neoadjuvant chemotherapy for osteosarcoma of the extremity: long-term results of the Rizzoli's 4th protocol. Eur J Cancer. 2001;37:2030–9.
65. Chou AJ, Kleinerman ES, Krailo MD, et al. Addition of muramyl tripeptide to chemotherapy for patients with newly diagnosed metastatic osteosarcoma: a report from the Children's Oncology Group. Cancer. 2009;115:5339–48.
66. Fagioli F, Aglietta M, Tienghi A, et al. High-dose chemotherapy in the treatment of relapsed osteosarcoma: an Italian Sarcoma Group Study. J Clin Oncol. 2002;20:2150–6.
67. Kasper B, Lehnert T, Bernd L, et al. High-dose chemotherapy with autologous peripheral blood stem cell transplantation for bone and soft-tissue sarcomas. Bone Marrow Transplant. 2004;34:37–41.
68. Letourneau PA, Xiao L, Harting MT, et al. Location of pulmonary metastasis in pediatric osteosarcoma is predictive of outcome. J Pediatr Surg. 2011;46:1333–7.
69. Bacci G, Fabbri N, Balladelli A, et al. Treatment and prognosis for synchronous multifocal osteosarcoma in 42 patients. J Bone Joint Surg Br. 2006;88:1071–5.
70. Kager L, Zoubek A, Kastner U, et al. Skip metastases in osteosarcoma: experience of the Cooperative Osteosarcoma Study Group. J Clin Oncol. 2006;24:1535–41.
71. Longhi A, Fabbri N, Donati D, et al. Neoadjuvant chemotherapy for patients with synchronous multifocal osteosarcoma: results in eleven cases. J Chemother. 2001;13:324–30.
72. Gelderblom H, Jinks RC, Sydes M, et al. Survival after recurrent osteosarcoma: data from 3 European Osteosarcoma Intergroup (EOI) randomized controlled trials. Eur J Cancer. 2011; 47:895–902.

73. Rejin K, Aykan OA, Omer G, et al. Intraabdominal metastasis in osteosarcoma: survey and literature review. Pediatr Hematol Oncol. 2011;28:609–15.
74. Berrak SG, Pearson M, Berberoğlu S, et al. Highdose ifosfamide in relapsed pediatric osteosarcoma: therapeutic effects and renal toxicity. Pediatr Blood Cancer. 2005;44:215–9.
75. Kung FH, Pratt CB, Vega RA, et al. Ifosfamide/etoposide combination in the treatment of recurrent malignant solid tumors of childhood. A Pediatric Oncology Group Phase II study. Cancer. 1993;71:1898–903.
76. Massimo B, Giovanni G, Stefano F, et al. Phase 2 trial of two courses of cyclophosphamide and etoposide for relapsed high risk osteosarcoma patients. Cancer. 2009;115:2980–7.
77. Qi WX, He AN, Tang LN, et al. Efficacy and safety of gemcitabine docetaxel combination therapy for recurrent or refractory highgrade osteosarcoma in China: a retrospective study of 18 patients. Jpn J Clin Oncol. 2012;42:427–31.
78. Grignani G, Palmerini E, Dileo P, et al. A phase II trial of sorafenib in relapsed and unresectable highgrade osteosarcoma after failure of standard multimodal therapy: an Italian Sarcoma Group study. Ann Oncol. 2012;23:508–16.
79. Ferrari S, Briccoli A, Mercuri M, et al. Postrelapse survival in osteosarcoma of the extremities: prognostic factors for long-term survival. J Clin Oncol. 2003;21:710–5.
80. Bielack SS, Kempf-Bielack B, Branscheid D, et al. Second and subsequent recurrences of osteosarcoma: presentation, treatment, and outcomes of 249 consecutive Cooperative Osteosarcoma Study Group patients. J Clin Oncol. 2009;27:557–65.
81. Saylors RL, Stine KC, Sullivan J, et al. Cyclophosphamide plus topotecan in children with recurrent or refractory solid tumours: a pediatric oncology group (POG) phase II study. J Clin Oncol. 2001;19:3463–9.
82. Leu KM, Ostruszka LJ, Shewach D, et al. Laboratory and clinical evidence of synergistic cytotoxicity of sequential treatment with gemcitabine followed by docetaxel in the treatment of sarcoma. J Clin Oncol. 2004;22:1706–12.
83. Laverdiere C, Kolb EA, Supko JG, et al. Phase II study of ecteinascidin 743 in heavily pretreated patients with recurrent osteosarcoma. Cancer. 2003;98:832–40.
84. Kleinerman ES. Biologic therapy for osteosarcoma using liposome encapsulated muramyl tripeptide. Hematol Oncol Clin North Am. 1995;9:927–38.
85. Meyers PA, Schwartz CL, Krailo MD, et al. Osteosarcoma: the addition of muramyl tripeptide to chemotherapy improves overall survival. A report from the Children's Oncology Group. J Clin Oncol. 2008;26:633–8.
86. Anderson PM, Markivic SN, Sloan JA, et al. Aerosol granulocyte macrophage-colony stimulating factor: a low toxicity, lung-specific biological therapy in patients with lung metastases. Clin Cancer Res. 1999;5:2316–23.
87. Densmore CL, Kleinerman ES, Gautam A, et al. Growth suppression of established human osteosarcoma lung metastases in mice by aerosol gene therapy with PEI- *p53* complexes. Cancer Gene Ther. 2001;8:619–27.
88. Verschraegen CF, Gilbert BE, Loyer E, et al. Clinical evaluation of the delivery and safety of aerosolized liposomal 9-nitro-20(S)-camptothecin in patients with advanced pulmonary malignancies. Clin Cancer Res. 2004;10:2319–26.
89. Bielack SS, Smeland S, Whelan J, et al. MAP plus maintenance pegylated interferon α2b (MAPIFN) versus MAP alone in patients (pts) with resectable highgrade osteosarcoma and good histologic response to preoperative MAP: first results of the EURAMOS1 good response randomization. Clin Oncol. 2013; 31(Suppl 15):Abstract A-LBA 10504.
90. Loeb DM, Garrett-Mayer E, Hobbs RF, et al. Dose finding study of 153 Sm EDTMP in patients with poor prognosis osteosarcoma. Cancer. 2009;115:2514–22.
91. Ewing J. Diffuse endotelioma of bone. Proc N Y Pathol Soc. 1921;21:17–24.
92. Grier HE, Krailo MD, Tarbell NJ, et al. Addition of ifosfamide and etoposide to standard chemotherapy for Ewing's sarcoma and primitive neuroectodermal tumor of bone. N Engl J Med. 2003;348:694–701.
93. Donaldson SS, Torrey M, Link MP, et al. A multidisciplinary study investigating radiotherapy in Ewing's sarcoma: end results of POG #8346. Pediatric Oncology Group. Int J Radiat Oncol Biol Phys. 1998;42:125–35.

94. Ferrari S, Mercuri M, Rosito P, et al. Ifosfamide and actinomycinD, added in the induction phase to vincristine, cyclophosphamide and doxorubicin, improve histologic response and prognosis in patients with non-metastatic Ewing's sarcoma of the extremity. J Chemother. 1998;10:484–91.
95. Paulussen M, Craft AW, Lewis I, et al. Results of the EICESS92 Study: two randomized trials of Ewing's sarcoma treatment cyclophosphamide compared with ifosfamide in standard risk patients and assessment of benefit of etoposide added to standard treatment in high risk patients. J Clin Oncol. 2008;26(27):4385–93.
96. Jürgen's C, Weston C, Lewis I, et al. Safety assessment of intensive induction with vincristine, ifosfamide, doxorubicin, and etoposide (VIDE) in the treatment of Ewing tumors in the EURO-E.W.I.N.G. 99 clinical trial. Pediatr Blood Cancer. 2006;47:22–9.
97. Womer RB, West DC, Krailo MD, et al. Randomized controlled trial of interval compressed chemotherapy for the treatment of localized Ewing sarcoma: a report from the Children's Oncology Group. J Clin Oncol. 2012;30:4148–54.
98. Krasin MJ, Davidoff AM, Rodriguez Galindo C, et al. Definitive surgery and multiagent systemic therapy for patients with localized Ewing sarcoma family of tumors: local outcome and prognostic factors. Cancer. 2005;104:367–73.
99. Smith MA, Ungerleider RS, Horowitz ME, et al. Influence of doxorubicin dose intensity on response and outcome for patients with osteogenic sarcoma and Ewing's sarcoma. J Natl Cancer Inst. 1991;83:1460–70.
100. Kolb EA, Kushner BH, Gorlick R, et al. Long-term event-free survival after intensive chemotherapy for Ewing's family of tumors in children and young adults. J Clin Oncol. 2003;21: 3423–30.
101. Granowetter L, Womer R, Devidas M, et al. Dose-intensified compared with standard chemotherapy for non-metastatic Ewing sarcoma family of tumors: a Children's Oncology Group Study. J Clin Oncol. 2009;27:2536–41.
102. Kushner BH, Meyers PA. How effective is dose intensive/myeloablative therapy against Ewing's sarcoma/primitive neuroectodermal tumor metastatic to bone or bone marrow? The Memorial Sloan Kettering experience and a literature review. J Clin Oncol. 2001;19: 870–80.
103. Marina N, Meyers PA. High-dose therapy and stem cell rescue for Ewing's family of tumors in second remission. J Clin Oncol. 2005;23:4262–4.
104. Burdach S. Treatment of advanced Ewing tumors by combined radio chemotherapy and engineered cellular transplants. Pediatr Transplant. 2004;8 Suppl 5:67–82.
105. McTiernan A, Driver D, Michelagnoli MP, et al. High dose chemotherapy with bone marrow or peripheral stem cell rescue is an effective treatment option for patients with relapsed or progressive Ewing's sarcoma family of tumours. Ann Oncol. 2006;17: 1301–5.
106. Burdach S, Meyer-Bahlburg A, Laws HJ, et al. High dose therapy for patients with primary multifocal and early relapsed Ewing's tumors: results of two consecutive regimens assessing the role of total body irradiation. J Clin Oncol. 2003;21:3072–8.
107. Meyers PA, Krailo MD, Ladanyi M, et al. High dose melphalan, etoposide, total body irradiation, and autologous stem cell reconstitution as consolidation therapy for high-risk Ewing's sarcoma does not improve prognosis. J Clin Oncol. 2001;19:2812–20.
108. Oberlin O, Rey A, Desfachelles AS, et al. Impact of high dose busulfan plus melphalan as consolidation in metastatic Ewing tumors: a study by the Société Française des Cancers de l'Enfant. J Clin Oncol. 2006;24:3997–4002.
109. Hawkins D, Barnett T, Bensinger W, et al. Busulfan, melphalan, and thiotepa with or without total marrow irradiation with hematopoietic stem cell rescue for poor-risk Ewing-Sarcoma-Family tumors. Med Pediatr Oncol. 2000;34:328–37.
110. Rosenthal J, Bolotin E, Shakhnovits M, et al. High dose therapy with hematopoietic stem cell rescue in patients with poor prognosis Ewing family tumors. Bone Marrow Transplant. 2008;42:311–8.
111. Burdach S, Thiel U, Schöniger M, et al. Total body MRI-governed involved compartment irradiation combined with high-dose chemotherapy and stem cell rescue improves long-term

survival in Ewing tumor patients with multiple primary bone metastases. Bone Marrow Transplant. 2010;45:483–9.
112. Gaspar N, Rey A, Bérard PM, et al. Risk adapted chemotherapy for localized Ewing's sarcoma of bone: the French EW93 study. Eur J Cancer. 2012;48:1376–85.
113. Drabko K, Raciborska A, Bilska K, et al. Consolidation of first line therapy with busulphan and melphalan, and autologous stem cell rescue in children with Ewing's sarcoma. Bone Marrow Transplant. 2012;47:1530–4.
114. Thiel U, Wawer A, Wolf P, et al. No improvement of survival with reduced versus high intensity conditioning for allogeneic stem cell transplants in Ewing tumor patients. Ann Oncol. 2011;22:1614–21.
115. Paulussen M, Ahrens S, Dunst J, et al. Localized Ewing tumor of bone: final results of the cooperative Ewing's Sarcoma Study CESS 86. J Clin Oncol. 2001;19:1818–29.
116. Oberlin O, Deley MC, Bui BN, et al. Prognostic factors in localized Ewing's tumours and peripheral neuroectodermal tumours: the third study of the French Society of Paediatric Oncology (EW88 study). Br J Cancer. 2001;85:1646–54.
117. Denecke T, Hundsdörfer P, Misch D, et al. Assessment of histological response of paediatric bone sarcomas using FDG PET in comparison to morphological volume measurement and standardized MRI parameters. Eur J Nucl Med Mol Imaging. 2010;37:1842–53.
118. Lin PP, Jaffe N, Herzog CE, et al. Chemotherapy response is an important predictor of local recurrence in Ewing sarcoma. Cancer. 2007;109:603–11.
119. Fernández CH, Lindberg RD, Sutow WW, Samuels ML. Localized Ewing's sarcoma – treatment and results. Cancer. 1974;34:143–8.
120. Tepper J, Glaubiger D, Lichter A, et al. Local control of Ewing's sarcoma of bone with radiotherapy and combination chemotherapy. Cancer. 1980;46:1969–73.
121. Dahlin DC, Coventy MD, Scanlon PW. Ewing's sarcoma: a critical analysis of 165 cases. J Bone Joint Surg Am. 1962;43:185–92.
122. Krasin MJ, Rodriguez-Galindo C, Davidoff AM, et al. Efficacy of combined surgery and irradiation for localized Ewings sarcoma family of tumors. Pediatr Blood Cancer. 2004;43(3): 229–36.
123. Bacci G, Longhi A, Briccoli A, et al. The role of surgical margins in treatment of Ewing's sarcoma family tumors: experience of a single institution with 512 patients treated with adjuvant and neoadjuvant chemotherapy. Int J Radiat Oncol Biol Phys. 2006;65:766–72.
124. Wagner TD, Kobayashi W, Dean S, et al. Combination short course preoperative irradiation, surgical resection, and reduced field high dose postoperative irradiation in the treatment of tumors involving the bone. Int J Radiat Oncol Biol Phys. 2009;73:259–66.
125. Yock TI, Krailo M, Fryer CJ, et al. Local control in pelvic Ewing sarcoma: analysis from INT0091. A report from the Children's Oncology Group. J Clin Oncol. 2006;24:3838–43.
126. Suit HD. Role of therapeutic radiology in cancer of bone. Cancer. 1975;35:930–5.
127. Kuttesch Jr JF, Wexler LH, Marcus RB, et al. Second malignancies after Ewing's sarcoma: radiation dose dependency of secondary sarcomas. J Clin Oncol. 1996;14:2818–25.
128. Rombi B, DeLaney TF, MacDonald SM, et al. Proton radiotherapy for pediatric Ewing's sarcoma: initial clinical outcomes. Int J Radiat Oncol Biol Phys. 2012;82:114–28.
129. Nesbit Jr ME, Gehan EA, Burget EO, et al. Multimodal therapy for the management of primary, nonmetastatic Ewing's sarcoma of bone: a long-term follow up of the First Intergroup study. J Clin Oncol. 1990;8:1664–74.
130. Shuck A, Hofmann J, Rube C, et al. Radiotherapy in Ewing's sarcoma and PNET of the chest wall: results of the trials CESS 81, CESS 86 and EICESS 92. Int J Radiat Oncol Biol Phys. 1998;42:1001–6.
131. Shankar AG, Pinkerton CR, Atra A, et al. Local therapy and other factors influencing site of relapse in patients with localised Ewing's sarcoma. Eur J Cancer. 1999;35:1698–704.
132. Rosito P, Mancini AF, Rondelli R, et al. Italian Cooperative Study for the treatment of children and young adults with localized Ewing sarcoma of bone: a preliminary report of 6 years of experience. Cancer. 1999;86:421–8.
133. Yaw KM. Pediatric bone tumors. Semin Surg Oncol. 1999;16:173–83.

134. Dunst J, Jürgen's H, Sauer R, et al. Radiation therapy in Ewing's sarcoma: an update of the CESS 86 trial. Int J Radiat Oncol Biol Phys. 1995;32:919–30.
135. Scully SP, Temple HT, O'Keefe RJ, et al. Role of surgical resection in pelvic Ewing's sarcoma. J Clin Oncol. 1995;13:2336–41.
136. Ginsberg JP, Woo SY, Johnson ME, Hicks MJ, Horowitz ME. Ewing's sarcoma family of tumors: Ewing's sarcoma of bone and soft tissue and peripheral primitive neuroectodermal tumors. In: Pizzo P, Poplack D, editors. Principles and practice of pediatric oncology. 4th ed. Philadelphia: Lippincott Williams & Wilkins; 2002. p. 973–1016.
137. Givens SS, Woo SY, Huang LY, et al. Non metastatic Ewing's sarcoma: twenty years of experience suggest that surgery is a prime factor for successful multimodality therapy. Int J Radiat Oncol Biol Phys. 1999;14:1039–43.
138. Wang CC, Schultz MD. Ewing's sarcoma. N Engl J Med. 1953;248:371–6.
139. Hustu HO, Pinkel D, Pratt CB. Treatment of clinically localized Ewing's sarcoma with radiotherapy and chemotherapy. Cancer. 1972;30:1522–7.
140. Burgert EO, Nesbit ME, Garnsey LA, et al. Multimodal therapy for the management of nonpelvic, localized Ewing's sarcoma of bone: intergroup study IESS-II. J Clin Oncol. 1990;8:1514–24.
141. Hayes FA, Thompson EI, Parvey L, et al. Metastatic Ewing's sarcoma: remission induction and survival. J Clin Oncol. 1987;5:1199–204.
142. Jurgens H, Ahrens S, Frohlich B, et al. European Intergroup Cooperative Ewing's Sarcoma Study (EICESS-92): first results. Proc Am Soc Clin Oncol. 2000; 19:581a.
143. Oberlin O, Habrand JL, Zucker JM, et al. No benefit of ifosfamide in Ewing's sarcoma: a non-randomized study of FSPO. J Clin Oncol. 1992;10:1407–12.
144. Womer RB, Daller RT, Fenton JG, et al. Granulocyte colony stimulating factor permits dose intensification by interval compression in the treatment of Ewing's sarcomas and soft tissue sarcomas in children. Eur J Cancer. 2000;36:87–94.
145. Miser JS, Goldsby RE, Chen Z, et al. Treatment of metastatic Ewing sarcoma/primitive neuroectodermal tumor of bone: evaluation of increasing the dose intensity of chemotherapy. A report from the Children's Oncology Group. Pediatr Blood Cancer. 2007;49(7):894–900.
146. Ladenstein R, Pötschger U, Le Deley MC, et al. Primary disseminated multifocal Ewing sarcoma: results of the EuroEWING 99 trial. J Clin Oncol. 2010;28:3284–91.
147. Barker LM, Pendergrass TW, Sanders JE, et al. Survival after recurrence of Ewing's sarcoma family of tumors. J Clin Oncol. 2005;23:4354–62.
148. Bacci G, Longhi A, Ferrari S, et al. Pattern of relapse in 290 patients with no metastatic Ewing's sarcoma family tumors treated at a single institution with adjuvant and neoadjuvant chemotherapy between 1972 and 1999. Eur J Surg Oncol. 2006;32:974–9.
149. Wasilewski-Masker K, Liu Q, Yasui Y, et al. Late recurrence in pediatric cancer: a report from the Childhood Cancer Survivor Study. J Natl Cancer Inst. 2009;10:1709–20.
150. Michon J, Oberlin O, Demeocq F, et al. Poor results in metastatic Ewing's sarcoma treated according to the scheme of the St. Jude 1978–1985 study: a study of the FSPO. SIOP XXV Meeting. Med Pediatr Oncol. 1993;21:572.
151. Miser JS, Krailo MD, Tarbell NJ, et al. Treatment of metastatic Ewing's sarcoma or primitive neuroectodermal tumor of bone: evaluation of combination ifosfamide and etoposide. A Children's Cancer Group and Pediatric Oncology Group study. J Clin Oncol. 2004;22: 2873–6.
152. Paulino AC, Mai WY, Teh BS. Radiotherapy in metastatic Ewing sarcoma. Am J Clin Oncol. 2013;36:283–6.
153. Paulussen M, Ahrens S, Burdach S, et al. Primary metastatic (stage IV) Ewing tumor: survival analysis of 171 patients from the EICESS studies. European Intergroup Cooperative Ewing Sarcoma Studies. Ann Oncol. 1998;9:275–81.
154. Casey DL, Wexler LH, Meyers PA, et al. Radiation for bone metastases in Ewing sarcoma and rhabdomyosarcoma. Pediatr Blood Cancer. 2015;62:445–9.
155. EURO-EWING INTERGROUP EE99 (COGAEWS0331/NCT00020566) (Combination Chemotherapy With or Without Peripheral Stem Cell Transplantation, Radiation Therapy,

and/or Surgery in Treating Patients With Ewing Sarcoma): A randomized study for patients with pulmonary metastases only, which is evaluating standard chemotherapy and PBSC transplant vs standard chemotherapy and bilateral lung radiation.
156. Luksch R, Grignani G, Fagioli F, et al. Response to melphalan in upfront investigational window therapy for patients with metastatic Ewing's family tumours. Eur J Cancer. 2007;43(5):885–90.
157. Stahl M, Ranft A, Paulussen M, et al. Risk of recurrence and survival after relapse in patients with Ewing sarcoma. Pediatr Blood Cancer. 2011;57:549–53.
158. Rodriguez-Galindo C, Billups CA, Kun LE, et al. Survival after recurrence of Ewing tumors: the St Jude Children's Research Hospital experience, 1979–1999. Cancer. 2002;94:561–9.
159. Leavey PJ, Mascarenhas L, Marina N, et al. Prognostic factors for patients with Ewing sarcoma (EWS) at first recurrence following multimodality therapy: a report from the Children's Oncology Group. Pediatr Blood Cancer. 2008;51:334–8.
160. Hunold A, Weddeling N, Paulussen M, et al. Topotecan and cyclophosphamide in patients with refractory or relapsed Ewing tumors. Pediatr Blood Cancer. 2006;47(6):795–800.
161. Mora J, Cruz CO, Parareda A, et al. Treatment of relapsed/refractory pediatric sarcomas with gemcitabine and docetaxel. J Pediatr Hematol Oncol. 2009;31:723–9.
162. Fox E, Patel S, Wathen JK, et al. Phase II study of sequential gemcitabine followed by docetaxel for recurrent Ewing sarcoma, osteosarcoma, or unresectable or locally recurrent chondrosarcoma: results of Sarcoma Alliance for Research Through Collaboration Study 003. Oncologist. 2012;17:321.
163. Ferrari S, del Prever AB, Palmerini E, et al. Response to high dose ifosfamide in patients with advanced/recurrent Ewing sarcoma. Pediatr Blood Cancer. 2009;52(5):581–4.
164. Wagner LM, McAllister N, Goldsby RE, et al. Temozolomide and intravenous irinotecan for treatment of advanced Ewing sarcoma. Pediatr Blood Cancer. 2007;48:132–9.
165. Casey DA, Wexler LH, Merchant MS, et al. Irinotecan and temozolomide for Ewing sarcoma: the Memorial Sloan Kettering experience. Pediatr Blood Cancer. 2009;53:1029–34.
166. Raciborska A, Bilska K, Drabko K, et al. Vincristine, irinotecan, and temozolomide in patients with relapsed and refractory Ewing sarcoma. Pediatr Blood Cancer. 2013;60:1621–5.
167. Burdach S, van Kaick B, Laws HJ, et al. Allogeneic and autologous stemcell transplantation in advanced Ewing tumors. An update after longterm followup from two centers of the European Intergroup study EICESS. StemCell Transplant Programs at Düsseldorf University Medical Center, Germany and St. Anna Kinderspital, Vienna, Austria. Ann Oncol. 2000;11:1451–62.
168. Gardner SL, Carreras J, Boudreau C, et al. Myeloablative therapy with autologous stem cell rescue for patients with Ewing sarcoma. Bone Marrow Transplant. 2008;4:867–72.
169. Mitsiades N, Poulaki V, Mitsiades C, et al. Ewing's sarcoma family tumors are sensitive to tumor necrosis factor-related apoptosis-inducing ligand and express death receptor 4 and death receptor 5. Cancer Res. 2001;61:2704–12.
170. Zhou Z, Jia SF, Hung MC, et al. E1A sensitizes HER2/neu-over-expressing Ewing's sarcoma cells to topoisomerase II-targeting anticancer drugs. Cancer Res. 2001;61:3394–8.
171. González I, Andreu EJ, Panizo A, et al. Imatinib inhibits proliferation of Ewing tumor cells mediated by the stem cell factor/KIT receptor pathway, and sensitizes cells to vincristine and doxorubicin-induced apoptosis. Clin Cancer Res. 2004;10:751–61.
172. Malempati S, Weigel B, Ingle AM, et al. Phase I/II trial and pharmacokinetic study of cixutumumab in pediatric patients with refractory solid tumors and Ewing sarcoma: a report from the Children's Oncology Group. J Clin Oncol. 2012;30:256–62.
173. Jürgen's H, Daw NC, Geoerger B, et al. Preliminary efficacy of the antiinsulinlike growth factor type 1 receptor antibody figitumumab in patients with refractory Ewing sarcoma. J Clin Oncol. 2011;29:4534–40.
174. Pappo AS, Patel SR, Crowley J, et al. R1507, a monoclonal antibody to the insulin-like growth factor 1 receptor, in patients with recurrent or refractory Ewing sarcoma family of tumors: results of a phase II Sarcoma Alliance for Research through Collaboration study. J Clin Oncol. 2011;29:4541–7.

175. Tap WD, Demetri G, Barnette P, et al. Phase II study of ganitumab, a fully human anti type1 insulin like growth factor receptor antibody, in patients with metastatic Ewing family tumors or desmoplastic small round cell tumors. J Clin Oncol. 2012;30:1849–56.
176. Naing A, LoRusso P, Fu S, et al. Insulin growth factor receptor (IGF1R) antibody cixutumumab combined with the mTOR inhibitor temsirolimus in patients with refractory Ewing's sarcoma family tumors. Clin Cancer Res. 2012;18:2625–31.

Chapter 3
Molecular Biology of Pediatric Bone Sarcomas

Ana Patiño-García, Marta Zalacain-Díez, and Fernando Lecanda

Abstract Genetic studies can help in the diagnosis and treatment of pediatric bone sarcoma patients as well as in the determination of prognosis for these patients. New drugs and targeted therapies are currently under development as a result of recent advances in molecular biology.

Keywords Osteosarcoma • Ewing's sarcoma • Genetic alteration • Prognostic marker • Tumor suppressor gene • Oncogene • Translocation

3.1 Osteosarcoma

3.1.1 Genetic Alterations

The molecular pathways involved in osteosarcoma development are complex, have not been fully explored, and their implication in the development and prognosis of this childhood tumor are not well understood. Even though certain clinical markers are clearly associated with prognosis, the value of such markers is limited by the fact that they only become evident in advanced stages of the tumoral process: development of metastases, relapse and response to neo-adjuvant chemotherapy. It is becoming imperative to find early molecular markers that allow for a more rational use of chemotherapy, for the development of new effective treatments and for the stratification of patients according to risk [1].

A. Patiño-García, PhD (✉)
Department of Pediatrics, University Clinic of Navarra IdiSNA,
Navarra Institute for Health Research, Pio Xii 36, Pamplona, Navarra 31008, Spain
e-mail: apatigar@unav.es

M. Zalacain-Díez, PhD
Pediatrics Laboratory, University Clinic of Navarra, Pamplona, Navarra, Spain

F. Lecanda, PhD
Program in Solid Tumors and Biomarkers, Center for Applied Medical Research (CIMA), Pamplona, Spain

M. San-Julian (ed.), *Cañadell's Pediatric Bone Sarcomas: Epiphysiolysis before Excision*, DOI 10.1007/978-3-319-24220-0_3

In this chapter, we will give a concise description of the pathways most frequently associated with osteosarcoma development and of the associated molecular markers that have proved to be of prognostic value.

3.1.2 *Cell Cycle Control*

Alteration of the different components involved in cell cycle control, particularly components of the p53 and retinoblastoma (RB1) pathways, seems to be the hallmark of the carcinogenic process underlying pediatric osteosarcoma: an alteration in the p53 pathway, the RB1 pathway or both has been detected in most tumors [2].

3.1.2.1 The p53 Pathway

Alterations that lead to inactivation of the p53 tumor suppression gene are frequently found in sporadic human tumors. The result is a loss of control of the cell cycle and DNA repair mechanisms (Fig. 3.1). Although there is considerable published evidence suggesting that the p53 protein has a role in the development of both sporadic osteosarcomas and those associated with the Li–Fraumeni syndrome, [3, 4] the prognostic value of alterations in p53 has not been conclusively established [5, 6]. The p53 protein is a tumor suppressor that gets activated upon DNA damage, arresting proliferation and inducing senescence, differentiation or apoptosis. Losses and deletions at the TP53 locus, at 17p13.1, are detected in 30–40 % of cases in which p53 is altered, with an additional 10–40 % showing point mutations of the

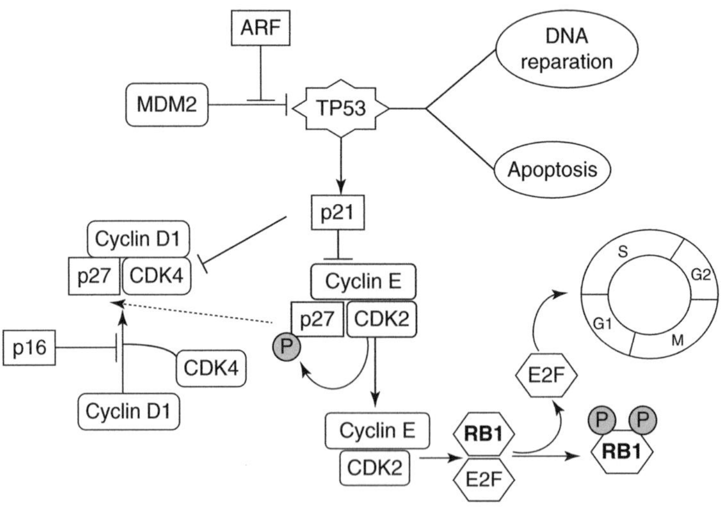

Fig. 3.1 Schematic representation of the cell cycle control mediated by TP53 and RB1

gene. P53 can also be post-translationally affected by MDM2, which either induces p53 degradation and/or down-regulates transcription. This latter type of alteration, being relatively infrequent, is an important marker of advanced stages of disease (metastasis and recurrences) [2].

3.1.2.2 The RB1 Pathway

The cell cycle control pathway that includes the retinoblastoma gene, RB1, is frequently altered in human tumors, especially in osteosarcomas [7] (Fig. 3.1). As described later, the loss of genetic material affecting the long arm of chromosome 13 (13q14) is a frequent genetic event in primary osteosarcomas, and this fact was interpreted to indicate the presence of a tumor suppressor gene at this chromosomal location. This suppressor has turned out to be RB1 [8].

The RB1 encodes a tumor suppressor protein, pRB, which regulates cell cycle progression (G1/S) by inhibiting E2F and other transcription factors of the same family. Cell cycle regulation involves cyclins, cyclin-dependent kinases (CDKs) and cyclin-dependent kinase inhibitors (CDKIs or CDKNs), and all of these genes and proteins, as key parts of the pRB pathway for cell cycle control, are often mutated or altered in osteosarcoma; examples include CDK4 amplification (10 % of cases), amplification of PRIM1 (40 %), deletion of 9p21, where CDKN2A/p16INK4, p14ARF and CDKN2B/p15INK4B are located (in about 5–20 %) [2].

About 20–70 % of osteosarcomas have a hemizygous deletion affecting the RB1 gene [9, 10]. About 30 % have structural rearrangements 18 and about 10 % have point mutations of the gene [11]. The presence of alterations at the RB1 locus can be considered as an early marker of malignancy and of unfavorable prognosis and, in addition, RB1 alterations are more frequently encountered in high-grade than in low-grade osteosarcomas [12, 13]. However, as with many of the molecular markers of this specific tumor, this prognostic association is not always found [14].

3.1.3 Growth Factors

1. *Members of the WNT Family* (*Wingless-Type*). The WNT signaling pathway controls normal bone formation during embryogenesis and bone homeostasis in the adult. Various publications describe research into this pathway in the context of the osteosarcoma model. Recent data suggest that the WNT pathway may have a paracrine and autocrine effect involved in the metastatic potential of osteosarcoma, [15, 16] although these data remain to be reproduced.
2. *Her-2/neu* (*Epidermal Growth Factor Receptor*). Overexpression of this tyrosine kinase is considered an indicator of poor prognosis in various types of carcinoma, since it is related with tumor growth and the metastatic process. Her-2 is

expressed in a proportion of osteosarcoma cases but, despite the implied involvement of Her-2 in osteosarcoma, neither normal nor pathological levels of Her-2 expression have been unequivocally established and consequently the prognostic value of Her-2 is still being researched; different reports present contradictory results. However, Her-2 remains an attractive therapeutic target. To date, at least one study of trastuzumab for the treatment of osteosarcoma has been completed, and although the findings suggest that trastuzumab can be safely used with chemotherapy in osteosarcoma, its therapeutic benefit remains uncertain. The authors conclude that definitive assessment of trastuzumab's potential role in treating osteosarcoma would require a randomized study of patients with Her-2-positive disease [17, 18].

There are many other genes of interest under investigation. One of these is ezrin, which is a prototypical member of the ERM (Ezrin/Radixin/Moesin) protein family. The encoded protein is involved in cell-to-cell interaction, in connecting the actin cytoskeleton and the plasma membrane and in signal transduction. Overexpression of ezrin promotes metastasis, probably by allowing metastatic cells to overcome the controls and limitations imposed on them during the metastatic cascade and by facilitating the cells' interaction with the environment of the secondary, metastatic, site: metastatic cells must rapidly adapt to their new environment in order to survive, and it seems that, through participation in processes such as the translation of new proteins and the generation of ATP, ezrin expression could be related to this cellular adaption [19].

The fact that the timing of the peak incidence of osteosarcoma overlaps with that of the pubertal growth spurt may indicate that insulin-like growth factor-I (*IGF-I*) and its receptor play a role in the pathogenesis of this disease. The IGF-I growth factor acts as a mitogen on both murine and human osteosarcoma cells, and osteosarcoma cell lines are dependent on IGF-I for *in vitro* growth. It has been hypothesized that even in osteosarcoma patients whose levels of IGF-I and its binding protein (IGFBP3) are not increased, other members of the IGF-I axis could be involved in the development and progression of osteosarcoma [20, 21].

3.1.4 Angiogenesis

The vascular endothelial growth factor (VEGF) stimulates microvascular growth and has a clear role in the development of certain tumors (such as those of the breast and colon) by increasing the supply of nutrients and blood to them. The use of anti-angiogenic agents (inhibitors of the VEGF pathway) is controversial in the case of osteosarcoma, and reports show contradictory results [22, 23]. Therefore, the utility of this and other related molecules (for example, pigment epithelium derived factor [PEDF]) as therapeutic targets in osteosarcoma have yet to be determined, as have the synergic effect of these molecules with chemotherapy. Studies are already in progress [24].

3.1.5 Matrix Metalloproteinases

Matrix metalloproteinases (MMPs) are enzymes that are physiologically involved in tissue remodeling and angiogenesis. Excessive production of MMPs, whether as a result of increased transcription of coding genes or as a result of a lack of inhibitors, is important in the process of invasion and metastasis. MMP9, a member of this family, seems to have a prominent role in bone remodeling diseases like osteosarcoma, and several publications have shown that MMP9 overexpression in osteosarcoma is a factor indicating poor prognosis (with an increase in metastatic potential and reduced overall 5-year survival) [25, 26]. MMP9 can be repressed by a variety of molecules, a fact that makes it an interesting target for attempts to decrease the invasive potential of tumor cells. Indeed, this effect has been demonstrated in animal models and cultured cells.

3.1.6 P Glycoprotein

P glycoprotein (P-gp), which is coded by the multidrug resistance 1 (MDR1) gene, is a membrane molecule involved in drug transport. For more than a decade, P-gp overexpression has been known to be a negative prognostic factor in osteosarcoma [27]. There are various reasons for this, one of them being that P-gp is what makes osteosarcoma cells resistant to doxorubicin, a prime cytostatic drug in the standard chemotherapy for this pediatric tumor [28]. Some authors have identified a link between P-gp and p53 overexpression. As described above, the p53 molecular pathway is another pathway frequently altered in osteosarcomas. According to this model, patients whose tumors have co-overexpression of P-gp and p53 would have significantly reduced survival and a more unfavorable Enneking stage [29].

3.1.7 Chromosomal Alterations

Conventional karyotype analyses show that, as a general rule, osteosarcomas have complex altered karyotypes with multiple numerical and structural aberrations; this is mostly due to an elevated rate of chromosomal instability (CIN) involved in the pathogenesis of osteosarcoma. The most frequently encountered alterations in primary tumors (as opposed to cell lines) are the duplication or gain of chromosome arms 1p, 1q, 6p, 8q, and 17p; and the loss of chromosomes or chromosome arms 3q, 6q, 9, 10, 13 (RB1 locus), 17p (TP53 locus), and 18q [30]. In general, regions frequently found to be deleted or lost are suspected to contain tumor suppressor genes, while genomic regions that are duplicated, gained or amplified are suspected to contain oncogenes [2, 31].

Metaphase comparative genomic hybridization (CGH) has proved a useful, high-resolution tool to unveil and characterize complex karyotypes, and studies based on CGH have identified high copy number regions or amplifications at 8q12–q21.3, 8q22–q23 (MYC gene) and at 17p11.2–17p12 [31]. The chromosomal regions that are more frequently gained or lost have been carefully identified and reviewed [32–34]. Work by Ozaki and colleagues establishes that the gain or loss of some of these regions, either as isolated aberrations or as specific combinations, might have prognostic value [35].

3.1.8 New Identification Studies, GWAS

Recently, new approaches such as genome-wide association studies (GWAS) have been applied to identify genes potentially involved in osteosarcoma. An international, multi-institutional collaborative study of osteosarcoma performed a GWAS including 941 osteosarcoma cases and 3291 cancer-free adult controls. The study found two regions of susceptibility: 2p25.2, an apparent desert region, and 6p21.3, containing the metabotropic glutamate receptor 4 (GRM4) gene. Although further studies are needed, GRM4 seems to be a significant gene in osteosarcoma and even a plausible candidate gene for the disease, and it is expressed in osteoblasts and osteoclasts. GRM4 has been implicated in intracellular signaling by inhibition of the cAMP cascade. In mice, a gene with similar function (Prkar1α) is an osteosarcoma tumor suppressor gene involved in tumorigenesis [36].

3.2 Ewing's Sarcoma Tumors

3.2.1 Introduction

Tumors within the Ewing's sarcoma family (EFTs) constitute the second most frequent type of bone-/soft- tissue sarcoma in children and adolescents [37, 38]. The family comprises classical Ewing's sarcoma, peripheral primitive neuroectodermal tumors, and Askin's tumor, all of which are highly aggressive and frequently metastatic [39]. Tumors often appear in tubular bones of the appendicular skeleton (58 %), although they also arise in the axial skeleton (33 %) and at extraosseous sites [40]. Histologically, Ewing's tumors are characterized by the presence of small round cells with prominent and regular nuclei containing inconspicuous nucleoli, indistinct cytoplasm [38] and various degrees of neural and endothelial differentiation [41].

Until the advent of differential molecular techniques, an unambiguous diagnosis required experienced pathological assessment. None of the markers used in conventional immunohistochemistry showed complete specificity. The transmembrane glycoprotein MIC2/CD99, the most specific marker so far, is expressed in more than 98 % of EFTs [42].

Other tumors, including rhabdomyosarcoma and lymphoblastic lymphoma, also have immunohistochemical markers. Depending on the degree of neuroectodermal differentiation, EFTs may express neural markers, including S-100 synaptophysin, neural-specific enolase, CD57 and various neurofilaments [43]. Currently, the best tools for diagnosis are fluorescence *in situ* hybridization and RT-PCR with a combination of primers targeting the underlying chromosomal translocations [44].

Much of the progress over the last few decades has concerned improved pathological definition and staging [45]. Despite a parallel improvement in treatment by multi-modal combination of surgery with chemo- and radio- therapy, the 5-year survival rate has remained close to 50 % for patients with primary tumors [46] and only 25 % for patients with lung metastasis; the prognosis for patients with bone or bone marrow metastasis is even worse [47]. The tumor also exhibits a strong tendency to metastasize through hematogenous spread to the lungs and frequently to the skeleton. In addition to the stage, location and size of the tumor, metastasis is a reliable indicator of poor prognosis.

3.2.2 Molecular Biology

The demonstration that fusion proteins were the "culprits" of the transforming events giving rise to hematological malignancies provided a strong rationale for research into the role of fusion proteins in other tumors. EFTs belong to a growing family of sarcomas characterized by specific reciprocal chromosomal translocations, which generate fusion genes: the neoplasm has a relatively simple cytogenetic background [48]. At present, more than 15 different fusion proteins have been identified in EFTs. Chromosomal translocation t(11;22) q(24;q12) produces gene fusions between the amino terminus domain of EWS and the C-terminal region of a member belonging to the ETS family of transcription factors. Fusions resulting from this translocation give rise to transcription factors that function in an aberrant manner and can drive transformation in a permissive cellular context.

In 85 % of Ewing's tumors, it is the Friend Leukemia Integration 1 transcription factor (FLI-1) that is the EWS partner that accounts for the different fusion subtypes observed [49]. Depending on the juxtaposed exons assembled by EWS and FLI-1 breakpoints, several subtypes have been described. Most tumors contain EWS/FLI-1 fusion types 1 (60 %) and 2 (25 %), which have been associated with different clinical features and prognosis [50, 51]

The FLI-1 gene displays a restricted pattern of expression: it is expressed mainly in hematopoietic cells, and to a lesser degree in heart, lung and ovaries [52]. During development, FLI-1 is also expressed in cells of neural crest-derived mesenchymal lineage and endothelial cells, which is consistent with its known role in angiogenesis and hematopoiesis [53].

In contrast to FLI-1, the EWS gene encodes a ubiquitously expressed protein that belongs to the TET family of RNA binding proteins [49, 54]. The TET family also includes TAFII68 (or TAF15) [55, 56] and FUS (or TLS), [57] both of which share similar structural domains with EWS and have been found to form gene fusions with non-ETS transcription factors, giving rise to non-Ewing sarcomas such as myxoid liposarcomas, [58] myxoid chondrosarcomas [59] and desmoplastic small round-cell tumors, [60] with different histopathological features. EWS contains three arginine–glycine–glycine (RGG) rich motifs that participate in RNA synthesis and processing through interaction with proteins of the basal transcription machinery; these proteins include TFIID, RNA polymerase II [61, 62] and coactivators such as CBP/p300 [55, 54]. In addition, proteins in the TET family interact with splicing proteins. Indeed, EWS/FLI-1 has been shown to bind with the splicing factor U1C and subsequently to modulate splicing activity [62–64]. EWS interaction with other proteins has also been described, for example, with BARD1, although the relevance, if any, of this to tumorigenesis has not been elucidated [65].

Most research into EWS has focused on its function as a transcription factor. The amino terminal domain of EWS contains a glutamine-rich N-terminal region containing a potent transcriptional activation domain [66, 67] that, when fused to the DNA-binding domain of FLI-1, generates an aberrant but active transcription factor capable of specifically binding DNA [68]. Since the majority of fusion subtypes do not encompass the RGG domain, there has been less research into the effects of EWS–ETS fusions on RNA synthesis. All members of the ETS family of transcription factors are characterized by a common DNA-binding domain. Fusions of EWS with other ETS family members have been described, [69] including fusions with ERG (in 10 % of Ewing's tumors) [70] and with other, more rare, partners such as ETV1, [71] ETV4 [72] and FEV [73]. The fact that different combinations of EWS/ETS give rise to Ewing's tumors of similar histopathology suggests that the potent transactivation domain of EWS, through interaction with other unknown proteins, is critical for transformation.

Complementary to this view, the DNA binding domains of ETS proteins are highly homologous and all recognize targets containing a similar core sequence. Therefore, despite their differences, all EWS–ETS fusion proteins can be expected to act in a similar manner that involves disruption of a tightly regulated pattern of gene transcription, resulting ultimately in the formation of Ewing's tumors.

3.2.3 The Oncoprotein EWS/FLI-1 as a Paradigm

The discovery of EWS/FLI-1 underscores the attractiveness of an approach to research based on seeking to reveal common mechanisms in many tumors arising from specific translocations. Depending on the cellular background, EWS/FLI-1 induces a variety of responses that include transformation, senescence, differentiation, and cell lineage commitment. The presence of neural markers in Ewing's tumor cells and the diverse sites of tumor origin have frequently led to the assumption or hypothesis that EFTs develop out of a cell type that possesses the potential to differentiate into multiple lineages.

In vitro experiments revealed that the chimeric EWS/FLI-1 acts as a potent repressor of normal cell fate. In murine primary marrow-derived stromal cells, EWS/FLI-1 represses osteogenic and adipogenic programs [74, 75]. Similarly, myogenic differentiation was suppressed by the chimeric protein in a murine multipotent mesenchymal cell line [74]. In contrast, in other cellular backgrounds, EWS/FLI-1 dictates cell lineage commitment by redirecting cells towards a neural-like phenotype [76]. Differentiation towards the neuroectodermal phenotype typical of Ewing's tumors, with the acquisition of a small round cell morphology, has been obtained in a fibroblastic cell line [77]. Similarly, in neuroblastoma, Hela, and rhabdomyosarcoma cell lines, the forced expression of EWS-FLI1 resulted in the acquisition of neural phenotypic traits [78]. Consistent with the role of FLI-1 during development, in a separate rhabdomyosarcoma cell line, the expression of neural crest phenotypic markers was induced by EWS/FLI-1 [79].

In addition to repression of normal cell fate, EWS/FLI-1 is thought to induce cell specific oncogenesis in a transformation-permissive cellular background. However, many cell lines, including Rat-1 fibroblasts, Ncm1, CTR, and the NIH 3 T3-derived cell line YAL-7, have been found to be refractory to transformation [80]. Single-step oncogenesis has been reported in murine primary cells [66, 77, 81, 82]. This finding can be attributed to a better transformation potential of rodent cells compared to human cells [83, 84]. In a study by Castillero-Trejo et al., tumorogenicity increased with cell passage in culture and other secondary events, including p53 deletion [81]. Murine bone-derived cells expressing EWS/FLI-1 showed formation of sarcomatous tumors in syngeneic mice. Riggi et al. reported that a single event of transduction with EWS/FLI-1 was sufficient to reconstitute the hallmarks of Ewing sarcoma genesis in a murine model [82]. In contrast, Riggi et al. were unable to reproduce the corresponding findings in primary human cells [85]. Studies of a human model have recently provided strong experimental evidence that the originating cell type is of mesenchymal lineage [86].

Why is it easier to induce tumorigenesis in mouse cells than in human cells? In the mouse, background tumor suppressor pathways, including p16/p19 and p53, may be overcome by unknown factors. In human cells, however, additional mutations may be required to circumvent the strong tumor suppressor program. Indeed, other cytogenetic events [87] and additional mutations have been found in 20–30 % [88–90] of human Ewing's tumors. An alternative suggestion recently put forward is that the cancer-initiating cells that are able to sustain tumor growth *in vivo* in humans may actually be deregulated progenitor cells present in adult tissues [91, 92]. It is possible that the target for the transformation event driven by EWS/FLI-1 is an as yet unidentified progenitor cell.

3.2.4 *Target Genes*

One of the main goals in the study of the genesis of Ewing sarcoma has been to identify downstream target genes regulated by EWS/FLI-1. Global transcriptome analysis in combination with other techniques has elucidated several genes involved in the genetic program driven by the fusion protein. The genes found are involved in neural differentiation, cell proliferation and anti-apoptotic functions. However, because the studies differ significantly in terms of cellular model, it has been difficult to discern which EWS/FLI-1-responsive genes are associated with the initiation and maintenance of tumors.

The most compelling identified target of EWS/FLI-1 is the gene coding for the homeodomain protein NKX2.2, [93] which is transcriptional repressor involved in neural cell differentiation. Induction of NKX2.2 is necessary for oncogenic transformation and represents a potential Ewing diagnostic marker. The protein's strong repressive function is mediated by a HDAC-dependent mechanism [93, 94].

Id2, a helix–loop–helix transcription factor without the DNA-binding domain, has been found to be upregulated by EWS/FLI-1 in Ewing's tumors. Through interaction with a variety of cell cycle proteins including p21 and Rb tumor suppressors, [95, 96] Id2 is able to promote cell proliferation. Other potential target genes transcriptionally upregulated by EWS/FLI-1 include PDGF-C, [97] which is expressed in more than 60 % of tumors, CCND1 [98, 99] and c-Myc [100, 101].

hTERT, the catalytic subunit of telomerase and one of the hallmarks of many Ewing's tumors, has been found to be upregulated in approximately 80 % of Ewing's samples. The upregulation is an indirect effect of EWS/FLI-1 [102] through the recruitment of an unknown ancillary protein. Similarly, key tumor suppressors such as p57, [100] p21 [103] and TGFBRII [104, 105] were found to be downregulated in Ewing's tumors. Interestingly, IGFBP-3 is a direct target of the fusion protein: EWS/FLI-1 binds to the IGFBP-3 promoter both *in vitro* and *in vivo*, [106] and the consequent repression leads to increased Akt activity and decreased apoptotic activity. Similarly, the IGF-1/IGF-1R axis, which is frequently required for Ewing's tumor cell growth, promotes cell survival through the Akt pathway [107, 108]. Different pharmacological strategies targeting IGF1R are currently being explored for the treatment of Ewing's tumors [109, 110].

Recently, the combination of the techniques of transcriptome analysis with high throughput chromatin immunoprecipitation analysis has validated previous research on EWS/FLI-1 by identifying previously reported genes (NKX2.2, ID2 and CCND1) and has also found additional relevant targets, including NROB1 [111–113] and GAS1. The role of these targets in Ewing sarcomagenesis is yet to be determined.

The complexity of the EWS/FLI-1 -induced program is underscored by the disruption of gene regulatory circuits as a direct result of induction or repression of enhancers: oncogenes are activated by a remodeling of the patterns of chromatin. Such oncogenes represent novel potential therapeutic targets, an example being the kinase VRK1 [114]. EWS/FLI-1 has also been shown to regulate alternative splicing [115] and to be itself regulated by a long piece of non-coding RNA: RNA-277 (Ewing sarcoma-associated transcript 1 [EWSAT1]) [116].

Massive DNA sequencing has revealed frequent somatic mutations in the following genes: STAG2 (17 %), CDKN2A (12 %), TP53 (7 %), EZH2, BCOR, and ZMYM3 (2.7 % each) [117, 118]. Interestingly, concurrent mutations in STAG2 and TP53 are associated with poor prognosis [118].

3.2.5 Future Directions

The experimental platforms developed in EFT research hold the potential to resolve many big questions regarding the development of both EFTs and a variety of other sarcomas. Despite the remarkable progress over the last two decades, there are still several areas that have not been rigorously addressed. Amongst these are the clear definition of the permissive cell and the specific time and micro-environment required for transformation. Similarly, the critical molecular events driven by the chimeric EWS/FLI-1 protein to initiate and maintain Ewing's tumors remain to be systematically dissected in an appropriate model. To this end, an animal model faithfully reproducing the spatiotemporal development of Ewing's sarcomas would be an invaluable tool. Only with precise knowledge at the cellular and molecular levels can we expect to elucidate the critical target gene or genes of the EWS/FLI-1 protein.

References

1. Clark JC, Dass CR, Choong PF. A review of clinical and molecular prognostic factors in osteosarcoma. J Cancer Res Clin Oncol. 2008;134:281–97.
2. Martin JM, Squire JA, Zielenska M. The genetics of osteosarcoma. Sarcoma. 2012;2012: 627254.
3. Soussi T, Leblanc T, Baruchel A, Schaison G. Germline mutations of the p53 tumor-suppressor gene in cancer-prone families: a review. Nouv Rev Fr Hematol. 1993;35:33–6.
4. Mirabello L, Yeager M, Mai PL, Gastier-Foster JM, Gorlick R, Khanna C, Patiño-Garcia A, Sierrasesúmaga L, Lecanda F, Andrulis IL, Wunder JS, Gokgoz N, Barkauskas DA, Zhang X, Vogt A, Jones K, Boland JF, Chanock SJ, Savage SA. Germline TP53 variants and susceptibility to osteosarcoma. J Natl Cancer Inst. 2015;107(7):djv101.
5. Kaseta MK, Khaldi L, Gomatos IP, et al. Prognostic value of bax, bcl-2, and p53 staining in primary osteosarcoma. J Surg Oncol. 2008;97:259–66.
6. Wunder JS, Gokgoz N, Parkes R, et al. TP53 mutations and outcome in osteosarcoma: a prospective, multicenter study. J Clin Oncol. 2005;23:1483–90.
7. Belchis DA, Gocke CD, Geradts J. Alterations in the rb, p16, and cyclin d1 cell cycle control pathway in osteosarcomas. Pediatr Pathol Mol Med. 2000;19:377–89.
8. Yamaguchi T, Toguchida J, Yamamuro T, et al. Allelotype analysis in osteosarcomas: frequent allele loss on 3q, 13q, 17p, and 18q. Cancer Res. 1992;52:2419–23.
9. Wadayama B, Feugeas O, Guriec N, et al. Loss of heterozygosity of the RB gene is a poor prognostic factor in patients with osteosarcoma. J Clin Oncol. 1996;14:467–72.
10. Benassi MS, Molendini L, Gamberi G, et al. Alteration of pRb/p16/cdk4 regulation in human osteosarcoma. Int J Cancer. 1999;84:489–93.
11. Wadayama B, Toguchida J, Shimizu T, et al. Mutation spectrum of the retinoblastoma gene in osteosarcomas. Cancer Res. 1994;54:3042–8.
12. Patiño-García A, Piñeiro ES, Díez MZ, Iturriagagoitia LG, Klüssmann FA, Ariznabarreta LS. Genetic and epigenetic alterations of the cell cycle regulators and tumor suppressor genes in pediatric osteosarcomas. J Pediatr Hematol Oncol. 2003;25:362–7.
13. Wunder JS, Czitrom AA, Kandel R, Andrulis IL. Analysis of alterations in the retinoblastoma gene and tumor grade in bone and soft-tissue sarcomas. J Natl Cancer Inst. 1991;83:194–200.
14. Heinsohn S, Evermann U, Zur Stadt U, Bielack S, Kabisch H. Determination of the prognostic value of loss of heterozygosity at the retinoblastoma gene in osteosarcoma. Int J Oncol. 2007;30:1205–14.

15. Chen K, Fallen S, Abaan HO, Hayran M, et al. WNT10b induces chemotaxis of osteosarcoma and correlates with reduced survival. Pediatr Blood Cancer. 2008;51:349–55.
16. Hoang BH, Kubo T, Healey JH, et al. Expression of LDL receptor-related protein 5 (LRP5) as a novel marker for disease progression in high-grade osteosarcoma. Int J Cancer. 2004;109:106–11.
17. Gill J, Geller D, Gorlick R. HER-2 involvement in osteosarcoma. Adv Exp Med Biol. 2014;804:161–77.
18. Ebb D, Meyers P, Grier H, Bernstein M, Gorlick R, Lipshultz SE, Krailo M, Devidas M, Barkauskas DA, Siegal GP, Ferguson WS, Letson GD, Marcus K, Goorin A, Beardsley P, Marina N. Phase II trial of trastuzumab in combination with cytotoxic chemotherapy for treatment of metastatic osteosarcoma with human epidermal growth factor receptor 2 overexpression: a report from the children's oncology group. J Clin Oncol. 2012;30:2545–51.
19. Ren L, Khanna C. Role of ezrin in osteosarcoma metastasis. Adv Exp Med Biol. 2014;804: 181–201.
20. Chavez Kappel C, Velez-Yanguas C, Hirschfeld S, Helman LJ. Human osteosarcoma cell lines are dependent on insulin-like growth factor for in vitro growth. Cancer Res. 1994;54: 2803–7.
21. Rodriguez-Galindo C, Poquette CA, Daw NC, Tan M, Meyer WH, Cleveland JL. Circulating concentrations of IGF-I and IGFBP-3 are not predictive of incidence or clinical behavior of pediatric osteosarcoma. Med Pediatr Oncol. 2001;36:605–11.
22. Ek ET, Ojaimi J, Kitagawa Y, Choong PF. Does the degree of intratumoral microvessel density and VEGF expression have prognostic significance in osteosarcoma. Oncol Rep. 2006;16:17–23.
23. Kreuter M, Bieker R, Bielack SS, et al. Prognostic relevance of increased angiogenesis in osteosarcoma. Clin Cancer Res. 2004;10:8531–7.
24. Stempak D, Gammon J, Halton J, Moghrabi A, Koren G, Baruchel S. A pilot pharmacokinetic and antiangiogenic biomarker study of celecoxib and low-dose metronomic vinblastine or cyclophosphamide in pediatric recurrent solid tumors. J Pediatr Hematol Oncol. 2006;28: 720–8.
25. Foukas AF, Deshmukh NS, Grimer RJ, Mangham DC, Mangos EG, Taylor S. Stage-IIB osteosarcomas around the knee A study of MMP-9 in surviving tumor cells. J Bone Joint Surg Br. 2002;84:706–11.
26. Kido A, Tsutsumi M, Iki K, et al. Overexpression of matrix metalloproteinase (MMP)-9 correlates with metastatic potency of spontaneous and 4-hydroxyaminoquinoline 1-oxide (4-HAQO)-induced transplantable osteosarcomas in rats. Cancer Lett. 1999;137:209–16.
27. Pakos EE, Ioannidis JP. The association of P-glycoprotein with response to chemotherapy and clinical outcome in patients with osteosarcoma A meta-analysis. Cancer. 2003;98(3): 581–9.
28. Baldini N, Scotlandi K, Serra M, et al. P-glycoprotein expression in osteosarcoma: a basis for risk-adapted adjuvant chemotherapy. J Orthop Res. 1999;17:629–32.
29. Park YB, Kim HS, Oh JH, Lee SH. The co-expression of p53 protein and P-glycoprotein is correlated to a poor prognosis in osteosarcoma. Int Orthop. 2001;24:307–10.
30. Sandberg AA, Bridge JA. Updates on the cytogenetics and molecular genetics of bone and soft tissue tumors: osteosarcoma and related tumors. Cancer Genet Cytogenet. 2003;145: 1–30. 32.
31. Squire JA, Pei J, Marrano P, et al. High-resolution mapping of amplifi cations and deletions in pediatric osteosarcoma by use of CGH analysis of cDNA microarrays. Genes Chromosomes Cancer. 2003;38:215–25.
32. Forus A, Weghuis DO, Smeets D, Fodstad O, Myklebost O, Geurts van Kessel A. Comparative genomic hybridization analysis of human sarcomas: II. Identification of novel amplicons at 6p and 17p in osteosarcomas. Genes Chromosomes Cancer. 1995;14:15–21.
33. Tarkkanen M, Karhu R, Kallioniemi A, et al. Gains and losses of DNA sequences in osteosarcomas by comparative genomic hybridization. Cancer Res. 1995;55:1334–8.

34. Zielenska M, Marrano P, Thorner P, et al. High-resolution cDNA microarray CGH mapping of genomic imbalances in osteosarcoma using formalin-fi xed paraffi n-embedded tissue. Cytogenet Genome Res. 2004;107:77–82.
35. Ozaki T, Schaefer KL, Wai D, et al. Genetic imbalances revealed by comparative genomic hybridization in osteosarcomas. Int J Cancer. 2002;102:355–65.
36. Savage SA, Mirabello L, Wang Z, Gastier-Foster JM, Gorlick R, Khanna C, Flanagan AM, Tirabosco R, Andrulis IL, Wunder JS, Gokgoz N, Patiño-Garcia A, Sierrasesúmaga L, Lecanda F, Kurucu N, Ilhan IE, Sari N, Serra M, Hattinger C, Picci P, Spector LG, Barkauskas DA, Marina N, de Toledo SR, Petrilli AS, Amary MF, Halai D, Thomas DM, Douglass C, Meltzer PS, Jacobs K, Chung CC, Berndt SI, Purdue MP, Caporaso NE, Tucker M, Rothman N, Landi MT, Silverman DT, Kraft P, Hunter DJ, Malats N, Kogevinas M, Wacholder S, Troisi R, Helman L, Fraumeni Jr JF, Yeager M, Hoover RN, Chanock SJ. Genome-wide association study identifies two susceptibility loci for osteosarcoma. Nat Genet. 2013;45:799–803.
37. Gurney JG, Davis S, Severson RK, Fang JY, Ross JA, Robison LL. Trends in cancer incidence among children in the U.S. Cancer. 1996;78:532–41.
38. Arndt CA, Crist WM. Common musculoskeletal tumors of childhood and adolescence. N Engl J Med. 1999;341:342–52.
39. de Alava E, Gerald WL. Molecular biology of the Ewing's sarcoma/primitive neuroectodermal tumor family. J Clin Oncol. 2000;18:204–13.
40. Grier HE. The Ewing family of tumors Ewing's sarcoma and primitive neuroectodermal tumors. Pediatr Clin North Am. 1997;44:991–1004.
41. Franchi A, Pasquinelli G, Cenacchi G, et al. Immunohistochemical and ultrastructural investigation of neural differentiation in Ewing sarcoma/PNET of bone and soft tissues. Ultrastruct Pathol. 2001;25:219–25.
42. Kovar H, Dworzak M, Strehl S, et al. Overexpression of the pseudoautosomal gene MIC2 in Ewing's sarcoma and peripheral primitive neuroectodermal tumor. Oncogene. 1990;5:1067–70.
43. Ushigome SMR, Sorensen PH. Ewing sarcoma/Primitive Neuroectodermal Tumor (PNET). In: Christopher DM, Fletcher KKU, Fredrik M, editors. Pathology and genetics of tumors of soft tissue and Bone World Health Organization classification of tumors. Lyon: Pathology and Genetics of Tumors of Soft Tissue and Bone International Agency for Research on Cancer; 2002.
44. Peter M, Gilbert E, Delattre O. A multiplex real-time PCR assay for the detection of gene fusions observed in solid tumors. Lab Invest. 2001;81:905–12.
45. Burchill SA. Ewing's sarcoma: diagnostic, prognostic, and therapeutic implications of molecular abnormalities. J Clin Pathol. 2003;56:96–102.
46. Paulussen M, Ahrens S, Craft AW, et al. Ewing's tumors with primary lung metastases: survival analysis of 114 (European Intergroup) Cooperative Ewing's Sarcoma Studies patients. J Clin Oncol. 1998;16:3044–52.
47. Cotterill SJ, Ahrens S, Paulussen M, et al. Prognostic factors in Ewing's tumor of bone: analysis of 975 patients from the European Intergroup Cooperative Ewing's Sarcoma Study Group. J Clin Oncol. 2000;18:3108–14.
48. Mackall CL, Meltzer PS, Helman LJ. Focus on sarcomas. Cancer Cell. 2002;2:175–8.
49. Delattre O, Zucman J, Plougastel B, et al. Gene fusion with an ETS DNA-binding domain caused by chromosome translocation in human tumors. Nature. 1992;359:162–5.
50. de Alava E, Kawai A, Healey JH, et al. EWS-FLI1 fusion transcript structure is an independent determinant of prognosis in Ewing's sarcoma. J Clin Oncol. 1998;16:1248–55.
51. Zoubek A, Dockhorn-Dworniczak B, Delattre O, et al. Does expression of different EWS chimeric transcripts define clinically distinct risk groups of Ewing tumor patients. J Clin Oncol. 1996;14:1245–51.
52. Ben-David Y, Giddens EB, Letwin K, Bernstein A. Erythroleukemia induction by Friend murine leukemia virus: insertional activation of a new member of the ets gene family, Fli-1, closely linked to c-ets-1. Genes Dev. 1991;5:908–18.

53. Melet F, Motro B, Rossi DJ, Zhang L, Bernstein A. Generation of a novel Fli-1 protein by gene targeting leads to a defect in thymus development and a delay in friend virus-induced erythroleukemia. Mol Cell Biol. 1996;16:2708–18.
54. Ohno T, Ouchida M, Lee L, Gatalica Z, Rao VN, Reddy ES. The EWS gene, involved in Ewing family of tumors, malignant melanoma of soft parts and desmoplastic small round cell tumors, codes for an RNA binding protein with novel regulatory domains. Oncogene. 1994;9:3087–97.
55. Bertolotti A, Lutz Y, Heard DJ, Chambon P, Tora L. hTAF(II)68, a novel RNA/ssDNA-binding protein with homology to the pro-oncoproteins TLS/FUS and EWS is associated with both TFIID and RNA polymerase II. EMBO J. 1996;15:5022–31.
56. Aman P, Panagopoulos I, Lassen C, et al. Expression patterns of the human sarcoma-associated genes FUS and EWS and the genomic structure of FUS. Genomics. 1996;37: 1–8.
57. Shing DC, McMullan DJ, Roberts P, et al. FUS/ERG gene fusions in Ewing's tumors. Cancer Res. 2003;63:4568–76.
58. Crozat A, Aman P, Mandahl N, Ron D. Fusion of CHOP to a novel RNA-binding protein in human myxoid liposarcoma. Nature. 1993;363:640–4.
59. Labelle Y, Zucman J, Stenman G, et al. Oncogenic conversion of a novel orphan nuclear receptor by chromosome translocation. Hum Mol Genet. 1995;4:2219–26.
60. Ladanyi M, Gerald W. Fusion of the EWS and WT1 genes in the desmoplastic small round cell tumor. Cancer Res. 1994;54:2837–40.
61. Petermann R, Mossier BM, Aryee DN, Khazak V, Golemis EA, Kovar H. Oncogenic EWS-Fli1 interacts with hsRPB7, a subunit of human RNA polymerase II. Oncogene. 1998;17: 603–10.
62. Yang L, Chansky HA, Hickstein DD. EWS. Fli-1 fusion protein interacts with hyperphosphorylated RNA polymerase II and interferes with serine-arginine protein-mediated RNA splicing. J Biol Chem. 2000;275:37612–8.
63. Knoop LL, Baker SJ. The splicing factor U1C represses EWS/FLI-mediated transactivation. J Biol Chem. 2000;275:24865–71.
64. Knoop LL, Baker SJ. EWS/FLI alters 5′ ¢ -splice site selection. J Biol Chem. 2001;276: 22317–22.
65. Spahn L, Petermann R, Siligan C, Schmid JA, Aryee DN, Kovar H. Interaction of the EWS NH2 terminus with BARD1 links the Ewing's sarcoma gene to a common tumor suppressor pathway. Cancer Res. 2002;62:4583–7.
66. May WA, Gishizky ML, Lessnick SL, et al. Ewing sarcoma 11;22 translocation produces a chimeric transcription factor that requires the DNA-binding domain encoded by FLI1 for transformation. Proc Natl Acad Sci USA. 1993;90:5752–6.
67. Lessnick SL, Braun BS, Denny CT, May WA. Multiple domains mediate transformation by the Ewing's sarcoma EWS/FLI-1 fusion gene. Oncogene. 1995;10:423–31.
68. Janknecht R, Nordheim A. Gene regulation by Ets proteins. Biochim Biophys Acta. 1993;1155:346–56.
69. Huang HY, Illei PB, Zhao Z, et al. Ewing sarcomas with p53 mutation or p16/p14ARF homozygous deletion: a highly lethal subset associated with poor chemoresponse. J Clin Oncol. 2005;23:548–58.
70. Zucman J, Melot T, Desmaze C, et al. Combinatorial generation of variable fusion proteins in the Ewing family of tumors. EMBO J. 1993;12:4481–7.
71. Jeon IS, Davis JN, Braun BS, et al. A variant Ewing's sarcoma translocation (7;22) fuses the EWS gene to the ETS gene ETV1. Oncogene. 1995;10:1229–34.
72. Kaneko Y, Yoshida K, Handa M, et al. Fusion of an ETS-family gene, EIAF, to EWS by t(17;22)(q12;q12) chromosome translocation in an undifferentiated sarcoma of infancy. Genes Chromosomes Cancer. 1996;15:115–21.
73. Peter M, Couturier J, Pacquement H, et al. A new member of the ETS family fused to EWS in Ewing tumors. Oncogene. 1997;14:1159–64.

74. Torchia EC, Jaishankar S, Baker SJ. Ewing tumor fusion proteins block the differentiation of pluripotent marrow stromal cells. Cancer Res. 2003;63:3464–8.
75. Gonzalez I, Vicent S, de Alava E, Lecanda F. EWS/FLI-1 oncoprotein subtypes impose different requirements for transformation and metastatic activity in a murine model. J Mol Med. 2007;85:1015–29.
76. Gershon TR, Oppenheimer O, Chin SS, Gerald WL. Temporally regulated neural crest transcription factors distinguish neuroectodermal tumors of varying malignancy and differentiation. Neoplasia. 2005;7:575–84.
77. Teitell MA, Thompson AD, Sorensen PH, Shimada H, Triche TJ, Denny CT. EWS/ETS fusion genes induce epithelial and neuroectodermal differentiation in NIH 3 T3 fibroblasts. Lab Invest. 1999;79:1535–43.
78. Rorie CJ, Thomas VD, Chen P, Pierce HH, O'Bryan JP, Weissman BE. The Ews/Fli-1 fusion gene switches the differentiation program of neuroblastomas to Ewing sarcoma/peripheral primitive neuroectodermal tumors. Cancer Res. 2004;64:1266–77.
79. Hu-Lieskovan S, Zhang J, Wu L, Shimada H, Schofield DE, Triche TJ. EWS-FLI1 fusion protein up-regulates critical genes in neural crest development and is responsible for the observed phenotype of Ewing's family of tumors. Cancer Res. 2005;65:4633–44.
80. Deneen B, Denny CT. Loss of p16 pathways stabilizes EWS/FLI1 expression and complements EWS/FLI1 mediated transformation. Oncogene. 2001;20:6731–41.
81. Castillero-Trejo Y, Eliazer S, Xiang L, Richardson JA, Ilaria Jr RL. Expression of the EWS/FLI-1 oncogene in murine primary bone-derived cells results in EWS/FLI-1-dependent, Ewing sarcoma-like tumors. Cancer Res. 2005;65:8698–705.
82. Riggi N, Cironi L, Provero P, et al. Development of Ewing's sarcoma from primary bone marrow-derived mesenchymal progenitor cells. Cancer Res. 2005;65:11459–68.
83. Tolar J, Nauta AJ, Osborn MJ, et al. Sarcoma derived from cultured mesenchymal stem cells. Stem Cells. 2007;25:371–9.
84. Rangarajan A, Hong SJ, Gifford A, Weinberg RA. Species- and cell type-specific requirements for cellular transformation. Cancer Cell. 2004;6:171–83.
85. Riggi N, Suva ML, Suva D, et al. EWS-FLI-1 expression triggers a Ewing's sarcoma initiation program in primary human mesenchymal stem cells. Cancer Res. 2008;68:2176–85.
86. Tirode F, Laud-Duval K, Prieur A, Delorme B, Charbord P, Delattre O. Mesenchymal stem cell features of Ewing tumors. Cancer Cell. 2007;11:421–9.
87. Szuhai K, Ijszenga M, Tanke HJ, Rosenberg C, Hogendoorn PC. Molecular cytogenetic characterization of four previously established and two newly established Ewing sarcoma cell lines. Cancer Genet Cytogenet. 2006;166:173–9.
88. Kovar H, Jug G, Aryee DN, et al. Among genes involved in the RB dependent cell cycle regulatory cascade, the p16 tumor suppressor gene is frequently lost in the Ewing family of tumors. Oncogene. 1997;15:2225–32.
89. Tsuchiya T, Sekine K, Hinohara S, Namiki T, Nobori T, Kaneko Y. Analysis of the p16INK4, p14ARF, p15, TP53, and MDM2 genes and their prognostic implications in osteosarcoma and Ewing sarcoma. Cancer Genet Cytogenet. 2000;120:91–8.
90. Lopez-Guerrero JA, Pellin A, Noguera R, Carda C, Llombart-Bosch A. Molecular analysis of the 9p21 locus and p53 genes in Ewing family tumors. Lab Invest. 2001;81:803–14.
91. Bonnet D, Dick JE. Human acute myeloid leukemia is organized as a hierarchy that originates from a primitive hematopoietic cell. Nat Med. 1997;3:730–7.
92. Jamieson CH, Weissman IL, Passegue E. Chronic versus acute myelogenous leukemia: a question of self-renewal. Cancer Cell. 2004;6:531–3.
93. Smith R, Owen LA, Trem DJ, et al. Expression profiling of EWS/FLI identifies NKX2.2 as a critical target gene in Ewing's sarcoma. Cancer Cell. 2006;9:405–16.
94. Owen LA, Kowalewski AA, Lessnick SL. EWS/FLI mediates transcriptional repression via NKX2.2 during oncogenic transformation in Ewing's sarcoma. PLoS One. 2008;3:e1965.
95. Fukuma M, Okita H, Hata J, Umezawa A. Upregulation of Id2, an oncogenic helix-loophelix protein, is mediated by the chimeric EWS/ets protein in Ewing sarcoma. Oncogene. 2003;22:1–9.

96. Nishimori H, Sasaki Y, Yoshida K, et al. The Id2 gene is a novel target of transcriptional activation by EWS-ETS fusion proteins in Ewing family tumors. Oncogene. 2002;21:8302–9.
97. Zwerner JP, May WA. PDGF-C is an EWS/FLI induced transforming growth factor in Ewing family tumors. Oncogene. 2001;20:626–33.
98. Matsumoto Y, Tanaka K, Nakatani F, Matsunobu T, Matsuda S, Iwamoto Y. Downregulation and forced expression of EWS-Fli1 fusion gene results in changes in the expression of G(1) regulatory genes. Br J Cancer. 2001;84:768–75.
99. Wai DH, Schaefer KL, Schramm A, et al. Expression analysis of pediatric solid tumor cell lines using oligonucleotide microarrays. Int J Oncol. 2002;20:441–51.
100. Dauphinot L, De Oliveira C, Melot T, et al. Analysis of the expression of cell cycle regulators in Ewing cell lines: EWS-FLI-1 modulates p57KIP2and c-Myc expression. Oncogene. 2001;20:3258–65.
101. Bailly RA, Bosselut R, Zucman J, et al. DNA-binding and transcriptional activation properties of the EWS-FLI-1 fusion protein resulting from the t(11;22) translocation in Ewing sarcoma. Mol Cell Biol. 1994;14:3230–41.
102. Takahashi A, Higashino F, Aoyagi M, et al. EWS/ETS fusions activate telomerase in Ewing's tumors. Cancer Res. 2003;63:8338–44.
103. Nakatani F, Tanaka K, Sakimura R, et al. Identification of p21WAF1/CIP1 as a direct target of EWS-Fli1 oncogenic fusion protein. J Biol Chem. 2003;278:15105–15.
104. Hahm KB. Repression of the gene encoding the TGF-beta type II receptor is a major target of the EWS-FLI1 oncoprotein. Nat Genet. 1999;23:481.
105. Im YH, Kim HT, Lee C, et al. EWS-FLI1, EWS-ERG, and EWS-ETV1 oncoproteins of Ewing tumor family all suppress transcription of transforming growth factor beta type II receptor gene. Cancer Res. 2000;60:1536–40.
106. Prieur A, Tirode F, Cohen P, Delattre O. EWS/FLI-1 silencing and gene profiling of Ewing cells reveal downstream oncogenic pathways and a crucial role for repression of insulin-like growth factor binding protein 3. Mol Cell Biol. 2004;24:7275–83.
107. Scotlandi K, Benini S, Nanni P, et al. Blockage of insulin-like growth factor-I receptor inhibits the growth of Ewing's sarcoma in athymic mice. Cancer Res. 1998;58:4127–31.
108. Scotlandi K, Avnet S, Benini S, et al. Expression of an IGF-I receptor dominant negative mutant induces apoptosis, inhibits tumorigenesis and enhances chemosensitivity in Ewing's sarcoma cells. Int J Cancer. 2002;101:11–6.
109. Scotlandi K, Maini C, Manara MC, et al. Effectiveness of insulin-like growth factor I receptor antisense strategy against Ewing's sarcoma cells. Cancer Gene Ther. 2002;9:296–307.
110. Manara MC, Landuzzi L, Nanni P, et al. Preclinical in vivo study of new insulin-like growth factor-I receptor-specific inhibitor in Ewing's sarcoma. Clin Cancer Res. 2007;13:1322–30.
111. Kinsey M, Smith R, Lessnick SL. NR0B1 is required for the oncogenic phenotype mediated by EWS/FLI in Ewing's sarcoma. Mol Cancer Res. 2006;4:851–9.
112. Garcia-Aragoncillo E, Carrillo J, Lalli E, et al. DAX1, a direct target of EWS/FLI1 oncoprotein, is a principal regulator of cell-cycle progression in Ewing's tumor cells. Oncogene. 2008.
113. Mendiola M, Carrillo J, Garcia E, et al. The orphan nuclear receptor DAX1 is up-regulated by the EWS/FLI1 oncoprotein and is highly expressed in Ewing tumors. Int J Cancer. 2006;118:1381–9.
114. Selvanathan SP, Graham GT, Erkizan HV, Dirksen U, Natarajan TG, Dakic A, Yu S, Liu X, Paulsen MT, Ljungman ME, Wu CH, Lawlor ER, Üren A, Toretsky JA. Oncogenic fusion protein EWS-FLI1 is a network hub that regulates alternative splicing. Proc Natl Acad Sci USA. 2015;112:E1307–16.
115. Marques Howarth M, Simpson D, Ngok SP, Nieves B, Chen R, Siprashvili Z, Vaka D, Breese MR, Crompton BD, Alexe G, Hawkins DS, Jacobson D, Brunner AL, West R, Mora J, Stegmaier K, Khavari P, Sweet-Cordero EA. Long noncoding RNA EWSAT1-mediated gene repression facilitates Ewing sarcoma oncogenesis. J Clin Invest. 2014;124:5275–90.
116. Brohl AS, Solomon DA, Chang W, Wang J, Song Y, Sindiri S, Patidar R, Hurd L, Chen L, Shern JF, Liao H, Wen X, Gerard J, Kim JS, Lopez Guerrero JA, Machado I, Wai DH,

Picci P, Triche T, Horvai AE, Miettinen M, Wei JS, Catchpool D, Llombart-Bosch A, Waldman T, Khan J. The genomic landscape of the Ewing Sarcoma family of tumors reveals recurrent STAG2 mutation. PLoS Genet. 2014;10:e1004475.

117. Tirode F, Surdez D, Ma X, Parker M, Le Deley MC, Bahrami A, Zhang Z, Lapouble E, Grossetête-Lalami S, Rusch M, Reynaud S, Rio-Frio T, Hedlund E, Wu G, Chen X, Pierron G, Oberlin O, Zaidi S, Lemmon G, Gupta P, Vadodaria B, Easton J, Gut M, Ding L, Mardis ER, Wilson RK, Shurtleff S, Laurence V, Michon J, Marec-Bérard P, Gut I, Downing J, Dyer M, Zhang J, Delattre O, Jude Children's Research Hospital–Washington University Pediatric Cancer Genome Project and the International Cancer Genome Consortium. Genomic landscape of Ewing sarcoma defines an aggressive subtype with co-association of STAG2 and TP53 mutations. Cancer Discov. 2014;4:1342–53.

118. Riggi N, Knoechel B, Gillespie SM, Rheinbay E, Boulay G, Suvà ML, Rossetti NE, Boonseng WE, Oksuz O, Cook EB, Formey A, Patel A, Gymrek M, Thapar V, Deshpande V, Ting DT, Hornicek FJ, Nielsen GP, Stamenkovic I, Aryee MJ, Bernstein BE, Rivera MN. EWS-FLI1 utilizes divergent chromatin remodeling mechanisms to directly activate or repress enhancer elements in Ewing sarcoma. Cancer Cell. 2014;26:668–81.

Chapter 4
Limb Salvage in Skeletally Immature Patients with Extremity Sarcoma

Mathew J. Most and Franklin H. Sim

Abstract The different types of limb salvage procedures can be classified as biologic (i.e. autograft, allograft), non-biologic (i.e. megaprosthesis, expandable prosthesis), or combination (i.e. allograft-prosthetic composite). Each of these types has its own indications, as well as advantages and disadvantages. In skeletally immature patients, there are several considerations to be into account.

Keywords Bone sarcoma • Limb salvage • Allograft • Megaprosthesis • Expandable prosthesis

4.1 Introduction

Primary bone and soft tissue sarcomas are rare in children [21, 22]. In the United States, the average annual incidence of cancer of the bone in children under the age of 20 is 8.7 per million. This amounts to approximately 650–700 new malignant bone tumors per year in children and adolescents. Almost two-thirds of these cases are of osteogenic sarcoma, and most of the remaining one-third are cases of Ewing's sarcoma [21]. Overall, these cases account for 6 % of all pediatric malignancies [27].

Over the last 30–40 years, great advances have been made in the diagnosis and treatment of these conditions. Improvements in imaging, chemotherapy, and surgical technique have increased 5-year survival from historical rates of 10–20 % to current rates of 60–70 % [3, 48]. This, in turn, has led to increasing interest in preserving a functional limb for the patient [36, 45, 48]. Forty years ago, approximately 80 % of pediatric patients with an extremity sarcoma would have been treated with an amputation. Now, 80–90 % of patients can undergo a limb-sparing procedure [27, 32].

M.J. Most, MD
Division of Orthopedic Oncology, Department of Orthopedics and Physical Rehabilitation, UMass Memorial Health Care, Worcester, MA, USA

F.H. Sim, MD (✉)
Department of Orthopedic Surgery, Mayo Clinic,
200 First Street SW, Rochester, MN 55905, USA
e-mail: sim.franklin@mayo.edu

M. San-Julian (ed.), *Cañadell's Pediatric Bone Sarcomas: Epiphysiolysis before Excision*, DOI 10.1007/978-3-319-24220-0_4

4.2 General Considerations

Limb salvage surgery in the pediatric population presents unique challenges. These include the smaller size of a young patient's skeleton; the growth potential of the unaffected leg and eventual limb length discrepancy; and the need for a durable reconstruction that can withstand the high activity levels and long life expectancies in these younger patients [33].

The most common locations for these malignant bone lesions include the distal femur, proximal tibia, and proximal humerus; approximately 75 % of these tumors occur near a physis [10]. Resection of these tumors therefore often entails excision of the physis (or multiple physes) as well, which can have a significant effect on the remaining growth of the salvaged extremity. In the lower extremity, 60–70 % of limb growth occurs around the knee (distal femoral and proximal tibial physes), and 80 % of the growth of the humerus occurs at the proximal physis [1, 4]. As such, after treatment of these tumors, a significant limb length discrepancy can develop.

Leg length discrepancies of less than 2 cm in the lower extremities are well-tolerated, with little to no functional or clinical significance. These can often be treated with shoe modifications (i.e. shoe lifts) alone. If a predicted limb length discrepancy will be less than 2 cm, the affected leg can be slightly over-lengthened by a centimeter or so at resection and reconstruction to compensate as well. In the still-growing child, predicted discrepancies of 2–4 cm can usually be treated with epiphysiodesis of the contralateral extremity or lengthening procedures on the involved side. However, predicted leg length differences of greater than 4 cm generally require other types of procedures, and often multiple interventions, to achieve similar ultimate limb lengths [17, 33].

Therefore, a relative contraindication to limb-sparing surgery is very immature skeletal age (<8 years old), as patients this young would have a very large anticipated limb-length discrepancy, likely requiring multiple operations over many years to minimize the length difference, with each procedure entailing the inherent risks of surgery [48]. However, San-Julian and colleagues reported on a series of 40 patients under the age of ten treated with physeal-sparing limb salvage for extremity sarcoma. Their overall survival rate was 75 % at final follow-up, with 90 % of the patients retaining their extremity [47]. Moreover, newer expandable prostheses, which do not require surgery or anesthesia to lengthen, may facilitate limb salvage in this age group.

4.3 Types of Limb Salvage Procedures

The types of limb salvage procedures can be classified as biologic (i.e. autograft, allograft), non-biologic (i.e. megaprosthesis, expandable prosthesis), or combination (i.e. allograft-prosthetic composite) [1]. Each of these types has its own indications, as well as advantages and disadvantages.

4.4 Biologic Reconstruction

Biologic reconstructions utilize autograft and/or allograft bone to fill in defects subsequent to tumor resection, and rely on bone to bone healing for ultimate stability. For metadiaphyseal tumors, often an intercalary resection and reconstruction can be performed (allograft, autograft, or combination), salvaging the joints above and below the tumor. If the tumor encroaches upon or involves the joint, then osteoarticular allograft remains an option for biologic reconstruction.

Another important consideration is the location of the tumor relative to the physes of the involved bone. If the tumor resection involves removal of one or more physes, then limb length discrepancy can be problematic if significant skeletal growth potential remains. This may have to be addressed with lengthening procedures on the involved side and/or epiphysiodesis or shortening procedures on the contralateral extremity.

4.4.1 Intercalary Allografts

Massive allografts have a long history of use in reconstruction after tumor resection in adult patients, with generally good results. A long term study of 104 intercalary allograft procedures performed at the Massachusetts General Hospital (adult and children) and published in 1997 reported an overall success rate of 84 % at an average follow-up of 5.6 years (Figs. 4.1 and 4.2) [42].

In 1995, Alman and colleagues reported a review of 26 pediatric and adolescent patients who underwent tumor resection and massive allograft reconstruction.

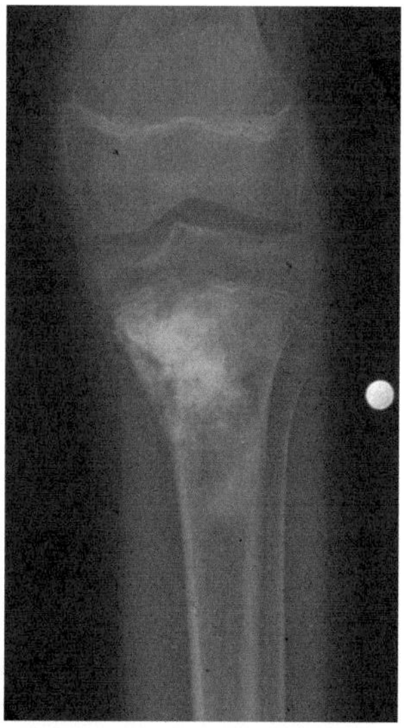

Fig. 4.1 Anteroposterior (AP) radiograph of the knee, demonstrating osteosarcoma of the proximal tibia in an 11 year-old

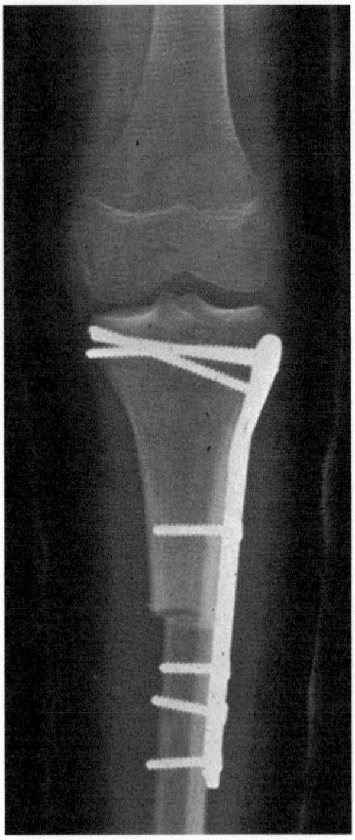

Fig. 4.2 The same patient as in Fig. 4.1, following resection of the proximal tibial osteosarcoma and reconstruction with an osteoarticular allograft

Eighteen of the 26 patients had an excellent or good result at final follow-up, and 88 % of patients with a lower extremity reconstruction that survived their disease retained their allograft at final follow-up. However, complication rates were high. At least one complication occurred in 77 % of the patients (not including limb-length discrepancy). Allograft fractures occurred in 54 %, and the infection rate was 12 %. Two of the three patients who developed infection went on to amputation. Four patients (15 %) developed a non-union; each was treated with an additional autologous bone grafting procedure, and each went on to heal within 12 months. A limb-length discrepancy over 2 cm occurred in 60 % of patients with lower extremity reconstruction. The authors concluded that, although the complication rate was higher than in adults, allograft reconstruction was a useful option in younger patients in whom limb-length discrepancy would be predicted to be mild, or those discrepancies that could be easily treated [2].

More recently, Musculo and colleagues published a series of 22 patients under the age of ten who had massive allografts placed after sarcoma resection (13 intercalary and 9 osteoarticular). At latest follow-up, three patients died of their disease, one patient had a subsequent amputation, and 18 patients were alive and had retained their limb. Fifteen of those 18 retained their original allograft. Eight complications occurred which required repeat surgeries (3 local recurrences, 3 fractures, 1 infection, and 1 nonunion); 4 of the 8 had their original allograft preserved. Mean Musculoskeletal Tumor Society (MSTS) functional scores and International Society of Limb Salvage radiographic scores were 27 % and 94 %, respectively. Four patients that had both physes preserved had no limb length discrepancy at final follow-up. Fourteen patients that had resection of one physis with their tumor had a mean leg length discrepancy of 2.1 cm at latest follow-up. The authors therefore concluded that allograft reconstruction was an acceptable technique in young children with extremity sarcoma [37].

4.4.2 *Osteoarticular Allografts*

Osteoarticular allografts tend to do less well than intercalary allografts, and this is generally due to degeneration of the allograft articular surface secondary to chondrocyte cell death and subchondral bone resorption and collapse [23, 35]. Musculo and colleagues reported on a series of 76 adult and pediatric patients with a tumor of the distal femur that underwent a resection and reconstruction with a distal femoral osteoarticular allograft. Overall allograft survival was 78 % at both 5 and 10 years, and the rate of allograft survival without the need for joint resurfacing was 71 % at both 5 and 10 years. However, 35 % of patients did have radiographic evidence of joint degeneration [38].

In another large series of osteoarticular allografts, Mnaymneh and co-authors reported on a series of 96 patients (adult and pediatric) who underwent distal femoral osteoarticular allograft reconstruction after resection of benign or malignant tumors. Overall complications included a fracture rate of 14 %, nonunion rate of 12 %, and infection rate of 6 %. Clinically significant arthritis developed in 10 %, and instability in 7 %. Significant differences were seen in the results based upon whether or not the patient had received chemotherapy. The overall complication rate in the chemotherapy group was 47 %, compared to 30 % in those patients who did not undergo chemotherapy. In patients who had received chemotherapy, the infection rate was 13 % (versus 2 % without chemotherapy), and the nonunion rate was 23 % (versus 6 %). The modified Mankin classification system was utilized to grade the functional results. Of the patients who did not receive chemotherapy, 70 % had good or excellent results, 26 % had fair results, and 4 % had poor results. In contrast, for those patients who underwent chemotherapy, only 53 % had good or excellent results, 37 % had fair results, and 10 % had poor results. Although the complication rates were high, the authors felt that osteoarticular allograft reconstruction was a viable option, in which most of the complications could be treated adequately [35].

4.4.3 *Autografts*

While the aforementioned studies, and others, show that massive allografts are useful in pediatric bone sarcoma reconstructions, these procedures are associated with relatively high complication rates. The three most common complications associated with massive allograft reconstruction include infection, nonunion, and fracture. These complications are likely related to the avascular status of the allograft bone [36]. In an effort to reduce these complication rates, free vascularized fibula autografts have been used to reconstruct segmental defects after sarcoma resection. The vascularized fibula graft brings well-perfused bone to the site that is capable of osteogenesis. However, being of smaller diameter, it usually lacks the mechanical strength of large allografts. The fibular autograft will grow, hypertrophy, and remodel over time, but this takes a considerable amount of time, and repeated stress fractures may require repetitive prolonged immobilization [36].

Chen and colleagues from the Memorial Sloan Kettering Cancer Center reported on a series of 25 consecutive patients (adult and pediatric) treated with a vascularized fibular free flap after limb-sparing resection of extremity sarcomas. All flaps survived to final follow-up. The infection rate was 12 %. Uncomplicated bony union occurred in 78 % within 6 months. After secondary bone grafting procedures, 93 % ultimately went on to union. According to MSTS functional scores, all patients who went on to union had good functional results. Eight patient (32 %) developed local recurrence or metastasis, and ultimately six died of their disease. Two of the pediatric patients in the series went on to develop significant leg length discrepancies, both of which had successful limb-lengthening procedures. Based on these results, including lower infection and nonunion rates, the authors recommended vascularized fibular autografts as the reconstruction of choice for long segmental bone defects after tumor resection [11].

4.4.4 Allograft/Autograft Combination

In order to combine the mechanical advantages of massive allograft with the biologic advantages of a vascularized fibula autograft, Capanna and colleagues described a technique of reconstruction that utilizes both a large structural allograft in conjunction with a vascularized fibula [9]. Moran and colleagues from the Mayo Clinic reported on a series of seven pediatric and adolescent patients with extremity sarcoma who were treated with limb salvage using this reconstructive technique (Figs. 4.3, 4.4a, b, and 4.5). The mean follow-up time was 36 months. All seven patients retained their limb at final follow-up. Fibular autograft healing occurred by an average of 4 months, while allograft –host healing tended to take longer, and averaged 9 months. Two cases required secondary bone grafting procedures to obtain union at the allograft-host junction. There were no infections noted during the study period. Two patients developed allograft fractures over 2 years after primary surgery. Both fractures were successfully treated with internal fixation (one also had bone grafting at the time of fracture repair). Four patients had significant limb length discrepancies – two patients with discrepancies less than 2.5 cm were treated with shoe lifts, while two patients with larger discrepancies were treated with contralateral epiphysiodesis and limb shortening procedures. According to the modified Mankin functional classification, there were four excellent results and three good results. These results led the authors to conclude that the Capanna technique is a reliable reconstructive option, and is especially well-suited for the younger

Fig. 4.3 AP x-ray of the tibia, showing a lytic lesion in the proximal tibia of a 14-year-old female with soft tissue extension. Biopsy showed osteosarcoma

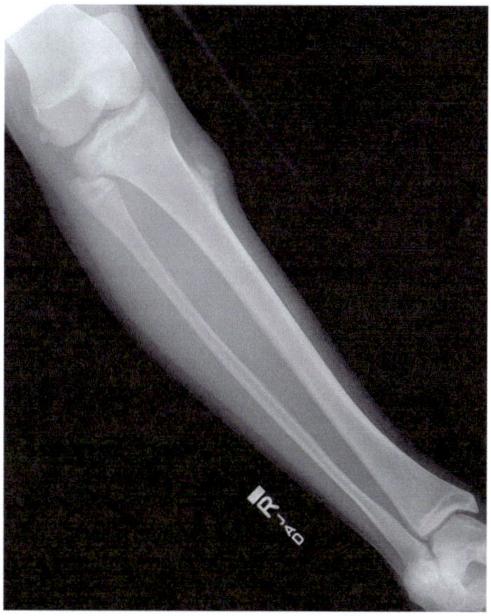

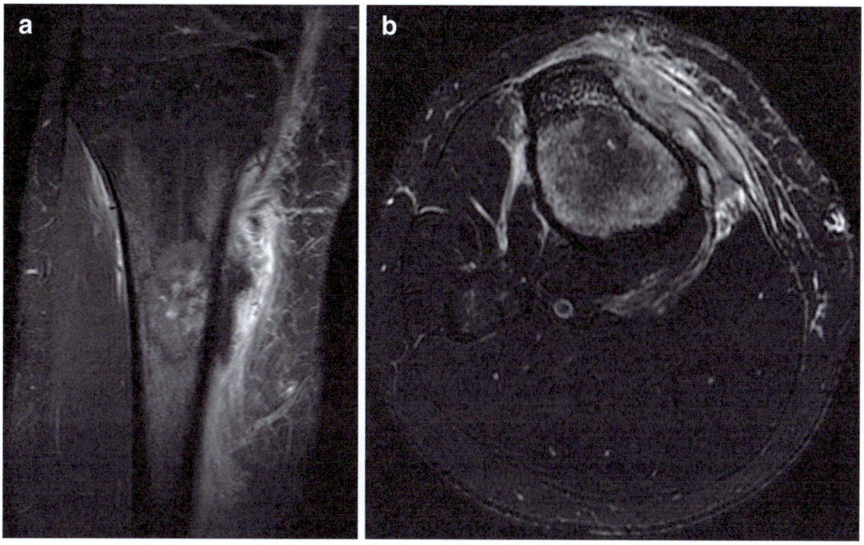

Fig. 4.4 (**a**, **b**) Coronal (**a**) and axial (**b**) MRI images of the patient in Fig. 4.3 following biopsy, showing medullary involvement and soft tissue extension

patient, whose higher activity demands and longer life span make allograft fracture and infection a more likely issue [36].

Cañadell and San-Julian have described an innovative technique that can improve the achievement of a safe surgical margin while helping to preserve the native joint surface in certain appropriately selected children. Most pediatric bone sarcomas occur in the metaphysis, but the physis can serve as a physical barrier to tumor

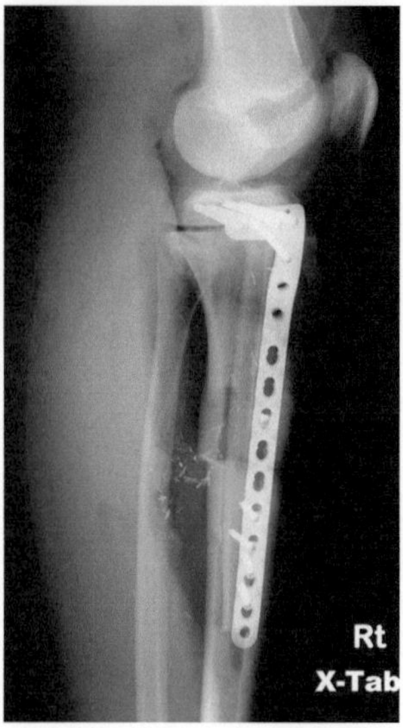

Fig. 4.5 Lateral x-ray of the patient in Figs. 4.3 and 4.4, following resection through the epiphysis sparing the articular surface. Reconstruction was carried out with an intercalary allograft and intramedullary vascularized fibular graft. A locking plate was utilized for fixation

spread. Cañadell and San-Julian have been able to achieve preservation of the epiphysis by performing epiphysiolysis with an external fixator to provide distraction across the physis of 1–1.5 mm per day. This can be performed while the child is receiving his or her neoadjuvant chemotherapy. High quality imaging is required to determine the exact margins of tumor extension [8].

4.5 Prosthetic Reconstruction

Non-biologic reconstruction after resection of an extremity sarcoma involves the placement of a prosthesis to replace the resected bone. The advantages of this technique include better initial fixation which can allow earlier weight-bearing, more predictable function, and lower risk of early complications [1]. Current implants incorporate a modular design, which allows the prosthesis to be assembled to match the defect created at the time of surgery. Additionally, a variety of stem lengths and diameters allow for greater intraoperative flexibility, with cemented and uncemented designs available. Prosthetic designs exist to replace the proximal humerus, proximal femur, distal femur, entire femur, and proximal tibia.

4.5.1 Standard Prostheses

In older children, who are nearing the end of their skeletal growth, a standard, static, adult-type endoprosthesis can be employed, if the expected leg-length discrepancy will be less than 2–3 cm [1]. Additionally, in tumors that occur about the knee, some growth can still be obtained from the remaining physis (i.e. the proximal tibia in distal femur tumors, and vice versa), by placing an uncemented component through a central hole in the physis that would allow the prosthetic stem to slide as the bone continues to grow around it. The distal femoral or proximal tibial physis can then continue to grow without angular deformity, but at a slower rate. The proximal tibia can achieve approximately 80 % of normal growth compared to the contralateral leg, whereas the distal femur can achieve about 60 % [1, 18].

Standard non-expandable endoprostheses have been used for several decades in adult patients, and have also been utilized in pediatric patients who are nearing skeletal maturity. They have a very good overall track record. In a review of 25 patients (adult and pediatric) treated with a proximal femoral endoprosthetic hemi-arthroplasty, the 10-year prosthesis survival rate was 86 %. There was one deep infection that was successfully treated with irrigation and debridement and retention of the components; one prosthetic dislocation; and one local recurrence. Three patients had significant acetabular wear, and were planning to undergo acetabular replacement. In each case, the abductor tendons were affixed to the prosthetic trochanter. Some degree of Trendelenburg limp was present in 92 % of patients (mild, 56 %; moderate 16 %; severe, 20 %). Functional outcome was excellent or good in 68 %, fair in 28 %, and poor in 4 % [14].

4.5.2 *Expandable Prostheses*

Early endoprostheses were static devices that did not allow for lengthening or growth through the device itself. In order to minimize significant limb length discrepancies in younger patients, subsequent procedures were often required to either lengthen the ipsilateral extremity (i.e. distraction osteogenesis), or to slow the growth of or even shorten the contralateral extremity (i.e. epiphysiodesis, shortening osteotomy). In the 1970s and 1980s, endoprosthetic devices began to incorporate designs that would allow lengthening of the prosthesis itself to allow the affected limb to keep pace with the contralateral limb. The first advance that allowed lengthening was the introduction of modularity. A modular prosthesis could be lengthened by exchanging a mid-body segment of the prosthesis for a longer segment, without the need to revise the entire prosthesis. However, this expansion would require a sizable operative exposure, with excision of the pseudocapsule that forms around the prosthesis, in order to perform this type of exchange lengthening. Complications including neurovascular injury, joint stiffness, and infection were not uncommon with these procedures [15].

Later expandable prostheses incorporated designs that would allow for less invasive lengthening procedures over time. These designs worked via one of several mechanisms to allow lengthening, including exchangeable C-collars, ball-bearings, or worm drives. With several of these newer prostheses, expansion procedures could be performed in a percutaneous fashion through a stab incision under fluoroscopic guidance, whereby a screwdriver could be inserted into the lengthening mechanism to expand the prosthesis [1, 4, 6, 15, 18, 40].

In 2000, Eckardt and colleagues published a series of 32 endoprostheses that were implanted following malignant bone tumor resection, which could be lengthened by exchanging modular mid-body segments. Over the 12 years that encompassed the study period, four different prosthesis designs were employed. At the time of publication, half of the patients had undergone at least one lengthening exchange procedure. In the 16 patients that had at least one lengthening procedure, a total of 32 lengthening procedures were performed. Eighteen of the original 32 patients had a total of 27 complications. These complications included aseptic loosening (5 patients), temporary nerve palsy (4 patients), prosthesis collapse or mechanical failure (6 patients), and local recurrence (2 patients). There were no infections noted. Three patients required an operative intervention for knee flexion contractures [15].

Proximal tibia replacements are often associated with even higher rates of complications, most often due to problems with wound breakdown and infection, and due to the challenges in restoring the extensor mechanism. The group from Birmingham, England reported on a series of expandable proximal tibial prostheses in 20 patients in 2000. Five patients died of their disease, and four others underwent above-knee amputation for complications (2 for local recurrence and 2 for infection). There were seven infections, of which five seemed directly related to open lengthening procedures. The authors determined the risk of infection to be 5.1 % per lengthening procedure, and at 10 years the overall risk of infection was 68 %. The patients in the study underwent an average of ten operations, from initial biopsy and prosthesis implant, to lengthenings and procedures to address complications (i.e. knee and ankle manipulations, contracture releases, periprosthetic fractures). However, at final analysis, the average MSTS score was 83 %, and the mean leg length discrepancy was 10 mm. Most patients had a mild to moderate extensor lag, as well as some limitation in knee flexion, which is not dissimilar from the results found in proximal tibial endoprosthetic reconstruction in adults [18].

Even with the development of percutaneous lengthening techniques, patients still required anesthesia, and the multiple operative procedures increased the risk of infection. In order to obviate the need for repeated surgical procedures, the newest expandable endoprosthetic models have incorporated non-invasive lengthening mechanisms [1, 5, 20, 40].

One type of non-invasive lengthening method utilizes external electromagnetic energy to allow the release of potential energy stored within a spring inside the prosthesis, which allows for expansion (Repiphysis Limb Salvage System, Wright Medical Technology, Arlington, TN, USA; formerly known as the Phenix prosthesis) [40]. Lengthening can be performed on an outpatient basis, without anesthesia or an incision required. Generally, the prosthesis is lengthened between 6 and 10 mm per expansion (Figs. 4.6a, b, and 4.7).

Another non-invasive expandable prosthesis involves a magnet, a gearbox, and a telescoping screw (Juvenile Tumor System, Stanmore Implants Worldwide, Stanmore, United Kingdom). The magnet is activated by an external electromagnetic force, which then initiates the gearbox, which in turn drives the threaded screw to lengthen the prosthesis [20]. Like the Repiphysis, the Stanmore prosthesis can be

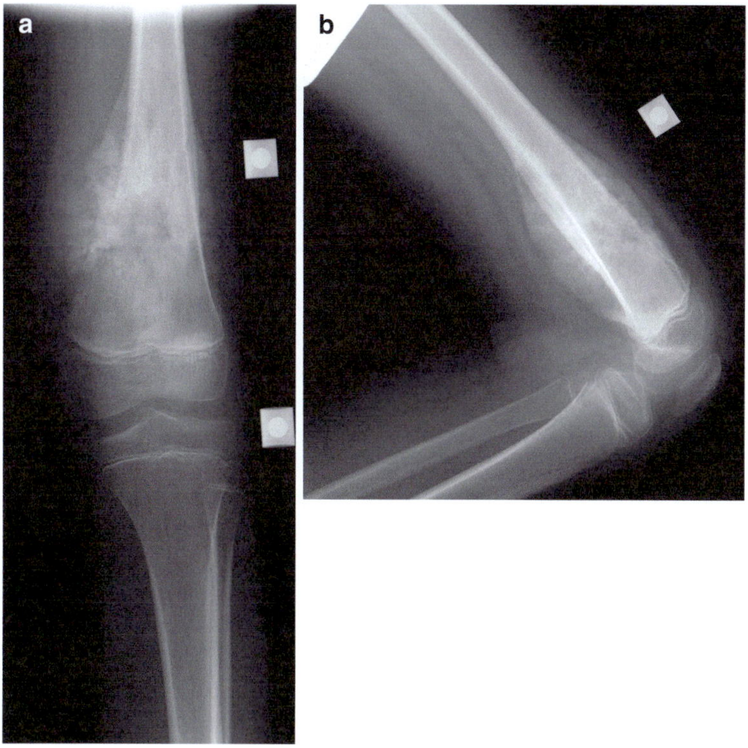

Fig. 4.6 (**a**, **b**) AP (**a**) and lateral (**b**) x-rays of the distal femur, showing Ewing's sarcoma in this 8-year-old patient. Note the large soft tissue mass

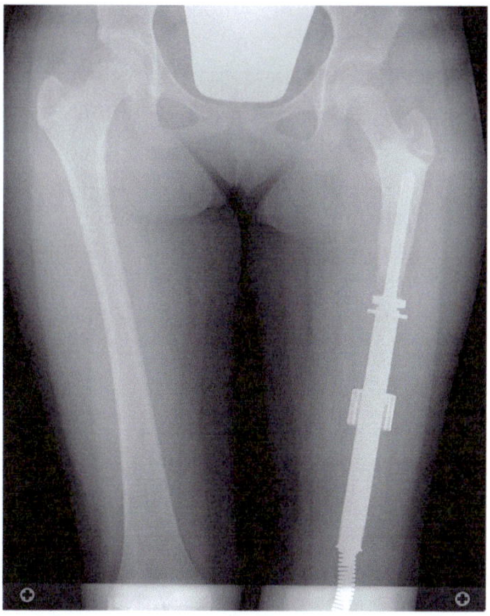

Fig. 4.7 AP scanogram x-ray of the patient in Fig. 4.6, after resection of the distal femur and reconstruction with a Repiphysis noninvasive expandable prosthesis

lengthened in the outpatient setting, without any incisions or anesthesia necessary (Fig. 4.8a, b).

Neel and colleagues reported on their experience with the Repiphysis prosthesis in 2003. Eighteen prostheses were implanted in 15 patients. Three patients in the study had to have their prosthesis revised to a new expandable prosthesis due to failure of the electromagnetic expansion portion failed. One patient underwent an above-knee amputation 10 months after surgery for an arterial thrombosis. There were eight revisions in seven patients, mostly due to either prosthesis failure or fracture. A total of 60 lengthenings have been performed, with all but two performed on an outpatient basis, and with an average of 8.5 mm of length gained at each procedure. There were no neurovascular injuries or significant loss of range of motion after any lengthening procedure. There were no deep infections. The average MSTS functional score at final follow-up in surviving patients was 90 %. All three of the patients that had achieved skeletal maturity by the time of publication had leg length discrepancies of less than 10 mm [40].

Cipriano and colleagues reported their experience with the Repiphysis prosthesis in 2014. They also noted a high complication and revision rate (12 patients had 37 implant related complications requiring 15 reoperations). Half of the patients had to undergo revision of the prosthesis for aseptic loosening. Furthermore, they noted severe peri-implant bone loss, which often limited subsequent revision options. While only one patient developed a deep infection, they saw frequent problems with arthrofibrosis, flexion contractures, extensor lags, and patellar maltracking. Contrary to Neel's study reporting excellent MSTS scores, Cipriano's patients only achieved a mean MSTS score of 67 % [12].

In 2006, Gupta and colleagues published their experience with the Stanmore prosthesis. In their early experience, this prosthesis was implanted into seven patients. Lengthenings were performed on an outpatient basis without anesthesia. The average length gained per procedure was 4 mm, with patients undergoing anywhere between one and 14 lengthening procedures. No neurovascular compromise was seen. One patient developed a 25° knee flexion contracture, which was treated successfully with manipulation under anesthesia and serial casting. There were no instances of deep infection, implant failure, aseptic loosening, or local tumor recurrence [20]. Their medium term results were subsequently published in 2012, incorporating 55 patients between 2002 and 2009, with mean follow-up of 41.2 months. Their complication rate was 29.1 % overall, with six deep infections (10.9 %). Three patients had a mechanical failure of the extension mechanism. Ultimately ten patients underwent a revision of their prosthesis (18.2 %). The mean MSTS score was 82.3 %, and Toronto Extremity Salvage score (TESS) was 92.3 %. Ten out of the 11 patients who had reached skeletal maturity at the time of publication had equal leg lengths, and 9 of the 11 had full hip and knee range of motion [44].

Hwang and colleagues published their experience with the Stanmore prosthesis in 2012 as well. They reported on 34 patients over 7 years, with an average follow-up of 44 months. Three patients had a local recurrence and went on to amputation. There were two mechanical failures for implant breakage, one at the sliding component and one at the lengthening mechanism. Six patients developed a deep infection

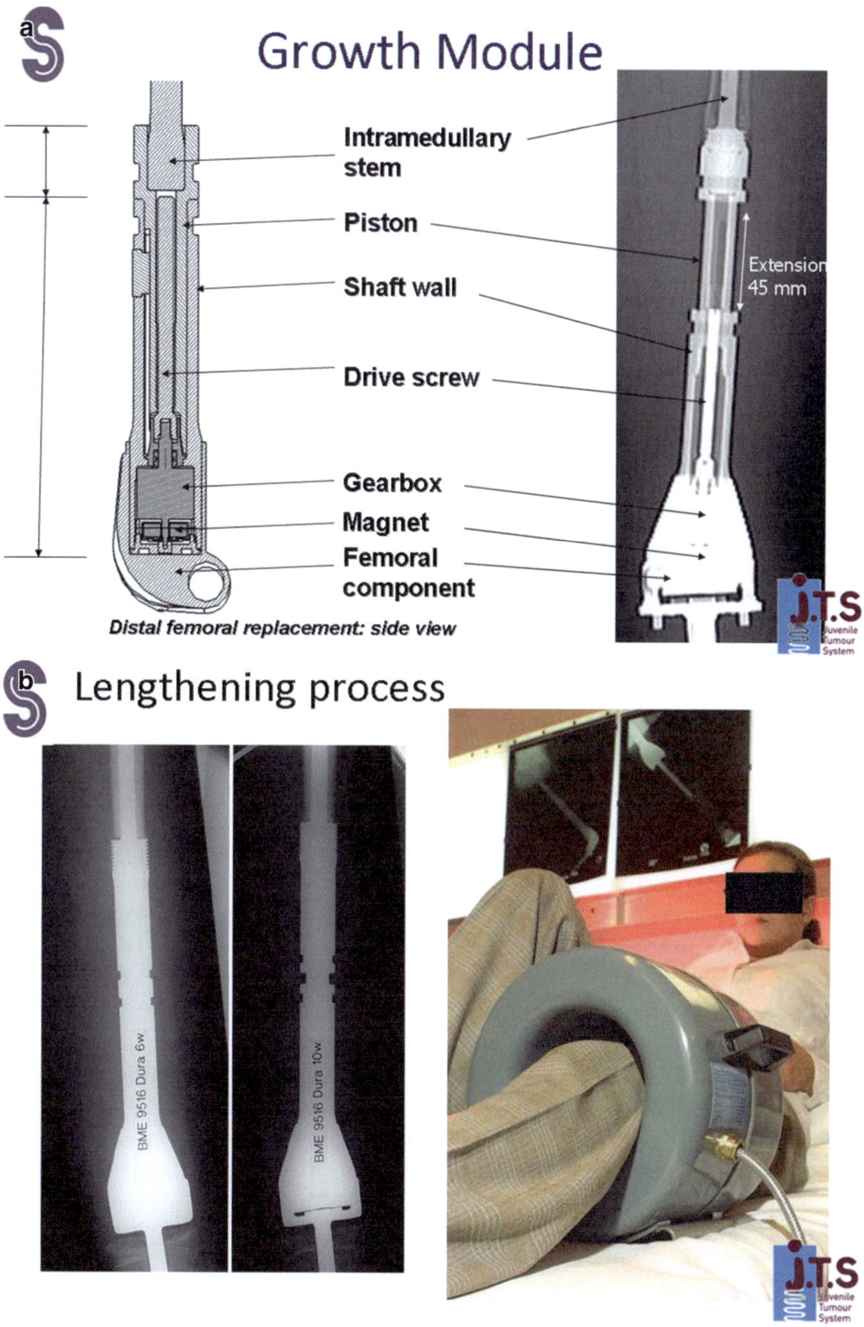

Fig. 4.8 (**a**, **b**) Stanmore method for lengthening of expandable prosthesis

(18 %). Eleven of 32 patients required subsequent surgery, with five patients going on to amputation (3 for local recurrence and 2 for infection). Despite the high complication rate, the mean MSTS score at latest follow-up was 85 % [28].

Some groups have sought to compare older invasive expandable prosthesis designs with newer non-invasive ones. Henderson and colleagues published their 13 year experience with expandable prostheses at a single institution, incorporating 39 patients. Three different implants were utilized. Early patients were treated with open expansion involving 1 cm incremental lengthening by placing a metal spacer secured by a locking clip (12 patients). As prosthesis design improved, subsequent patients had a minimally invasive expandable prosthesis placed, which could be lengthened by inserting a screwdriver through a stab incision under fluoroscopy to actuate the lengthening mechanism (18 patients). More recently, as non-invasive expandable prostheses became available, nine patients had a Stanmore Juvenile Tumor System prosthesis placed. The overall complication rate was 42 %, with 10 out of 26 surviving patients requiring revision surgery (38 %). There were three deep infections, all of which occurred after a surgical lengthening procedure; there were no deep infections in the Stanmore group, though they had the shortest follow-up time. The mean MSTS score was 87 % and the mean Pediatric Outcomes Data Collection Instrument (PODCI) score was 85.8. The authors concluded that patients undergoing expandable prosthesis placement after malignant bone tumor resection have good physical and emotional function, but that complication rates remain high. In those patients that had reached skeletal maturity, the mean leg length discrepancy was 7 mm [24].

The group from the Rizzoli Institute published a report of 32 children treated with expandable prostheses at their institution over a 14 year period from 1996 to 2010. They also used three different prostheses over the course of the study. Ten patients received a minimally invasive growing prosthesis (Kotz Growing Prosthesis, Stryker, UK). From 2002 to 2007, 15 patients received the Repiphysis prosthesis. Since 2009, seven patients had the Stanmore prosthesis implanted. Overall survival of the primary prosthesis was 78 % and 66 % at 48 and 72 months, respectively. When analyzed by prosthesis, survival of the Kotz prosthesis was 90 % at 48 and 72 months; survival of the Repiphysis prosthesis was only 60 % at 48 months and 32 % at 72 months; and survival of the Stanmore implant was 100 % at 48 months. Seven failed Repiphysis prostheses were revised to a Kotz Growing Prosthesis, for a total of 39 prostheses in their study. The overall complication rate was 51.3 %, with complications occurring in 20 of the 39 implants. Nine revision surgeries were performed (4 for aseptic loosening, 3 for infection, and 2 for prosthesis breakage). Three other patients were anticipated to require revision surgery in the near future, two for aseptic loosening and one for hip subluxation. The mean MSTS score was 79 %, and there were no statistically significant differences in MSTS scores between the different prostheses. Of the nine patients that had reached skeletal maturity, three had equal leg lengths while six had discrepancies of 15–30 mm [46].

In 2014, Ness and colleagues published a study comparing the functional outcomes after non-invasive expandable prosthesis placement versus standard modular non-expandable prostheses in children. They had a total of 42 patients, with 29 receiving a standard adult-type non-expandable modular prosthesis, and 13 patients having a Repiphysis implanted. Obviously, there was a significant difference in the age of the patients in the two groups, as younger patients with significant remaining skeletal growth had an expandable prosthesis, while older patients who were already skeletally mature or were felt to have the potential for less than 4 cm of discrepancy received a modular non-expandable prosthesis. There were no significant differences found between the two groups when comparing complication/revision rates or functional outcomes. In the modular prosthesis group, 14/29 patients (48 %) required a total of 26 repair or revision procedures (5 for periprosthetic fracture and 21 for loosening or hardware failure). In the Repiphysis group, 6/13 patients (46 %) underwent a total of 13 repairs or revisions (one for fracture and 12 for loosening). The authors did not specifically report their infection rates or overall patient, limb, or prosthesis survival rates. There was no difference between the two groups when assessing MSTS scores (modular prosthesis 69 % versus Repiphysis 73 %), TESS scores (85.23 for the modular prosthesis group and 87.00 for Repiphysis group), or Functional Mobility Assessment scores (46.90 in the modular prosthesis patients and 49.15 in the Repiphysis patients). This led the authors to conclude that patients with newer non-invasive expandable prostheses do just as well functionally as patients with traditional non-expandable devices [41].

4.6 Biologic-Prosthetic Combinations

In order to combine some of the advantages of biologic and prosthetic reconstruction, the technique of allograft prosthetic composite (APC) reconstruction was devised (Figs. 4.9a, b, 4.10a, b, 4.11, and 4.12a, b). This technique utilizes bulk allograft to replace the missing bone, combined with more standard arthroplasty implants to replace the joint surface. This allows for more options, especially with regards to joint stability and constraint. By resurfacing the joint, the potential for cartilage degradation and joint degeneration 5–10 years after implantation is eliminated [13]. Another advantage of this technique, especially in the proximal femur, proximal tibia, and proximal humerus, is the presence of allograft soft tissue tendon that is still attached at its insertion on the allograft bone. The patient's remaining native hip abductors, knee extensor mechanism, or rotator cuff can then be reconstructed via more reliable soft tissue to soft tissue repair, allowing for potentially improved stability and function [23].

The APC technique can be utilized in the proximal humerus, proximal or distal femur, or proximal tibia. In general, the long stem of the selected prosthetic component is cemented into the allograft, and then ideally press-fit into the remaining host bone. Cement is utilized in the allograft in order to achieve immediate stability as well as longer term stability (since bony ingrowth from the avascular allograft is unlikely); and to minimize the risk of fracturing the allograft from overstuffing it to obtain a stable press-fit [23]. Press-fit fixation in the host bone can minimize the risk of aseptic loosening.

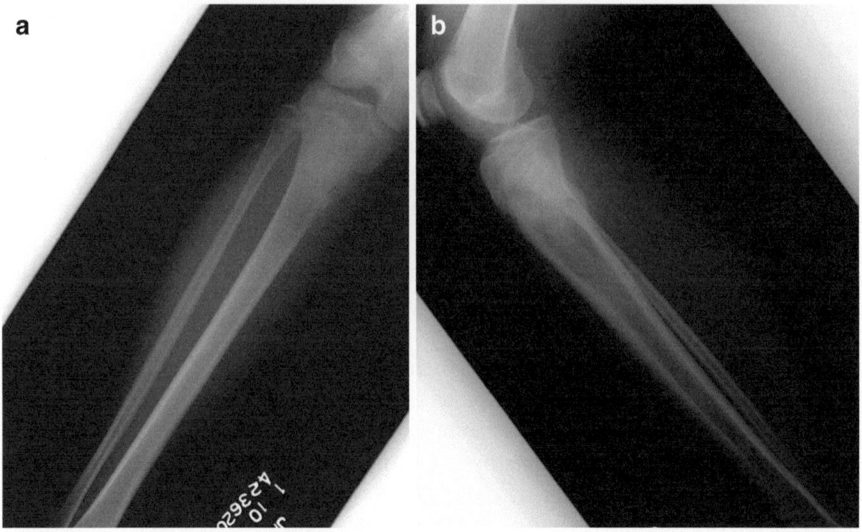

Fig. 4.9 (**a**, **b**) AP (**a**) and lateral (**b**) x-rays of the tibia demonstrating a mixed lytic and sclerotic lesion in the proximal tibia. Biopsy revealed osteosarcoma

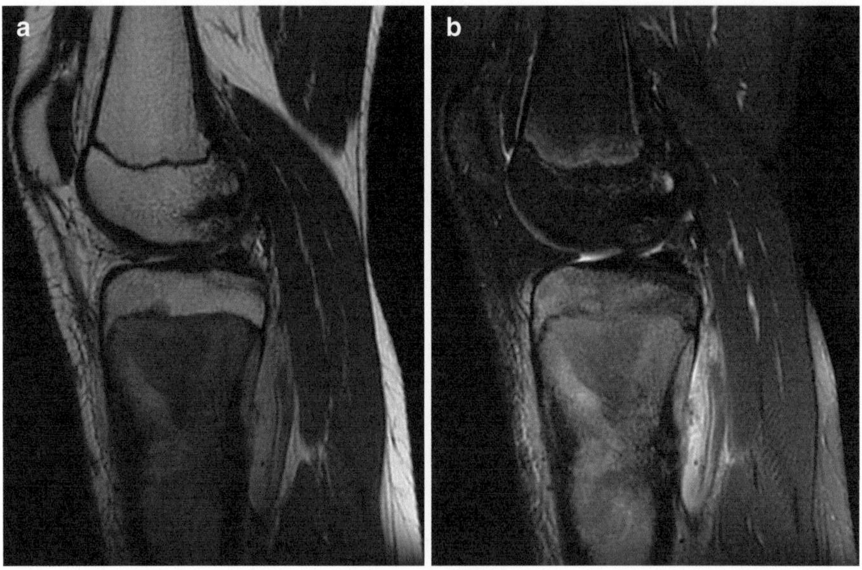

Fig. 4.10 (**a**, **b**) T_1 (**a**) and T_2 (**b**) weighted sagittal MRI images of the patient in Fig. 4.8 showing the lesion extending to the physis

In a review of 22 patients who underwent APC reconstruction after tumor resection, with an average follow-up of 45.1 months, Hejna and Gitelis found an overall survival rate of 73 %, and an average MSTS functional score of 94.3 %. There were

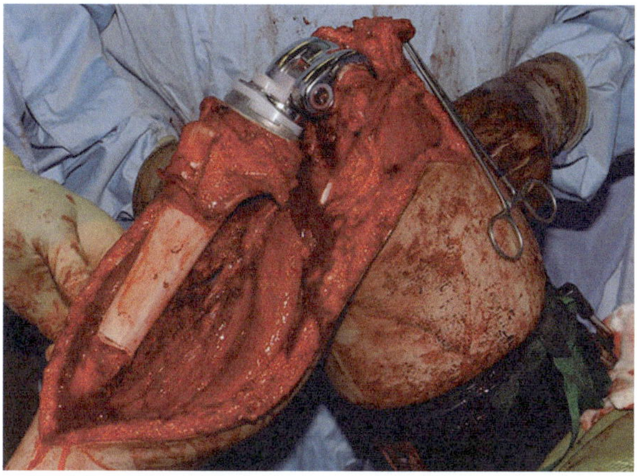

Fig. 4.11 Intraoperative photograph of the patient in Figs. 4.8 and 4.9 showing reconstruction with allograft prosthetic composite

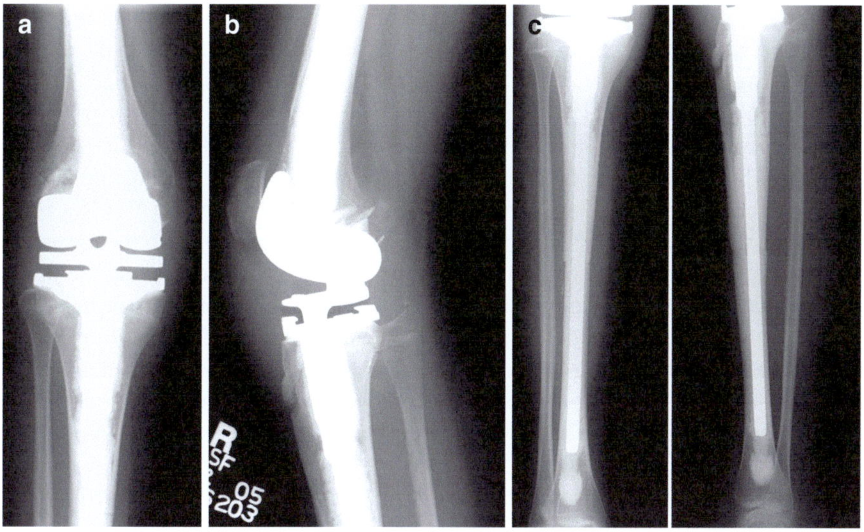

Fig. 4.12 (**a-c**) AP (**a**) and lateral (**b**) x-rays of the knee, and AP and lateral x-rays of the tibia (**c**) from the patient in Figs. 4.8, 4.9, and 4.10, following allograft prosthetic reconstruction

5 allograft-host junction non-unions, four of which healed after subsequent bone grafting procedures [13, 23].

4.7 Modified Amputations

In some instances, complete limb salvage may not be feasible for a particular patient. This may be due to very large predicted limb-length discrepancies that would require multiple procedures to correct; difficulty in obtaining size-matched implants or allografts; or social issues that potentially preclude the frequent and long-term follow-up required after limb salvage reconstruction. If an amputation is chosen for definitive treatment, than the level of amputation chosen should be as distal as possible while still ensuring local control of the tumor. Often, this would require a hip disarticulation or high above-knee amputation. However, the ability to preserve a longer residual limb facilitates external prosthetic fitting, which in turn enhances patient function. As such, several types of modified amputation procedures have been described to retain as much residual limb as possible. These include the Van Nes rotationplasty, the tibia turnplasty, and the tibia-hindfoot osteomusculocutaneous rotationplasty [7, 13, 43, 48].

4.7.1 Van Nes Rotationplasty

Of the three modified amputation techniques listed, the Van Nes rotationplasty leaves the longest residual stump, provides an effective "knee joint", and is a viable alternative to above-knee amputations in select patients [7]. It was first performed in 1930 by Borggreve for a patient with tuberculosis of the hip; it was later performed in 1932 by Demel and Gold and in 1950 by Van Nes for congenital femoral deficiencies [16, 30, 31]. The procedure has been employed in the treatment of malignant tumors of the femur since the 1970s [7, 25]. In order to perform a successful Van Nes rotationplasty, the sciatic nerve must be preserved; the vascular supply to the lower leg must be salvaged or reconstructed. The tumor is widely excised, leaving the distal lower leg attached by its neurovascular supply. The remaining tibia, with the attached foot, is then rotated 180° and transposed to the remaining distal femur. Tibiofemoral osteosynthesis is achieved using internal fixation devices (Figs. 4.13a, b, 4.14, 4.15, 4.16, and 4.17). The foot now faces posteriorly, with the remaining, functional ankle joint serving to replace the knee, with the foot acting as a below-knee amputation level stump [7, 25, 30, 48].

In a study of 12 patients that underwent rotationplasty following resection of a malignant tumor, Cammisa and colleagues reported that functional scores for the rotationplasty patients were statistically equal to those patients that underwent endoprosthetic reconstruction, and statistically better than those patients that underwent above-knee amputation. Disease-free survival was similar for all three groups. One patient had a nonunion at the tibiofemoral junction, which was successfully treated with an intramedullary nail and bone grafting. There were three infections (2 superficial and 1 deep). All complications resolved after treatment, with no functional or long term consequences. The authors therefore felt that Van Nes rotationplasty was an attractive option for reconstruction after tumor resection, and that it was superior to above-knee amputation [7].

Hillmann and colleagues published a report comparing endoprosthetic replacement to rotationplasty in 67 patients, both adults and children, with malignant tumors of the distal femur or proximal tibia. Endoprosthetic replacement was performed in 34 patients, and rotationplasty in 33. There was no statistically significant

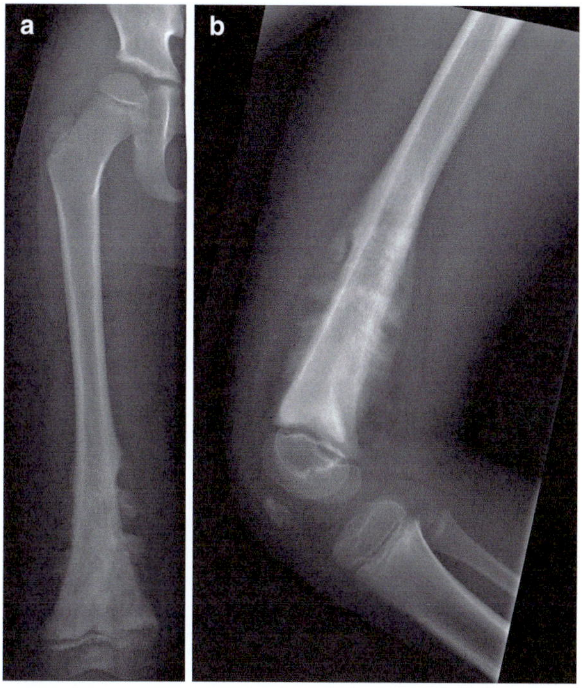

Fig. 4.13 (**a**, **b**) AP x-ray of the femur (**a**) and lateral x-ray of the distal femur (**b**) showing osteosarcoma in a 7 year-old boy

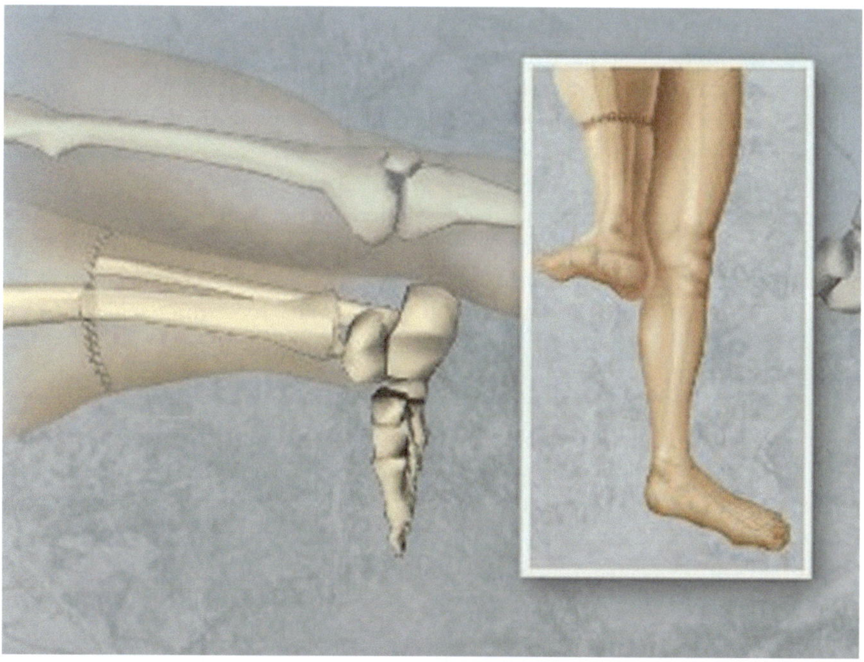

Fig. 4.14 An illustration of rotationplasty. The tibia is rotated 180° and fused to the femur

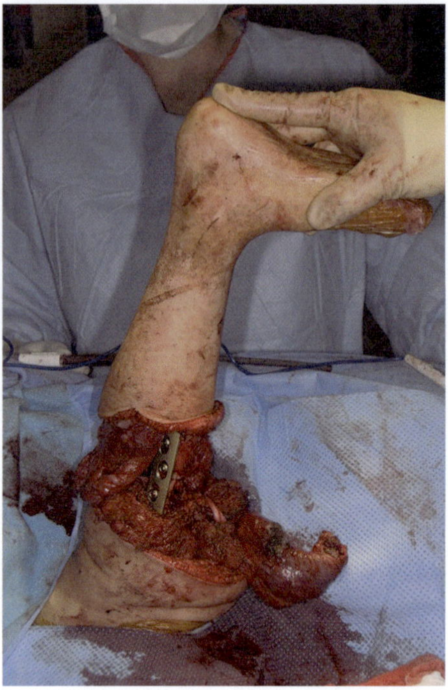

Fig. 4.15 Intraoperative photograph during rotationplasty procedure. The foot has been rotated 180°. A plate is utilized for fixation of the tibia and femur

difference in the mean MSTS functional score between the two groups (rotationplasty 24; endoprosthesis 25; $p = 0.47$). Fewer patients in the rotationplasty required gait aids for walking long distances. Subjective quality of life scores were significantly higher in the rotationplasty group, and daily activity restriction secondary to pain was significantly lower in the rotationplasty group. The authors did note that cosmetic appearance is likely the biggest drawback concerning rotationplasty [25]. However, several authors feel that the durability and functional advantage of rotationplasty justify the bizarre appearance [16, 25]. Others reported that patients were not as bothered by the appearance, and that they considered the procedure to be limb sparing (as opposed to an amputation) since the foot was retained. These patients felt that that improved function and mobility more than outweighed the appearance [29, 31].

In an excellent review of rotationplasty published in 1997, Kotz reviewed his experience in 40 patients for whom he performed this procedure. Thirty of the patients were followed for at least 3 years. There were no local recurrences; six patients died of metastatic disease. All patients were ambulating without gait aids, and most reported being able to participate in sports activities. Utilizing the MSTS functional scoring system, the results were excellent in 68 %, good in 28.5 %, and fair in 3.5 %; there were no poor results. Postoperative complications included four patients with vascular thrombosis (three were able to be revascularized; one had to undergo amputation after failure to recanalize the vessels). There were two cases of pseudoarthrosis at the tibiofemoral junction, both successfully treated with bone grafting and revision

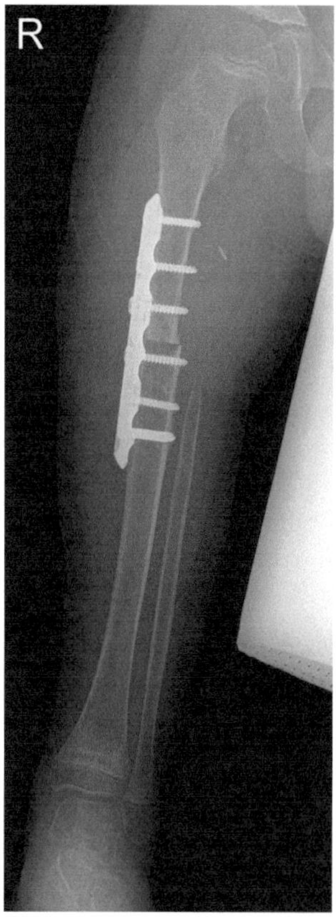

Fig. 4.16 AP radiograph of the right lower extremity showing osteosynthesis of the femur and tibia

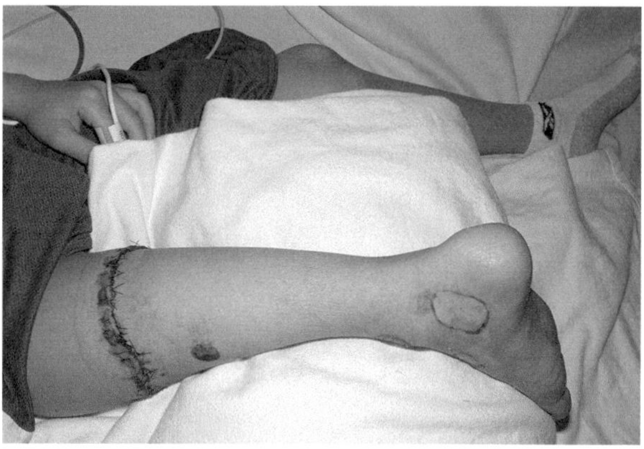

Fig. 4.17 Clinical photograph of rotated foot following wound closure after rotationplasty procedure

internal fixation. There were two cases of sciatic paresis, one of which resolved spontaneously. Kotz concluded that, although the indications for rotationplasty were decreasing with advances in extendable endoprostheses for children, there was still a role for rotationplasty in specific instances. For instance, proximal tibia tumors for which an amputation would require a below-knee amputation with a very short stump; or in tumors located more proximally in the femur. There is also still a role for rotationplasty in developing countries, where endoprostheses are often unobtainable, and where the infection rate after arthroplasty is unacceptably high [30].

In their review of limb salvage surgery for skeletally immature patients, Finn and Simon concluded that rotationplasty offers no compromise of oncologic outcome compared to above-knee amputation. While the complication rate after rotationplasty is higher than that for amputation, it compares favorably to the rates for other forms of limb salvage. Additionally, objective data shows that function is significantly improved over above-knee amputation [16].

When considering someone for rotationplasty, patient selection and preoperative education are critical. The procedure must not compromise the oncologic margins, and the sciatic nerve must be preserved in order for the foot to function as a surrogate knee. The blood supply to the lower leg and foot must be able to be preserved or reconstructed. Additionally, it is important to educate patients beforehand regarding the anticipated function and physical appearance of the residual limb. It can help to have patients and families view photos or videos that demonstrate the results of rotationplasty, or to even be able to meet with or speak to patients who have previously undergone the procedure [30].

4.7.2 Tibial Turnplasty

The tibia turnplasty, or turn-up procedure, offers another alternative to a high above-knee amputation. It can be used in the management of long distal femoral bone loss, particularly to salvage multiple previous biologic or endoprosthetic reconstruction failures or infections. Often times, in these patients, such a proximal level for above-knee amputation would not leave a sufficient stump to allow for a functional external prosthesis. Therefore, in order to lengthen the stump and improve prosthetic fitting, remaining tibia can be used as a vascularized autograft. The tibia is rotated 180° on its posterior tibial neurovascular pedicle, such that the distal tibia can be fixed to the remaining femoral stump. In a skeletally immature patient, if the proximal tibial physis can be preserved, then there can be continued longitudinal growth of the stump as well [34].

McDonald, Scott, and Eckardt reviewed their use of the tibial turn-up procedure in seven patients, three of whom were skeletally immature. Successful osteosynthesis was achieved in all patients, and all were able to ambulate with an above-knee amputation prosthesis. Two patients had post-operative wound complications. One patient ultimately went on to hemipelvectomy subsequent to recurrent tumor. The authors concluded that the tibial turnplasty could be useful to restore femoral stump length in patients who would otherwise require high above-knee amputations, but that it was perhaps best reserved for patients who have had multiple prior surgical failures, deep infections, or those who would be opposed to the appearance of a Van Nes rotationplasty [34].

4.7.3 Tibia-Hindfoot Osteomusculocutaneous Rotationplasty

In patients with significant tumor involvement or bone loss of the proximal femur, reconstruction options can include endoprosthetic reconstruction, allografts, or allograft-prosthetic composites. In some instances, however, reconstruction may not be possible, for instance if prior reconstructive efforts have been complicated by repeated deep infections. In these cases, often times a hip disarticulation amputation is required. A hip disarticulation is quite disabling and cosmetically disfiguring, and function with an external prosthesis can be challenging. In order to treat instances such as this, a new procedure was designed that would allow the distal lower extremity to be rotated up as a vascularized autograft on its posterior tibia neurovascular bundle to replace the proximal femur. Skin and soft tissue could be brought up with the bone to fill in any defects as an osteomusculocutaneous flap. The talus and calcaneus are kept with the distal tibia, via their ligamentous attachments. The distal tibia and hindfoot are then rotated 180° in the sagittal plane and 90° in the transverse plane to allow the calcaneal tuberosity to be placed into the acetabulum. The acetabulum is first reamed much like it would be for a hip arthroplasty; the calcaneal tuberosity can be prepared using the reamers that are usually utilized for the femoral head in hip resurfacing procedures. The calcaneal tuberosity is then inserted into the prepared acetabulum, and large screws are placed to facilitate calcaneopelvic fusion. Some "hip joint" motion can then be preserved via the intact tibiotalar and subtalar joints, and the tibia serves as an above-knee amputation stump [43].

Peterson, Koch, and Wood reported on the performance of this type of rotationplasty (also called a hip-ankle, or Hankle, rotationplasty) in two patients at the Mayo Clinic. Although in their report both patients required this procedure due to extensive loss of the proximal femur and pre-existing deep infection, the procedure could have oncologic indications in skeletally immature patients. In the series from Mayo, both patients had successful reconstruction with this technique, and were able to ambulate pain free on standard above-knee amputation prostheses [43].

4.8 Long Term Outcomes

Many studies have been published reporting on the long term outcomes in pediatric patients who were treated for extremity sarcomas. Many of these studies compare various techniques with one another. Generally, the oncologic and functional results after limb salvage compare favorably to those after amputation [12, 39, 49].

In a review published in 2002, Nagarajan and colleagues reported that, while survival is equivalent in limb salvage and amputation procedures, complications tend to be more frequent in the limb salvage group. Additionally, the long term outcomes with regards to function and quality of life do not appear to be substantially different [39]. However, they noted that limb salvage procedures remain the current practice at most tertiary centers, despite the "higher complication rate, questionable long term durability, and equivocal improved function and quality of life" [39].

In contrast, Rougraff, et al. in a multi-center study of patients with distal femoral osteosarcoma, reported higher average MSTS functional scores for patients that underwent limb salvage as opposed to those who had amputation. There were no differences between the groups in overall survival or post-operative disease-free periods. There was a higher rate of reoperation in the limb salvage group, but there were no significant differences in the patient's acceptance of the post-operative state, the ability to ambulate, or the amount of pain. There also were no apparent differences in psychosocial outcomes [45].

Despite the more frequent need for reoperation in limb salvage patients (whether for complications or for limb lengthening procedures), Wilkins and Miller found that average MSTS functional scores were similar in those limb salvage patients that required at least one subsequent operation compared to those who required no further surgical intervention. In their study of 36 patients with minimum 2 year follow-up, they found that 26 patients needed at least one reoperation (total 54 reoperations performed), while only ten patients did not need further surgery. There were no significant differences in functional scores in the reoperation group when comparing before and after reoperation, and no differences between the two groups [49].

Hopyan and colleagues also compared the functional outcomes in pediatric patients who underwent either limb salvage, rotationplasty, or amputation procedures for bone sarcoma. They found that average MSTS functional scores were significantly higher in the limb-sparing group compared to the above-knee amputation group. Additionally, although not statistically significant, the average Toronto Extremity Salvage Scores tended to be higher in the limb-sparing group. They found no significant differences in any psychosocial factors between the three groups [26].

Another factor for surgeons and patients to consider when choosing between limb salvage and amputation is cost effectiveness. Grimer and colleagues evaluated the costs associated with endoprosthetic limb salvage and compared that to those associated with amputation, in 1997 prices. They found that, even when adjusting for ongoing limb salvage costs relating to predicted rates of revision surgery (i.e. for aseptic loosening, infection, or implant failure), the overall 20-year cost of amputation is significantly higher. This is likely due to the high cost of sophisticated artificial limbs, the need for regular new prosthesis fabrication, the patient's desire to have a spare prosthesis available as well as specialized prosthesis for activities such as running or swimming, and others [19].

4.9 Conclusions

Significant multidisciplinary advances have been made in the ways in which we diagnose and treat sarcomas of the extremities. Five-year survival rates have approximately tripled over the last 30 years, but have now seemed to have reached a plateau. Surgical techniques have also advanced considerably over this time period.

The great majority of patients with extremity sarcoma are now candidates for limb salvage surgery instead of amputation.

Many different techniques exist to reconstruct a limb after resection of a malignant bone tumor. Each of these techniques has its own advantages and disadvantages. Ultimately, no one procedure will be right for every tumor in every anatomic location in every patient. Each patient must be evaluated on a case-by-case basis. Multiple factors must be considered and prioritized – the patient's life, the extremity, its function, potential leg length differences, and cosmetic appearance. Additionally, social, socioeconomic, and cultural factors must be accounted for in order to achieve the best outcome for the patient and his or her family [48]. Only when all of these factors are thoroughly evaluated and discussed, can an appropriate treatment plan be devised and embarked upon.

References

1. Abudu A, Grimer R, Tillman R, Carter S. The use of prostheses in skeletally immature patients. Orthop Clin North Am. 2006;37:75–84.
2. Alman BA, De Bari A, Krajbich JI. Massive allografts in the treatment of osteosarcoma and Ewing sarcoma in children and adolescents. J Bone Joint Surg Am. 1995;77-A:54–64.
3. Arndt CA, Crist WM. Common musculoskeletal tumors of childhood and adolescence. N Engl J Med. 1999;341:342–52.
4. Ayoub KS, Fiorenza F, Grimer RJ, Tillman RM, Carter SR. Extensible endoprostheses of the humerus after resection of bone tumors. J Bone Joint Surg Br. 1999;81-B:495–500.
5. Baumgart R, Hinterwimmer S, Krammer M, Meunsterer O, Mutschler W. The bioexpandable prosthesis: a new perspective after resection of malignant bone tumors in children. J Pediatr Hematol Oncol. 2005;27:452–5.
6. Belthur MV, Grimer RJ, Suneja R, Carter SR, Tillman RM. Extensible endoprostheses for bone tumors of the proximal femur in children. J Pediatr Orthop. 2003;23:230–5.
7. Cammisa FP, Glasser DB, Otis JC, Kroll MA, Lane JM, Healey JH. The Van Nes tibial rotationplasty: a functionally viable reconstructive procedure in children who have a tumor of the distal end of the femur. J Bone Joint Surg Am. 1990;72-A:1541–7.
8. Cañadell J, Forriol F, Cara JA, San-Julian M. Removal of metaphyseal bone tumours with preservation of the epiphysis. Physeal distraction before excision. In: Cañadell J, San-Julian M, Cara JA, editors. Surgical treatment of malignant bone tumours. Pamplona: Ediciones Universidad de Navarra; 1995. p. 153–60.
9. Capanna R, Bufalini C, Campanacci C. A new technique for reconstruction of large metadiaphyseal bone defects: a combined graft (allograft shell plus vascularized fibula). Orthop Traumatol. 1993;2:159–77.
10. Cara JA, Cañadell J. Limb salvage for malignant bone tumors in young children. J Pediatr Orthop. 1994;14:112–8.
11. Chen CM, Disa JJ, Lee HY, Mehrara BJ, et al. Reconstruction of extremity long bone defects after sarcoma resection with vascularized fibula flaps: a 10-year review. Plast Reconstr Surg. 2007;119:915–24.
12. Cipriani CA, Gruzinova IS, Frank RM, Gitelis S, Virkus WW. Frequent complications and severe bone loss associated with the Repiphysis expandable distal femoral prosthesis. Clin Orthop Relat Res. 2014;473(3):831–8. doi:10.1007/s11999-014-3564-3.
13. DiCaprio MR, Friedlaender GE. Malignant bone tumors: limb sparing versus amputation. J Am Acad Orthop Surg. 2003;11:25–37.

14. Donati D, Zavatta M, Gozzi E, Giacomini S, Campanacci L, Mercuri M. Modular prosthetic replacement of the proximal femur after resection of a bone tumour: a long-term follow-up. J Bone Joint Surg Br. 2001;83-B:1156–60.
15. Eckardt JJ, Kabo JM, Kelly CM, Ward WG, et al. Expandable endoprosthesis reconstruction in skeletally immature patients with tumors. Clin Orthop. 2000;373:51–61.
16. Finn HA, Simon MA. Limb-salvage surgery in the treatment of osteosarcoma in skeletally immature individuals. Clin Orthop. 1991;262:108–18.
17. Gonzalez-Herranz P, Burgos-Flores J, Ocete-Guzman JG, et al. The management of limb-length discrepancies in children after treatment of osteosarcoma and Ewing's sarcoma. J Pediatr Orthop. 1995;15:561–5.
18. Grimer RJ, Belthur M, Carter SR, Tillman RM, Cool P. Extendible replacements of the proximal tibia for bone tumours. J Bone Joint Surg Br. 2000;82-B:255–60.
19. Grimer RJ, Carter SR, Pynsent PB. The cost-effectiveness of limb salvage for bone tumors. J Bone Joint Surg Br. 1997;79-B:558–61.
20. Gupta A, Meswania J, Pollock R, Cannon SR, et al. Non-invasive distal femoral expandable endoprosthesis for limb-salvage surgery in pediatric tumours. J Bone Joint Surg Br. 2006; 88-B:649–54.
21. Gurney J, Swensen A, Bulterys M, et al. Malignant bone tumors. In: Ries LA, Smith MA, Gurney JG, editors. Malignant bone tumors. Cancer Statistics Branch, National Cancer Institute, SEER Program; 1999. p. 99–110.
22. Gurney JG, Young JL, Roffers SD, et al. Soft tissue sarcomas. In: Ries LA, Smith Ma, Gurney JG, editors. Soft tissue sarcomas. Cancer Statistics Branch, National Cancer Institute, SEER Program; 1999. p. 11–123.
23. Hejna MJ, Gitelis S. Allograft prosthetic composite replacement for bone tumors. Semin Surg Oncol. 1997;13:18–24.
24. Henderson ER, Pepper AM, Marulanda G, Binitie OT, Cheong D, Letson GD. Outcome of lower-limb preservation with an expandable endoprosthesis after bone tumor resection in children. J Bone Joint Surg Am. 2012;94:537–47.
25. Hillmann A, Hoffmann C, Gosheger G, Krakau H, Winkelmann W. Malignant tumor of the distal part of the femur of proximal part of the tibia: endoprosthetic replacement or rotationplasty. J Bone Joint Surg Am. 1999;81-A:462–8.
26. Hopyan S, Tan JW, Graham HK, Torode IP. Function and upright time following limb salvage, amputation, and rotationplasty for pediatric sarcoma of bone. J Pediatr Orthop. 2006;26:405–8.
27. Hosalkar HS, Dormans JP. Limb sparing surgery for pediatric musculoskeletal tumors. Pediatr Blood Cancer. 2004;42:295–310.
28. Hwang N, Grimer RJ, Carter SR, Tillman RM, Abudu A, Jeys LM. Early results of a non-invasive extendible prosthesis for limb salvage surgery in children with bone tumors. J Bone Joint Surg Br. 2012;94-B:265–9.
29. Jacobs PA. Limb salvage and rotationplasty for osteosarcoma in children. Clin Orthop. 1984;188:217–22.
30. Kotz R. Rotationplasty. Semin Surg Oncol. 1997;13:34–40.
31. Kotz R, Salzer M. Rotation-plasty for childhood osteosarcoma of the distal part of the femur. J Bone Joint Surg Am. 1982;64-A:959–69.
32. Kumta SM, Cheng JCY, Li CK, et al. Scope and limitations of limb-sparing surgery in childhood sarcomas. J Pediatr Orthop. 2002;22:244–8.
33. Lewis VO. Limb salvage in the skeletally immature patient. Curr Oncol Rep. 2005;7:285–92.
34. McDonald DJ, Scott SM, Eckardt JJ. Tibial turn-up for long distal femoral bone loss. Clin Orthop. 2001;383:214–20.
35. Mnaymneh W, Malinin TI, Lackman RD, Hornicek FJ, et al. Massive distal femoral osteoarticular allografts after resection of bone tumors. Clin Orthop. 1994;303:103–15.
36. Moran SL, Shin AY, Bishop AT. The use of massive bone allograft with intramedullary free fibula flap for limb salvage in a pediatric and adolescent population. Plast Reconstr Surg. 2006;118:413–9.
37. Musculo DL, Ayerza MA, Aponte-Tinao L, Farfalli G. Allograft reconstruction after sarcoma resection in children younger than 10 years old. Clin Orthop. 2008;466(8):1856–62.

38. Musculo DL, Ayerza MA, Aponte-Tinao LA, Ranalletta M. Use of distal femoral osteoarticular allografts in limb salvage surgery. J Bone Joint Surg Am. 2005;87-A:2449–55.
39. Nagarajan R, Neglia JP, Clohisy DR, Robison LL. Limb salvage and amputation in survivors or pediatric lower extremity bone tumors: what are the long term implications? J Clin Oncol. 2002;20:4493–501.
40. Neel MD, Wilkins RM, Rao BN, Kelly CM. Early multicenter experience with a noninvasive expandable prosthesis. Clin Orthop. 2003;415:72–81.
41. Ness KK, Neel MD, Kaste SC, Billups CA, Marchese VG, Rao BN, Daw NC. A comparison of function after limb salvage with non-invasive expandable or modular prostheses in children. Eur J Cancer. 2014;50:3212–20.
42. Ortiz-Cruz E, Gebhardt MC, Jennings LC, Springfield DS, Mankin HJ. The results of transplantation of intercalary allografts after resection of tumors. J Bone Joint Surg Am. 1997; 79-A:97–106.
43. Peterson CA, Koch LD, Wood MB. Tibia-hindfoot osteomusculocutaneous rotationplasty with calcaneopelvic arthrodesis for extensive loss of bone from the proximal part of the femur: a report of two cases. J Bone Joint Surg Am. 1997;79-A:1504–9.
44. Picardo NE, Blunn GW, Shekkeris AS, Meswania J, Aston WJ, et al. The medium-term results of the Stanmore non-invasive extendible endoprosthesis in the treatment of paediatric bone tumours. J Bone Joint Surg Br. 2012;94-B:425–30.
45. Rougraff BT, Simon MA, Kneisl JS, Greenberg DB, Mankin HJ. Limb salvage compared with amputation for osteosarcoma of the distal end of the femur. J Bone Joint Surg. 1994;76-A: 649–56.
46. Ruggieri P, Mavrogenis AF, Pala E, Romantini M, Manfrini M, Mercuri M. Outcome of expandable prostheses in children. J Pediatr Orthop. 2013;33:244–53.
47. San-Julian M, Dolz R, Garcia-Barrecheguren E, et al. Limb salvage in bone sarcomas in patients younger than age 10. J Pediatr Orthop. 2003;23:753–62.
48. Weisstein JS, Goldsby RE, O'Donnell RJ. Oncologic approaches to pediatric limb preservation. J Am Acad Orthop Surg. 2005;13:544–54.
49. Wilkins RM, Miller CM. Reoperation after limb preservation surgery for sarcomas of the knee in children. Clin Orthop. 2003;412:153–61.

Chapter 5
Location of Sarcomas Within Bone: The Growth Plate

Francisco Forriol, Mikel San-Julian, and José Cañadell†

Abstract Most malignant bone tumors are located in the metaphysis of the long bones, near to the growth plate. If the joint is preserved when a tumor is resected, the results in terms of future limb function are better. The growth plate can represent a barrier to tumoral spread. We describe the Cañadell technique, which can be of benefit to patients with metaphyseal tumors but whose physis is free from malignant cells, and which is based on epiphysiolysis by physeal distraction. Two prerequisites for Cañadell's technique are that the physis is unequivocally open and that the physis has not been invaded by the tumor.

Keywords Distraction • Limb salvage • Joint preservation • Growth plate • Bone tumor • Bone allograft

5.1 Pediatric Malignant Tumors Located in Long Bones

The most common tumors during childhood and adolescence are osteosarcoma and Ewing's sarcoma. In about 75 % of the cases of these two diseases, the lesions are located near to the growth plate. Advances in imaging technology, especially MRI, enable more reliable diagnosis, precise localization and determination of whether the growth plate has been infiltrated by the tumor. If the growth plate is free of malignant cells, it is possible to preserve the epiphysis and thereby achieve limb salvage without having to use a joint prosthesis or having to perform arthrodesis, two techniques that are always complicated in a child [10, 15, 43].

---

† Author was deceased at the time of publication

F. Forriol, MD, PhD (✉)
Department of Clinical Sciences, School of Medicine, University San Pablo – CEU, Campus de Monteprincipe, Boadilla del Monte, Madrid 28668, Spain
e-mail: fforriol@mac.com

M. San-Julian, MD, PhD
Department of Orthopaedic Surgery, University of Navarra, Pamplona, Navarra, Spain

J. Cañadell†, MD, PhD
Department of Orthopaedic Surgery, University of Navarra, Pamplona, Navarra, Spain

M. San-Julian (ed.), *Cañadell's Pediatric Bone Sarcomas: Epiphysiolysis before Excision*, DOI 10.1007/978-3-319-24220-0_5

Limb salvage includes two operative procedures. The first is tumor excision, the adequacy of which can be evaluated simply by the rate of local recurrence. To cure primary tumors it is necessary to perform en bloc resection of all macroscopic disease, including the biopsy scar. The degree of osteotomy required to allow a safe margin is determined on the basis of the intramedullary spread of tumor as revealed by imaging methods. There is no complete accordance among orthopedic surgeons about what constitutes a safe margin, but most consider 5 cm beyond the tumor as sufficient. Articular cartilage is thought to prevent tumor spread in most cases, and therefore can be considered as a safe margin. For this reason, in tumors involving the epiphysis, resection of the joint is adequate [6, 13–15, 27, 50, 59].

The second procedure in limb salvage is reconstruction. The selection of a method of reconstruction must consider the effects on function of any deformity secondary to tumor excision. Such deformity can be predicted by the amount of physeal cartilage removed. We believe that the choice of the type of reconstruction should be based on each patient's age, size, functional demands and personal wishes; the surgeon's experience is also an important factor. Patients with a primary tumor in the scapula, clavicle, proximal fibula or rib can be treated by simple resection and suffer only minimal functional impairment.

Resections requiring reconstruction can be subdivided into two major categories: diaphyseal resections and articular resections. Intercalary bone grafts are the most frequent treatment for diaphyseal resections when it is possible to preserve the epiphysis. Functional results with intercalary reconstruction after diaphyseal resection are better than those after articular resection (Fig. 5.1a, b). Compared with metallic implants, bone grafts offer many advantages, including tendinous

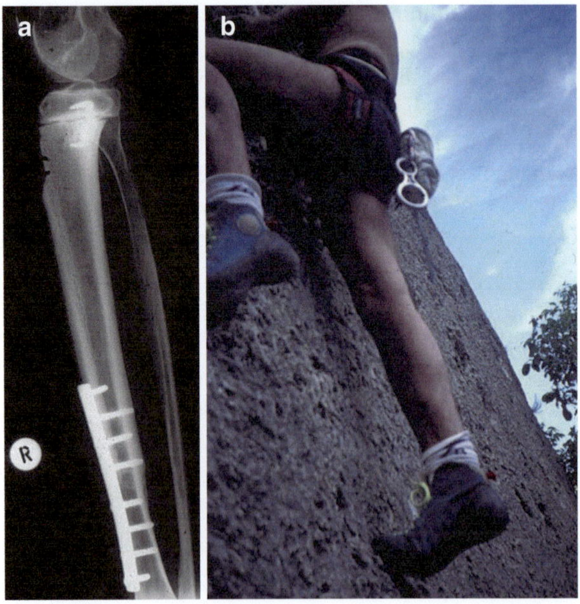

Fig. 5.1 (**a**) Intercalary reconstruction of the tibia by using an allograft after resection of an osteosarcoma. Note the holes for patellar tendon reattachment. (**b**) In this case, preservation of the epiphysis allowed the patient to do sporting activities such as climbing

reattachment, incorporation of the graft into the host bone and longevity [28, 44]. After resection with epiphyseal preservation, instead of a bone allograft, Fang et al. [22] have used a bone transport osteogenesis technique.

The growth plate has traditionally been considered to block the spread of a tumor, but this barrier is not impenetrable. In limb salvage procedures, although preserving the joint near the tumor enables better functional results, it is not possible to preserve the epiphysis in all cases. Articular resections pose the most complex problems of reconstruction in oncological surgery [15].

Magnetic resonance imaging (MRI) is an important tool in limb salvage procedures. Plain radiographs only indirectly show growth problems caused by physeal abnormalities and they do so long after damage has occurred. MRI, however, provides the resolution necessary to define many of the prenatal and postnatal stages of epiphyseal development *in vivo*. Differentiation between the different layers of the cartilage is well achieved with gadolinium enhancement that also identifies cartilage vascular canals. With MRI it is possible to differentiate epiphyseal cartilage, physeal cartilage, the zones of provisional calcification, physis of the secondary center of ossification, the perichondrium, vascularity of the cartilage canals, and hematopoietic and fatty marrow [6, 33, 50].

5.2 Morphology of Growth Plate

Physeal cartilage is the growth organ of the long bones. The cells of growth cartilage are chondrocytes, which direct the whole process of enchondral ossification and are responsible for controlling the extent of growth in the long bones during postnatal development. Endochondral ossification is a process involving chondrogenesis, chondrocyte hypertrophy, matrix mineralization, and vascularization followed by bone formation [26]. Morphologically, the growth plate is divided into zones of germinal cells, columnar cells, hypertrophic cells, and metaphyseal cells. In terms of function, we can refer to (1) the germinal zone; (2) the columnar zone with two well defined areas: the upper proliferating zone and the lower maturation zone; (3) the hypertrophic cell zone, with the upper 4/5 with a non-mineralized matrix and the lower 1/5 with a mineralized matrix; and (4) the outer reaches of the metaphysis [26].

Although the two most important states of a physeal chondrocyte are proliferation and hypertrophy, which includes the mineralization of the matrix before bone reabsorption during vascular invasion, a chondrocyte actually goes through several phases, each of which is characterized by a predominant functional activity. These phases occur synchronically: the youngest chondrocytes are proliferating cells, whilst the oldest are to be found in regions of vascular invasion. The upper hypertrophic zone is characterized by cells that have enlarged five- to tenfold implying a reduction in matrix volume relative to total tissue volume. The cells in this zone synthesize type X collagen [4], and the mineralized chondrocytes undergo apoptotic cell death [18]. The chondrocytes presumably trans-differentiate to osteocytes (although there is no evidence of *in vivo* one-step trans-differentiation) and then endothelial cells from the bone collar invade the terminal layer of apoptotic chondrocytes to form vascular channels [7]. These changes require a molecular interaction between vascular structures and cartilage; the two types of molecules involved in this process are proteases and growth factors [38, 48, 55]. In addition, the transition from cartilage to bone is highly regulated by transcriptional factors and local growth factors (Indian hedgehog (Ihh), Sox9, BMPs, and PTHrP) [29, 34, 36, 51, 58].

The mechanical properties of growth cartilage depend on the extracellular matrix, which is produced and maintained by the chondrocytes. In the case of many bone types, epiphyseal plates form, in some individuals, the greatest possible angle with the corresponding planes of shear strain. The space between the two plate surfaces is filled by growth cartilage, which, seen from the front, has a "V" shape. This arrangement minimizes the risk of shear strain separating the plates. Changes in tension in different areas of the periosteum may be a factor that leads to increased growth in certain parts of the physis [37].

In the event of injury that affects only the metaphyseal part of the growth cartilage, increased growth may be a temporary process which results in broadening of the physis. Good metaphyseal vascularization ensures rapid regeneration [39]. The epiphyseal part of the physis comprising the germinal layer is much more sensitive to trauma because such trauma not only disturbs the functional balance of the physis but can also bring about destruction of growth cartilage.

The three main sources of vascular supply to the metaphysis are (1) the feeder artery, which brings blood to the central metaphyseal area and has peripheral branches with small vessels that are distributed along the inside of the spongy bone and contributes up to 80 % of the blood; (2) the arteries penetrating the metaphysis; and (3) the arteries between the bone and the perichondrium. The central longitudinal branches reach the growth cartilage, resulting in a tree-like vascular pattern. A considerable number of metaphyseal vessels deriving from the articular arteries also contribute to the vascular supply of long bone metaphysis and growth cartilage. All these vessels end in vascular knots or clusters of capillaries just beneath the last intact transverse septum at the base of the cartilaginous part of the growth cartilage [9, 39].

The epiphysis receives its vascular supply from one or more vessels which penetrate the cartilage and branch out inside it. The epiphyseal vascular supply to growth cartilage is characterized by small arterial branches coming from the intra-epiphyseal arteries, which ramify to irrigate the proliferative layer of growth cartilage. However, arterial branches of the epiphyseal vessels do not extend into the cartilaginous part of the physis [26], and so the hypertrophic layer of growth cartilage is free of vascularization. The two most important circulatory systems, constituted respectively by epiphyseal and metaphyseal vessels, are separated both functionally and morphologically [13] (Fig. 5.2).

Vascular anastomoses between the epiphyseal and metaphyseal vessels across the growth plate occur physiologically only at the time of growth plate fusion at skeletal maturity [57].

Vascular invasion in general leads to the removal of cartilage, formation of bone marrow, and new bone formation and growth.

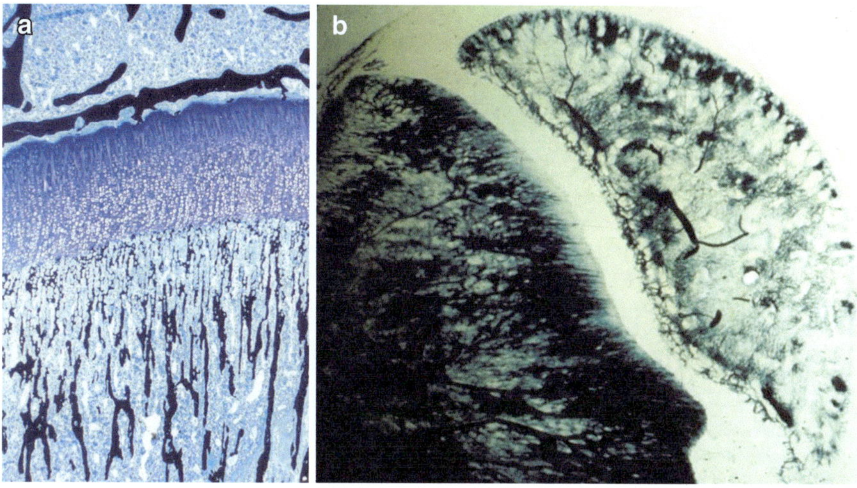

Fig. 5.2 (**a**) Indian ink injection and (**b**) Spaltenholz technique showing no vascular anastomoses between metaphyseal and epiphyseal vessels

5.3 Physeal Distraction in Orthopedic Surgery

Progressive lengthening is currently a common therapeutic method. Its history can be traced back to pioneering work in 1905 by Codivilla [16], whose technique was successively modified to make it simpler and more convenient for the patient, reducing the duration of treatment and the incidence of complications.

Distraction of the growth plate, physeal distraction or chondrodiastasis is a technique that has been used for bone lengthening and correction of angular deformity [11, 12, 30, 47] (Fig. 5.3). In animal models, growth plate distraction at a slow rate increases length by hyperplasia without causing epiphysiolysis; there is an increase in physeal cell activity demonstrable in the proliferating cell layer [3, 8, 17, 19, 35, 46, 52, 53]; Arriola et al. [5] found an increase in extension of the hypertrophic cell layer; and it has been suggested that the increase in physeal height may be caused by an increase of the metaphyseal blood supply [1, 2, 5, 17, 19, 21, 52]. Interruption of the metaphyseal vascular supply results in inhibited resorption in addition to a shortage of calcium in the hypertrophic chondrocytes.

When forces are applied in traction, epiphysiolysis (of type I according to Salter and Harris's classification) is always achieved. When diaphyseal-epiphyseal distraction is performed in a growing bone, breakage occurs in the zone of least resistance, that is, in the physis (Fig. 5.4). The fracture makes it possible to lengthen the bone in a single surgical operation and achieve rapid consolidation without the need for osteotomy or even section of the skin.

Fjeld and Steen [24] established that daily distraction of 0.25 % of bone length, over a period of between 5 and 9 days, brings about epiphyseal separations in animal models. In all experimental studies on physeal distraction, separation of the growth cartilage from the metaphysis has been observed [31, 32, 45, 49].

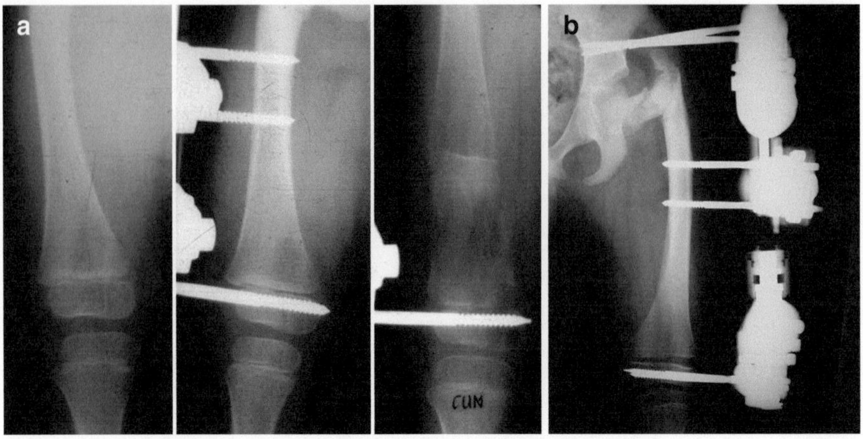

Fig 5.3 Physeal distraction has been widely used in orthopedics (**a**, **b**) as a bone lengthening procedure

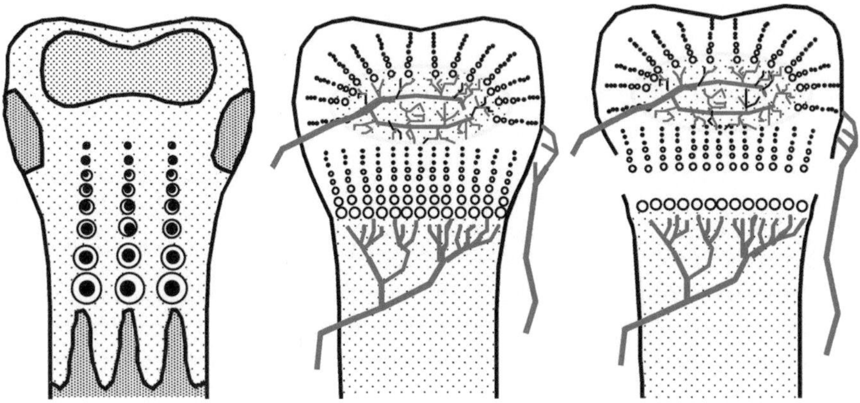

Fig. 5.4 Diagram showing the rupture in the metaphyseal part of a growth plate on application of the physeal distraction technique

In the course of the separation process, the periosteum breaks where the perichondrial ring inserts. This break produces a hematoma which fills the gap [23, 31, 32] and which is later replaced by fibrous tissue [40–42]. Newly formed bone deposition proceeds from the intact periosteum as well as from the epiphyseal and metaphyseal portions of the bone [40–42, 49, 54]. The characteristic pattern of grooves in the lengthening area, which can be seen by radiology, reflects the mineralization of the collagen fibers, which are arranged lengthways. Occasionally, a radiolucent area can be observed in the lengthening callus.

De Pablos and Cañadell [20, 21] demonstrated that distraction always produces epiphysiolysis, irrespective of the daily distraction rate. Their research established a relationship between morphological variations in the growth cartilage and the rate of distraction used. In sheep femora subject to lengthening at 0.5 mm/day, the

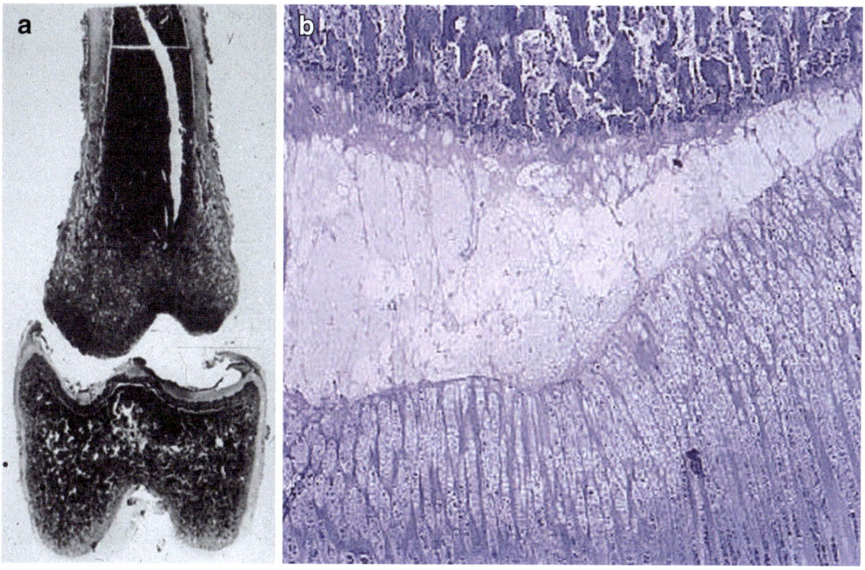

Fig. 5.5 These two histological images of an experimental epiphysiolysis in a lamb show the (**a**) disruption is produced through (**b**) the layer of degenerative cells of the growth plate. Most of the growth plate remains together with the epiphysis

cartilage remained normal (Fig. 5.5). However, femora lengthened by 1 mm/day, and particularly those lengthened by 2 mm/day, were found to have obvious injuries 45 days and 4 months later. Sledge and Noble [52] found that stimulation of the growth cartilage by applying distractional forces of 1–2 kg on the distal femoral physis in rabbits resulted in hyperplasia of the physis, with an increase in cell mitosis and a rise in polysaccharide sulfate synthesis. Spriggins et al. [53] used fixators equipped with instrumentation to study the forces of physeal distraction in rabbits. They detected two patterns of behavior. In one group of cases, the forces increased to maximum values of 20–32 N and then decreased until the next distraction. This indicates breakage of the growth cartilage, with the associated hyperplasia. In the other group of cases, lower forces with maximum values of 6–18 N were observed at the end of the distraction period. This indicates hyperplasia without bone fracture. Tercedor et al. [56] observed that in all physeal distractions there is an initial hyperplasic reaction in all the cell layers of the growth cartilage, and that this is followed by atrophy.

The so-called Cañadell technique is applied in certain cases of metaphyseal bone tumor in which there has been no invasion of the physis by the tumor and concerns physeal distraction of the distal extreme of the femur or the proximal end of the tibia. Cañadell's technique is indicated for pediatric bone sarcomas located in the metaphysis. The physis has to be open and the tumor must not have transgressed the physis [15]. If the tumor is in contact with part of the physis, physeal distraction can be tried, but because it is possible that tumor cells have crossed the physis, intraoperative histology is recommended [13]; if tumor cells are found in the physeal margin of the resection, surgical treatment is to be completed by transepiphyseal or epiphyseal resection. When the tumor has crossed the physis or if the tumor is in contact with all of the physis, the technique is contraindicated [15].

5.4 Technical Aspects of Physeal Distraction with a Unilateral External Fixator

The external fixator is of proven effectiveness in the treatment of fractures. As a consequence of direct experience, development and new designs, the indications for the external fixator have broadened far beyond the original basic indications. Nowadays, the external fixator is used by many departments in the treatment of limb fractures, as well as in cases of retarded consolidation, pseudoarthrosis, axial corrections and in limb lengthening.

On the basis of our experience, the stability of the external fixator should, at the outset, be greater than that of the bone. The stability can later be gradually reduced so that the weight of the load can be transmitted directly to the callus, thus stimulating bone formation. Surgical interventions involving an external fixator should be performed in the manner of corrective surgery and carefully planned to accommodate the technical specifications of the apparatus being used.

The surgical technique for distraction with an external fixator is not difficult. The mobility of the pin clamps and the fact that the length of the bar can be adjusted make use of the fixator straightforward. Once the size of fixator to be used has been chosen, the apparatus is placed alongside the bone that is to be lengthened, and the fixator adjusted according to the specific measurements of the particular bone.

Technically, physeal distraction does not differ greatly from lengthening procedure: the only important difference is that the two pins should be inserted at the level of the epiphysis, this frequently being distal in the femur or proximal in the tibia. The epiphyseal space requires that the pins be inserted one in front of the other, which means that these pins should be inserted perpendicularly relative to the diaphyseal pins. To carry out this particular procedure, all models of fixator apparatus include what is known as a T-piece. Pins should be 5 or 6 mm in diameter (4-mm pins are used only in very young children) and care should be taken to ensure that they enter neither too close to the joint cartilage nor too close to the growing cartilage [14, 25].

Limb saving surgery by physeal distraction can be used in young patients with an open epiphyseal plate. The advantages of the Cañadell technique are that it is simple surgically, it is effective, and it has relatively few complications [59]. Cañadell et al. [13, 15] and later San-Julian et al. [50] have reported good results with the Cañadell technique in terms of both underlying disease control and limb function; the technique was not associated with local recurrence even when the tumor was in close contact with the physis.

Yao et al. [59] reported on six patients, followed up for an average of 2.5 years (ranging from 1 to 5 years). Primary healing was obtained directly in five patients; the other patient suffered a superficial infection that was cured after a dressing change. Bone healing at the metaphysis junction took 6–9 months in five cases and

14 months in one case. Delayed union happened at the diaphysis junction in all patients. At the most recent follow-up, limb discrepancy was 1–3 cm in four patients and 3–5 cm in two patients; three patients had compensatory scoliosis; and two patients had claudication. Gao et al. [27] reported for the same patients that, despite a significant difference in limb length, the results according to the functional evaluation criteria of the International Society of Limb Salvage (ISOLS) were, at the most recent follow-up, fair in one case, good in two cases, and excellent in three cases.

References

1. Alberty A, Peltonen J, Ritsilä V. Effects of distraction and compression on proliferation of growth plate chondrocytes: a study on rabbits. Acta Orthop Scand. 1993;64:449–55.
2. Alberty A. Effects of physeal distraction on the vascular supply of the growth area: a microangiographical study in rabbits. J Pediatr Orthop. 1993;13:373–7.
3. Aldegheri R, Trivella G, Lavini F. Epiphyseal distraction. Chondrodiastasis. Clin Orthop Relat Res. 1989;241:117–27.
4. Alini M, Matsui Y, Dodge GR, Poole AR. The extracellular matrix of cartilage in the growth plate before and during calcification: changes in composition and degradation of type II collagen. Cal Tis Int. 1992;50:327–35.
5. Arriola F, Forriol F, Cañadell J. Histomorphometric study of growth plate subjected to different mechanical conditions (compression, tension and neutralization): an experimental study in lambs. J Pediatr Orthop. 2001;10B:334–8.
6. Betz M, Dumont CE, Fuchs B, Exner GU. Physeal distraction for joint preservation in malignant metaphyseal bone tumors in children. Clin Orthop Relat Res. 2012;470:1749–54.
7. Blumer MJ, Longato S, Fritsch H. Localization of tartrate-resistant acid phosphatase (TRAP), membrane type-1matrix metalloproteinases (MT1-MMP) and macrophages during early endochondral bone formation. J Anat. 2008;213:431–41.
8. Bright RW, Elmore SM. Physical properties of epiphyseal plate cartilage. Surg Forum. 1968;19:463–5.
9. Brighton CT. The growth plate. Orthop Clin North Am. 1984;15:571–95.
10. Campanacci L, Manfrini M, Colangeli M, Alí N, Mercuri M. Long-term results in children with massive bone osteoarticular allografts of the knee for high-grade osteosarcoma. J Pediatr Orthop. 2010;30:919–27.
11. Cañadell J, De Pablos J. Correction of angular deformities by physeal distraction. Clin Orthop Relat Res. 1992;283:98–105.
12. Cañadell J, de Pablos J. Breaking bony bridges by physeal distraction: a new approach. Int Orthop. 1985;9:223–9.
13. Cañadell J, Forriol F, Cara JA. Removal of metaphyseal bone tumours with preservation of the epiphysis: physeal distraction before excision. J Bone Joint Surg (Br). 1994;76-B:127–32.
14. Cañadell J, Forriol F. Use of mono-axial fixators in leg lengthening. In: Surgical techniques in orthopaedics and traumatology, Ed Scientifiques et Medicales. Paris: Elsevier SAS, 55-570-E-10; 2000, p. 1–5.
15. Cañadell J, San-Julian M. Pediatric bone sarcomas. Berlin: Springer; 2009.
16. Codivilla A. On the means of lengthening in the lower limbs, the muscles and the tissues which are shortened through deformity. Am J Orthop Surg. 1905;2:353–69.
17. Connolly JF, Huurman WW, Lippello L, Pankaj R. Epiphyseal traction to correct acquired growth deformities. Clin Orthop Relat Res. 1986;202:258–68.
18. Damron TA, Zhang M, Pritchard MR, Middleton FA, Horton JA, Margulies BM, et al. Microarray cluster analysis of irradiated growth plate zones following laser microdissection. Int J Radiat Oncol Biol Phys. 2009;74:949–56.

19. De Bastiani G, Aldegheri R, Renzi-Brivio L, Trivella G. Chondrodiastasis. Controlled symmetrical distraction of the epiphyseal plate. Limb lengthening in children. J Bone Joint Surg (Br). 1986;66-B:550–6.
20. De Pablos J, Cañadell J. Experimental physeal distraction in immature sheep. Clin Orthop Relat Res. 1990;250:73–80.
21. de Pablos J, Villas C, Cañadell J. Bone lengthening by physical distraction: an experimental study. Int Orthop. 1986;10:163–70.
22. Fang B, Yi C, Zhang H, Zhang QW, Li Y, Wei Q, He W. Combined epiphyseal preservation and autograft bone transfer in treatment of children osteosarcoma. Chin J Rep Reconstr Surg. 2013;27:45–9.
23. Fishbane BM, Riley LH. Continous transphyseal traction: experimental observations. Clin Orthop Relat Res. 1978;136:120–4.
24. Fjeld TO, Steen H. Limb lengthening by low rate epiphyseal distraction. An experimental study in the caprine tibia. J Orthop Res. 1988;6:360–8.
25. Forriol F, Cañadell J. Unilateral external fixation in reconstructive surgery. In: Asche G, Roth W, Schroeder L, editors. The external fixator. Standard indications, operating instructions and examples of frame configuration. Reinbeck: Einhorn-Presse Verlag; 2002. p. 175–89.
26. Forriol F, Shapiro F. Bone development interaction of molecular components and biophysical forces. Clin Orthop Relat Res. 2005;432:14–33.
27. Gao S, Cai Q, Yao W, Wang JQ, Zhang P, Wang CJ, et al. Epiphyseal distraction for preservation of epiphysis of osteosarcoma in children. Chin J Rep Reconstr Surg. 2012;26:1291–5.
28. Gebhardt MC, Flugstad DI, Springfield DS, Mankin HJ. The use of bone allografts for limb salvage in high-grade extremity osteosarcoma. Clin Orthop Relat Res. 1991;270:181–96.
29. Henry SP, Liang S, Akdemir KC, de Crombrugghe B. The postnatal role of Sox9 in cartilage. J Bone Miner Res. 2012;27:2511–25.
30. Ilizarov GA. The tension-stress effect on the genesis and growth tissue. Part II. The influence of the rate and frequency of distraction. Clin Orthop Relat Res. 1989;239:263–85.
31. Jani L. Die Distraktionepiphyseolyse: Tierexperimentelle Studie zum Problem der Beinverlängerung. Z Orthop. 1975;113:189–98.
32. Jani L. Tierexperimentelle Studie über Tibiaverlängerung durch Distrak-tionepiphyseolyse. Z Orthop. 1973;111:627–30.
33. Jaramillo D, Shapiro F. Growth cartilage: normal appearance, variants and abnormalities. Pediatr Musculoskelet MR Imaging. 1998;6:455–71.
34. Jing JJ, Ren Y, Zong Z, Liu CJ, Kamiya N, Mishina Y, et al. BMP receptor 1A determines the cell fate of the postnatal growth plate. Int J Biol Sci. 2013;9:895–906.
35. Kenwright J, Spriggins AJ, Cunningham JL. Response of the growth plate to distraction close to skeletal maturity: is fracture necessary? Clin Orthop Relat Res. 1990;250:61–72.
36. Kronenberg HM. Developmental regulation of the growth plate. Nature. 2003;423:332–6.
37. Kuijpers-Jagtman AM, Maltha JC, Bex JHM, Daggers JG. The influence of vascular and periosteal interferences on the histological structure of the growth plates of long bones. Anat Anz. 1987;164:245–54.
38. Liu Z, Lavine KJ, Hung IH, Ornitz DM. FGF18 is required for early chondrocyte proliferation, hypertrophy and vascular invasion of the growth plate. Dev Biol. 2007;302:80–91.
39. Magne D, Julien M, Vinatier C, Meri-Soussi F, Weiss P, Guicheux J. Cartilage formation in growth plate and arteries: from physiology to pathology. Bioessays. 2005;27:708–16.
40. Monticelli G, Spinelli R. Distraction epiphysiolysis as a method of limb lengthening. I. Experimental study. Clin Orthop Relat Res. 1981;154:254–61.
41. Monticelli G, Spinelli R. Distraction epiphysiolysis as a method of limb lengthening. II. Morphologic investigations. Clin Orthop Relat Res. 1981;154:262–73.
42. Monticelli G, Spinelli R. Distraction epiphysiolysis as a method of limb lengthening. III. Clinical applications. Clin Orthop Relat Res. 1981;154:274–85.
43. Muscolo DL, Ayerza M, Aponte-Tinao L, Ranalletta M. Partial epiphyseal preservation and intercalary allograft reconstruction in high-grade metaphyseal osteosarcoma of the knee. J Bone Joint Surg Am. 2005;87-A suppl 1:226–36.

44. Muscolo DL, Ayerza MA, Aponte-Tinao LA, Ranalletta M. Use of distal femoral osteoarticular allografts in limb salvage surgery: surgical technique. J Bone Joint Surg Am. 2006;88-A suppl 1:305–21.
45. Nakamura K, Matsushita T, Okazaki H, Nagano A, Kurokawa T. Attempted limb lengthening by physeal distraction. Clin Orthop Relat Res. 1991;267:306–11.
46. Noble J, Diamond R, Stirrat CR, Sledge CB. Breaking force of the rabbit growth plate and its application to epiphyseal distraction. Acta Orthop Scand. 1982;53:13–6.
47. Peltonen J, Alitalo I, Karaharju EO, Helio H. Distraction of the growth plate: experiments in pigs and sheep. Acta Orthop Scand. 1984;55:359–62.
48. Plumb DA, Ferrara L, Torbica T, Knowles L, Mironov Jr A, Kadler KE, et al. Collagen VII organises the pericellular matrix in the growth plate. PLoS One. 2011;6:29422.
49. Ring PA. Experimental bone lengthening by epiphyseal distraction. Br J Surg. 1958;46: 169–73.
50. San-Julian M, Aquerreta JD, Benito A, Cañadell J. Indications for epiphyseal preservation in metaphyseal malignant bone tumors of children: relationship between image methods and histological findings. J Pediatr Orthop. 1999;19:543–8.
51. Shu B, Zhang M, Xie R, Wang M, Jin H, Hou W, et al. BMP2, but not BMP4, is crucial for chondrocyte proliferation and maturation during endochondral bone development. J Cell Sci. 2011;124:3428–40.
52. Sledge CB, Noble J. Experimental limb lengthening by epiphyseal distraction. Clin Orthop Relat Res. 1978;136:111–9.
53. Spriggins AJ, Bader DL, Cunningham JL, Kenwright J. Distraction physiolysis in the rabbit. Acta Orthop Scand. 1989;60:154–8.
54. Steen H, Fjeld TO, Ronningen H, Langeland N, Gjerdet N, Bjerkreim I. Limb lengthening by epiphyseal distraction. An experimental study in the caprine femur. J Orthop Res. 1987;5: 592–9.
55. Takahara M, Naruse T, Takagi M, Orui H, Ogino T. Matrix metalloproteinase-9 expression, tartrate-resistant acid phosphatase activity, and DNA fragmentation in vascular and cellular invasion into cartilage preceding primary endochondral ossification in long bone. J Orthop Res. 2004;22:1050–7.
56. Tercedor J, Crespo V, Acosta F, Campos A, Fernandez E. Alargamiento tibial por distracción epifisaria proximal. Estudio experimental en conejos. Rev Ortop Traumatol. 1988;32IB:412–6.
57. Trueta J, Amato VP. The vascular contribution to osteogenesis. III. Changes in the growth cartilage caused by experimentally induced ischaemia. J Bone Joint Surg (Br). 1960;42-B:571–87.
58. Wuelling M, Vortkamp A. Chondrocyte proliferation and differentiation. Endocr Dev. 2011;21:1–11.
59. Yao W, Cai Q, Gao S, Wang JQ, Zhang P, Wang X. Epiphysis preserving by physeal distraction for treatment of femur osteosarcoma in children. Chin J Rep Reconstr Surg. 2013;27:423–7.

Chapter 6
A Histological Study of the Barrier Effect of the Physis Against Metaphyseal Osteosarcoma

Miguel Angel Idoate, Enrique de Alava, Julio de Pablos, Maria Dolores Lozano, Jesús Vazquez†, and José Cañadell†

Abstract In about half of the children affected by metaphyseal malignant bone tumors, the growth plate and epiphysis are not compromised by the tumor. Invasion of the epiphysis by the tumor seems to occur eventually but takes time.

Keywords Physis • Osteosarcoma • Barrier effect • Histology • Growth plate • Chemotherapy • Radiology • Invasion

6.1 Introduction

Osteosarcoma is a primary malignant bone tumor usually located in the metaphysis. It tends to infiltrate adjacent bone as well as soft tissue. Traditionally, the physis has been regarded as a barrier capable of blocking tumor extension [1, 5], and this idea has been strengthened by experimental studies carried out *in vitro,* which suggest

---

† Author was deceased at the time of publication

M.A. Idoate, MD, PhD (✉)
Department Pathology, University of Navarra Avda. Pio XII, Pamplona, Navarra 31008, Spain
e-mail: maidoate@unav.es

E. de Alava, MD, PhD
Department of Pathology, Virgen del Rocio University Hospital, Sevilla, Spain

J. de Pablos, MD, PhD
Department of Orthopaedic Surgery, Hospital San Juan de Dios, Pamplona, Navarra, Spain

M.D. Lozano, MD, PhD
Department of Pathology, Clínica Universidad de Navarra, Pamplona, Navarra, Spain

J. Vazquez†, MD, PhD
Department of Pathology, University of Navarra, Pamplona, Spain

J. Cañadell†, MD, PhD
Department of Orthopaedic Surgery, University of Navarra, Pamplona, Navarra, Spain

M. San-Julian (ed.), *Cañadell's Pediatric Bone Sarcomas: Epiphysiolysis before Excision*, DOI 10.1007/978-3-319-24220-0_6

the barrier effect is due to certain proteins in the physis that are inhibitory of angiogenesis [2, 10, 13, 15, 18]. In this respect, several molecules of possible relevance are different growth factors, such as fibroblast growth factor (FGF) and insulin-like growth factors (IGF) – which control growth of the epiphyseal growth plate growth – and bone morphogenetic proteins and the parathyroid hormone-related peptide [7, 14]. Doubts about the barrier function, however, have been raised by the fact that, in skeletally immature patients with osteogenic sarcoma, physeal invasion is observed to occur [4, 9, 11, 17, 19].

Knowledge of the frequency with which osteosarcoma invades the physis is important in assessment of tumor extension and in planning surgical resection.

In this study, the cases of a large series of skeletally immature patients with osteosarcoma were reviewed with the objective of clarifying how effective the physis is as a barrier to tumor spread. A particular objective was to assess any correlation between the pathological evaluation of the osteosarcoma in its relationship with the growth plate and the corresponding radiological findings. A principle observation made as a result of the study was that there were three different types or stages of behavior of osteosarcomas with regard to physeal invasion.

6.2 Materials and Methods

The series included 450 patients from whom a bone osteosarcoma was surgically removed and diagnosed by biopsy between 1979 and 2013. In order to ascertain tumor extension reliably at the time of diagnosis, all cases had been studied by conventional radiology and digital angiography, In the 1980s, the imaging method used was computerized axial tomography (CT); from the beginning of the 1990s, magnetic resonance imaging (MRI) was used. After histological diagnosis and previous to surgical resection, all patients but one received neoadjuvant chemotherapy, with intravenous doxorubicin, methotrexate, and cisplatin, which was administered intra-arterially.

In order to evaluate the reliability of basing the surgical decision about physis distraction on radiological imaging results, we studied in greater depth the cases in which the relationship of the tumor respect to the growth plate was doubtful. There were 170 such cases, of which a random selection of 38 were studied pathologically. This sub-sample was split into two groups according to whether or not it was considered appropriate to rule out a surgical approach of epiphyseal preservation after physeal distraction because the likelihood of physis invasion, as determined by the radiological evaluation, was too high.

Group I (n = 19):

Patients who received conservative surgery without physeal preservation. In 16 cases, the primary tumor was located in the distal *femur*, in two cases in the proximal *humerus* and in one case in the proximal *femur*. There were 12 girls and 7 boys. The mean age was 13 years, with a range between 9 and 17 years.

Group II (n = 19):

Patients who received conservative surgery with physeal and epiphyseal preservation after physeal distraction. In 13 cases the tumor was located in the *femur* and in 6 cases in the *tibia*. In all cases, on the basis of the above-mentioned imaging methods and prior to surgery, the epiphysis was deemed to be unaffected by the tumor. There were 4 girls and 15 boys. The mean age was 10.5 years (ranging from 4 to 15 years).

The specimens obtained by resection were studied macroscopically and microscopically. In all cases the histological stains applied were the H&E and Masson's trichrome. Multiple sections were taken from the metaphyseal area and, when included in the resection, from physeal and epiphyseal areas.

6.3 Results

Pathologically, the 38 osteosarcomas studied were of the following histological types: osteoblastic (31), chondroblastic (5), and fibroblastic (2). In all cases, as a result of the pre-operative chemotherapeutic treatment, the tumor tissue presented a highly altered histological picture at the time of resection. Most osteosarcomas showed a percentage of necrosis greater than 90 %. Only in cases in which osteosarcoma showed chondroblastic differentiation was the amount of tumoral necrosis lower. In some cases, there was only a dense mass of post-necrotic connective scar tissue within which histologically normal bone *trabeculae* could sometimes be seen (Fig. 6.1).

Physeal invasion was observed in 13 of the 38 resection specimens (34 %). Note that in all of these cases, on the basis of imaging the occurrence of physeal invasion had been considered to be uncertain. Of the 19 cases in Group I, 12 showed physeal invasion (63 %). There was one case (5 %) of physeal invasion in Group II. In the

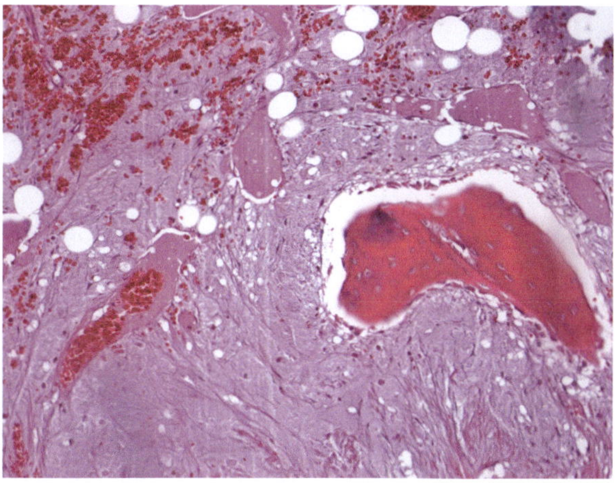

Fig. 6.1 A necrotic osteoblastic osteosarcoma post-chemotherapy can be observed in the border next to the physis (H&E, ×200)

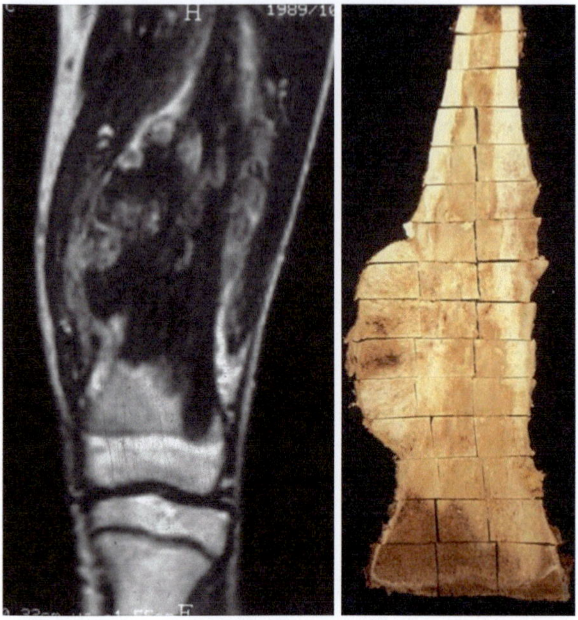

Fig. 6.2 *Left* MRI of an osteosarcoma that is apparently close to the physis. *Right* Macroscopically, an osteoblastic osteosarcoma that is destroying cortical bone and invading the medullar bone. The tumor is located several millimeters away from the growth plate

rest of the cases of Group I, tumors had a large contact area with the physis and had eroded it to some degree, but there was no demonstrable invasion. In Group II, most of the tumors were located at some distance from the physis; in two cases the tumors were close: at 3 mm and 5 mm from it; and in a further two cases the tumors were in contact with the growth plate, one of them with a large base of contact area but without invasion.

The average age at the time of tumor resection was 14.5 years for patients with epiphyseal involvement but 12.5 for patients without.

With regard to pathological findings, we observed the following three morphological growth patterns of tumor in relationship with the physis.

1. In 18 cases (47 %), between the tumor and the physis, there was a metaphyseal band of variable width (3–10 mm) within which there was no detectable neoplastic disease. Macroscopically, it was clear that the tumor was at a distance from the growth plate. In these cases, magnetic resonance images also indicated that the tumor was separate from the physis (Fig. 6.2). This disease-free metaphyseal zone had increased vascularization, which consisted of ectatic capillaries, and numerous osteoclastic cells flanking bone *trabeculae*, whose surfaces appeared undulate (Figs. 6.3 and 6.4). In these areas, there was often pronounced VEGF expression in both osteoblasts and osteoclasts (Fig. 6.5).
2. In eight cases (21 %) the tumor was in contact with the physis on the metaphyseal side. This contact without invasion was also suggested by MRI (Figs. 6.6 and 6.7). In the zone of contact, the physis appeared uniformly thinned, the hypertrophic and calcification zones having practically disappeared. To confirm non-invasion, a larger tissue sampling was obtained from these patients, but in no case was tumor observed in the epiphysis.

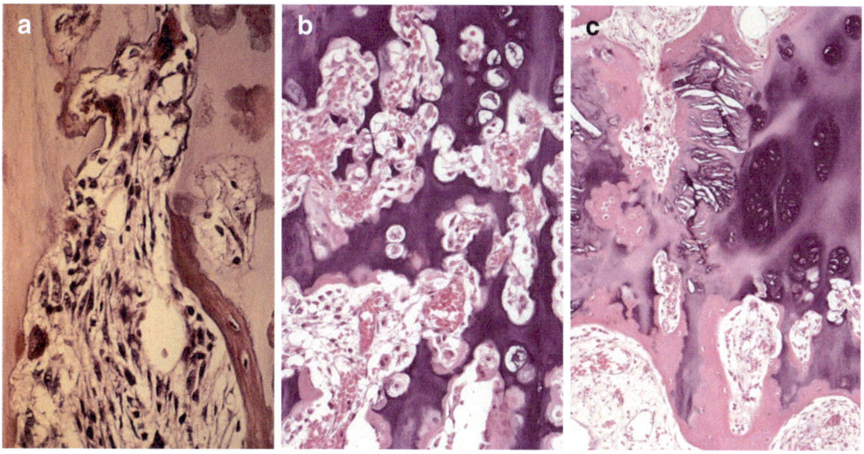

Fig. 6.3 (**a-c**) Osteoclastic activation accompanying fibrovascular proliferation in the femoral physis of a 10-year-old patient affected by osteosarcoma. The front edge of the tumor extends upwards to within 4 mm of the physis, which remains un-invaded (H&E, ×200)

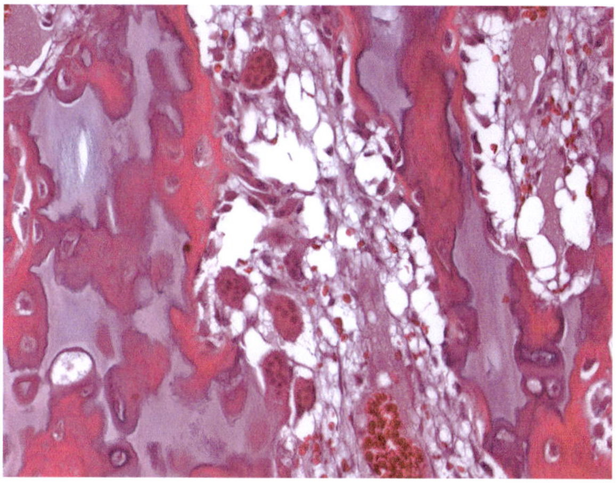

Fig. 6.4 A number of osteoclasts and osteoblasts are seen in the bone trabeculae in the growth plate. The osteoblasts have a hypertrophic aspect (H&E, ×200)

3. The third morphological picture was seen in the remaining 13 cases (32 %), where epiphyseal tumor invasion was observed. Macroscopically, the tumor was seen to be within the epiphysis, and this observation was corroborated by examination of the histological section (Fig. 6.8). Morphologically there were two patterns of physeal invasion. In the first pattern, epiphyseal areas were in close contact with the tumor but not completely invaded by it: tumor cells could be seen permeating the spaces between cartilaginous matrix columns next to dilated capillaries (Fig. 6.9). In the second pattern, in addition to the changes indicated above, there was perforation and thinning of the growth cartilage. The perforation was multi-focal, leaving dispersed islands of highly disorganized cartilage

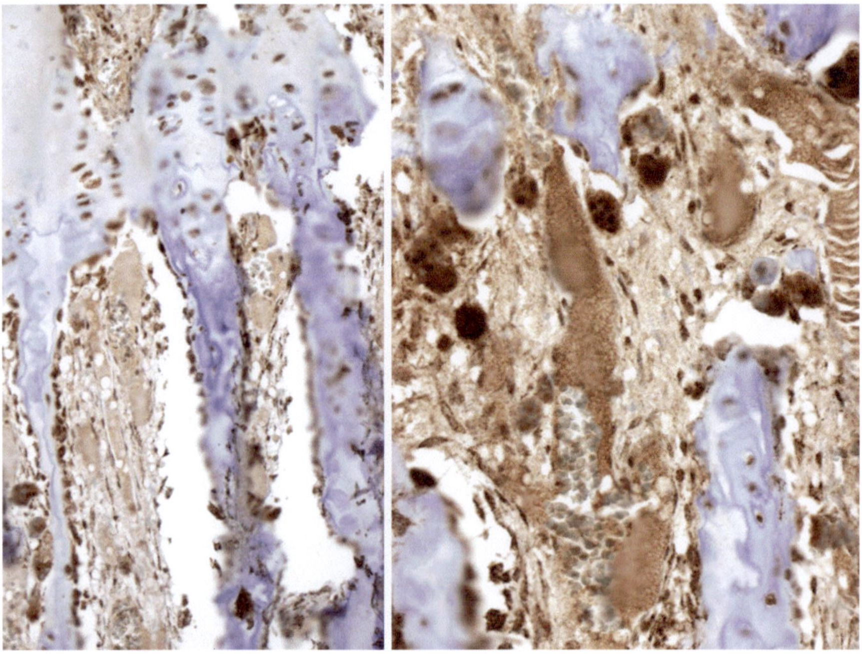

Fig. 6.5 A strong immunoreactivity against VEGF can be observed in the osteoclasts and osteoblasts in the physis. A high density of vessels can be distinguished (Immunohistochemistry, ×200)

within the tumor tissue (Fig. 6.10). In general, the extensions of tumor into the epiphysis appeared to have expanded evenly (Fig. 6.11). Some sections revealed paradoxical areas in which neoplastic tissue appeared on both sides of uncompromised growth cartilage; the apparent lack of connection can be explained by supposing that the plane of section did not cross the area of physeal involvement by the tumor (Fig. 6.12).

6.4 Discussion

Three types of behavior of an osteosarcoma in its relationship with the physis can be distinguished: tumoral contact with the physis, tumoral invasion of the physis, and tumoral trans-physeal invasion with involvement of the epiphysis. The clinical connotations of these growth patterns of remain to be determined, although it is probable that a large area of contact between a tumor and the growth plate is a risk factor for recurrence of tumor after physeal distraction. However, further studies are required to demonstrate that contact between tumor and physis is a contraindication for the technique of physeal distraction.

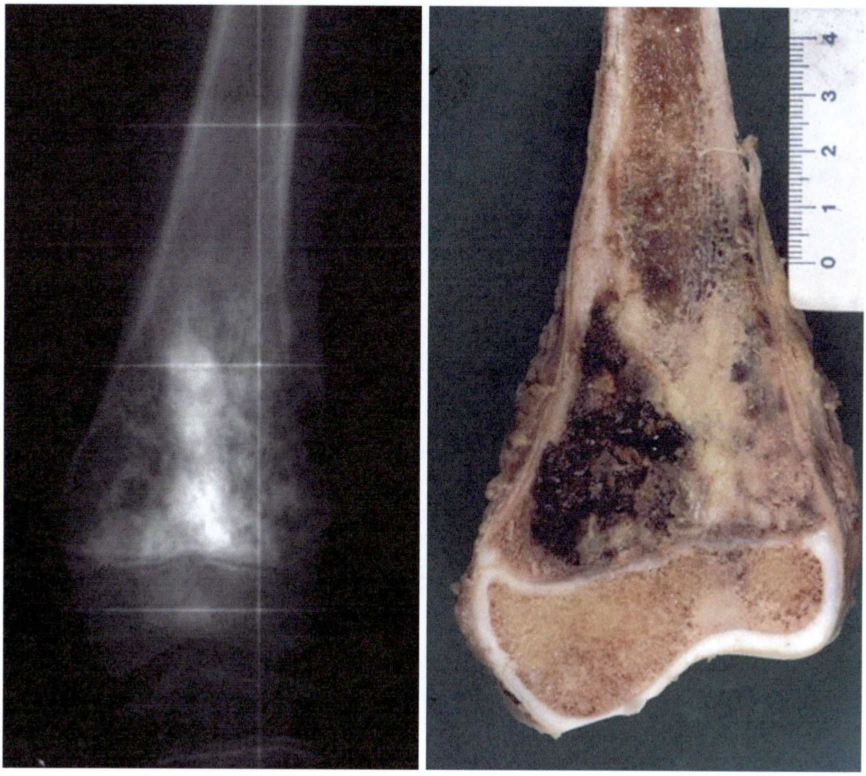

Fig 6.6 *Left* Radiography of a femoral osteosarcoma that shows that the tumor is in contact with the growth plate. *Right* An osteoblastic osteosarcoma in extensive contact with the physis; the histological study determined unequivocally that the tumor had not invaded the physis

The frequency of physeal invasion by the tumor in our series is lower than that in most series previously reported [9, 11, 17, 19]. Because physeal invasion by any metaphyseal osteosarcoma is likely to be a matter of time, differences in the frequency of physis invasion by osteosarcoma in different series can, in part, be explained by differences in the time elapsed between the diagnosis of patients and the evaluation of physeal invasion. In this respect, in our study we had the opportunity to evaluate consecutive MR images from several patients who did not receive any treatment for their tumor at or soon after the time of MRI (Fig. 6.13). These sequences of MR images show progressive osteosarcoma growth and, eventually, invasion of the physis. Conversely, an osteosarcoma's capacity for epiphyseal invasion was not found to have any clear relationship with its histological type.

From our results it can be concluded that it is valid to use radiological imaging as the basis for the decision on whether or not to undertake physeal distraction. In most cases in which conservative surgery was applied without physeal preservation, the resected material showed that the tumor had indeed invaded the physis or to be in extensive contact with it, and consequently the decision not to use physeal distraction

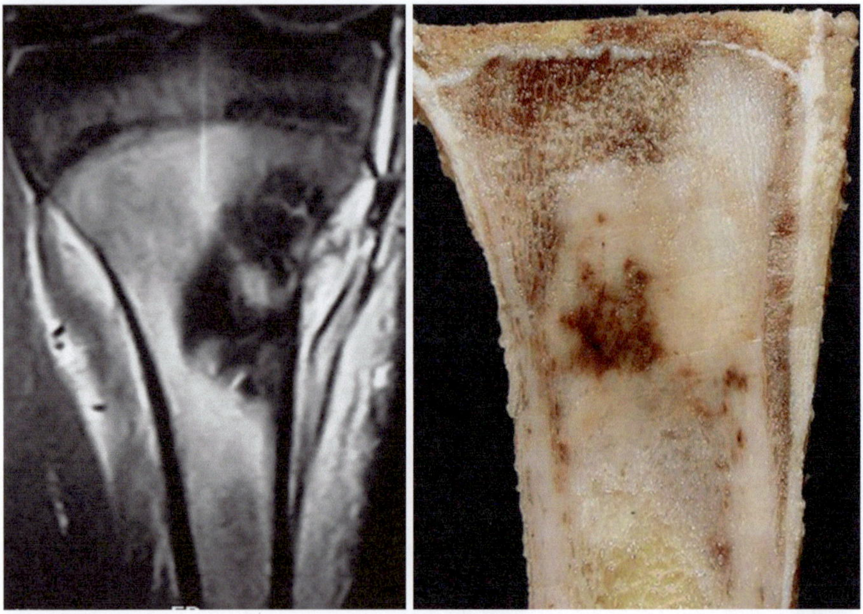

Fig. 6.7 *Left* In the MRI this tibial osteosarcoma seems to be in contact with the growth plate. *Right* However, macroscopically this osteoblastic osteosarcoma is found to be at a distance of 1 mm from the growth plate

was justified. There were, however, some case in which preservation of the physis was erroneously ruled out, while the physis was subsequently found not to have been transgressed by the tumor. From the clinical follow-up of all patients it was clear that only rarely did the tumor recur, and in the few cases when it did, it recurred in the diaphysis, not in the epiphysis. These data show that the radiological approach is valid for the decision on whether or not to carry out physeal distraction for a given patient.

The significant percentage of patients with epiphyseal invasion must surely raise doubts about the traditional notion of the physeal barrier. Two main theories have been proposed to explain how osteosarcoma, in its spread, is able to cross the physis [19]. According to the first, epiphyseal invasion takes place through the pre-existing trans-physeal vascular channels, which communicate the metaphysis with the epiphysis [9, 20]. However, Trueta and Morgan [21] and Brighton [3] observed that, from approximately 1.5–2 years of life until the age of skeletal maturity, the human epiphyseal and metaphyseal circulations are not connected in any way through the physis, which is hypertrophic. Most proliferating cartilage is practically avascular. The second theory is based on the possibility that the tumor induces an intense vascular response at its periphery, which favors its spread [8]. Our findings are concordant with such a mechanism. In fact, it has been demonstrated that osteoblasts [22] can synthesis VEGF, as we have observed in the physis next to the front edge of osteosarcoma. Vascular proliferation of the peritumoral stroma would favor tumor infiltration of the cellular columns of epiphyseal cartilage observed in our

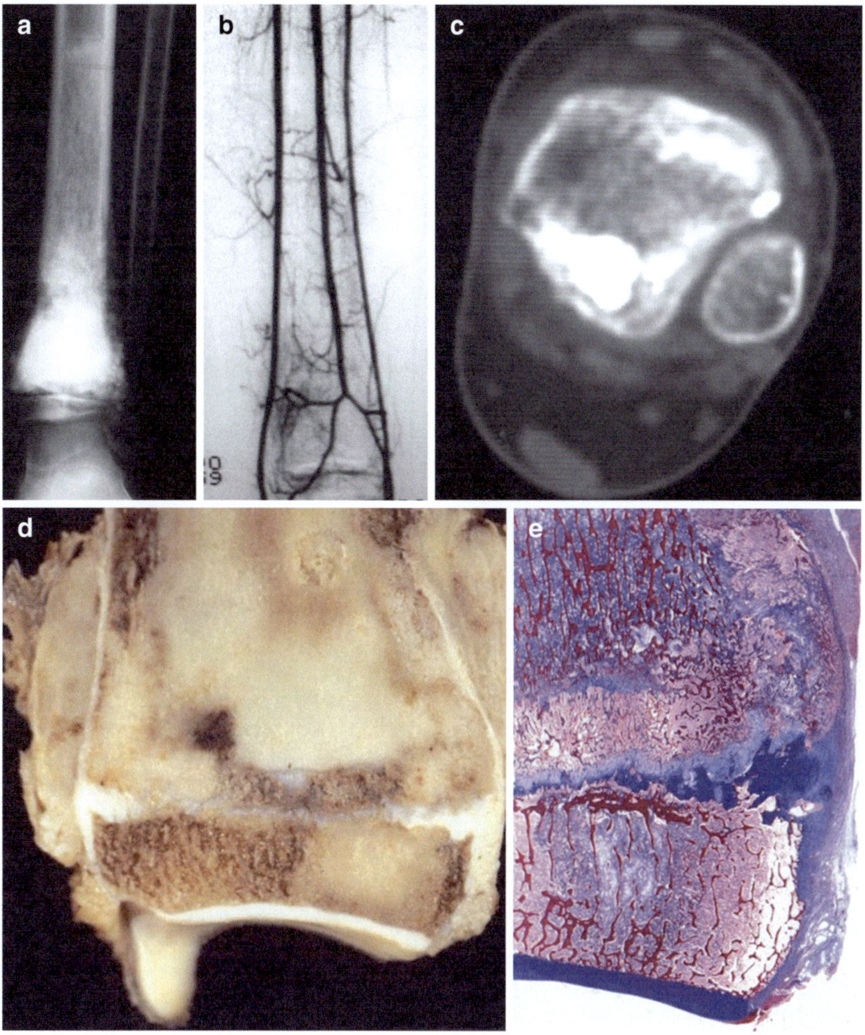

Fig. 6.8 (**a–c**) *Left* Osteosarcoma in the distal tibia. Angiography and CT scan showed invasion of the epiphysis. (Note that in the 1980s, MR imaging was not available). (**d**, **e**) This osteosarcoma is eroding the growth plate and invading the physis. In the histological cut stained with Masson trichrome, the osteoblastic osteosarcoma is clearly located in the epiphysis, but the location of physis invasion is not observed in this section

histological studies. The final effect of vascularization would depend on the balance between pro-angiogenic and antiangiogenic factors produced in the environment of osteosarcoma [12]. Several pro-angiogenic growth factors, such as FGF-2 and VEGF, produce their effect by linking to proteoglycans, such as heparan sulfate. Other molecules, such as syndecan or perlecan, regulate the vascular distribution [5, 12, 23]. As well as by vascularization, tumoral infiltration would also be

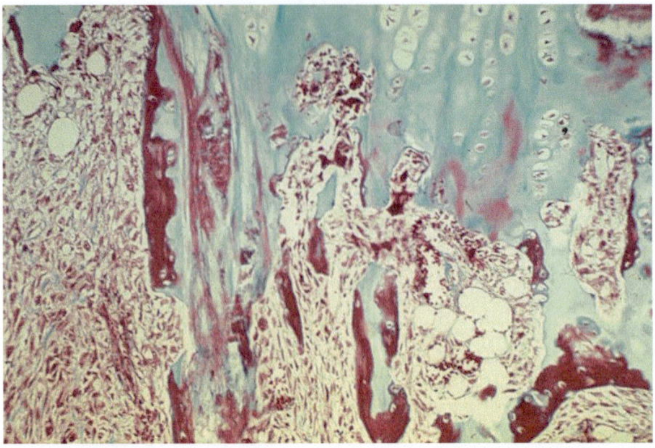

Fig. 6.9 Physeal invasion by an osteosarcoma in a 12-year-old boy. Tumor cells infiltrate as finger-like growths permeating the calcification and hypertrophic zones of the physeal cartilage (Masson's trichrome, ×40)

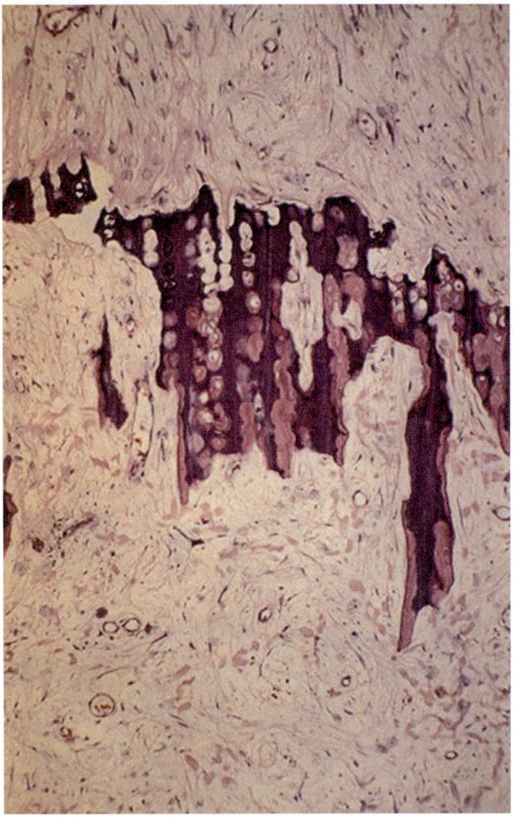

Fig. 6.10 The remains of physeal cartilage in the femur of an 8-year-old girl with metaphyseal osteoblastic osteosarcoma. The patient had received chemotherapy before resection of the tumor. Several islands of physeal cartilage can be seen surrounded by reparative tissue which occupies the whole thickness of the physis. This organization of tissue has substituted the necrotic tumor (H&E, ×100)

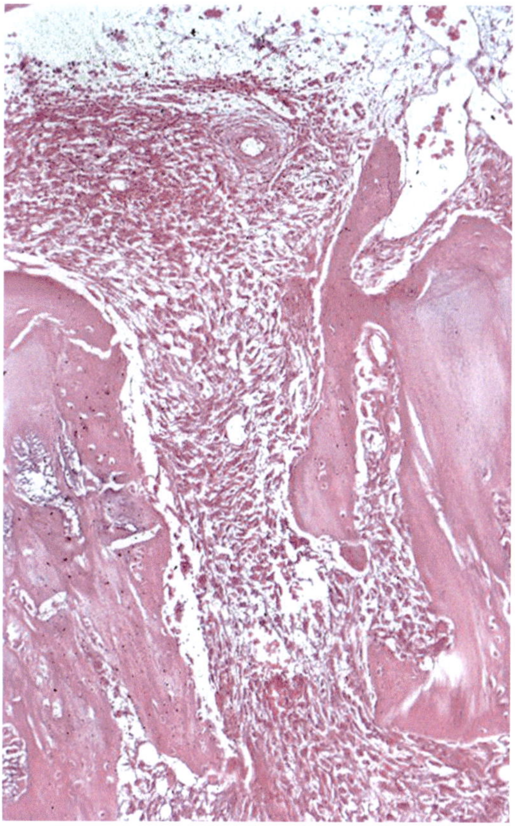

Fig. 6.11 Physeal tumor invasion in the form of finger-like projections in a 9-year-old girl with osteoblastic osteosarcoma. The periphery of the osteosarcoma was not necrotic despite pre-operative chemotherapy. This multi-focal type of growth is more difficult to detect radiologically (H&E, ×100)

enhanced by the osteoclastic reaction as a phenomenon that, hypothetically, could precede the progress of the tumor. This cellular reaction was seen in the free zone between the tumor and the physis. These findings have also been observed in a similar sequence of angiogenesis and osteoclastic activation in the growth plate [11].

Apart from via the trans-physeal route of epiphyseal invasion, another explanation of how the tumor gets into the epiphysis is to suppose that it can establish epiphyseal metastatic foci without alterations in the growth cartilage. This type of metastasis, so-called *skip metastasis*, has been observed to occur between various zones of a single bone [6] and even between adjacent bones of mature individuals without affecting the articular cartilage [16]. However, there was no evidence of such metastasis in our histological study.

Age is a factor which one might expect to influence trans-physeal spread of osteosarcoma. Physeal involution commences shortly before skeletal maturity and, as a result of this, at certain points, meta-physo-epiphyseal vascular communication is re-established. Theoretically, this factor would increase the possibility of an osteosarcoma invading the epiphysis.

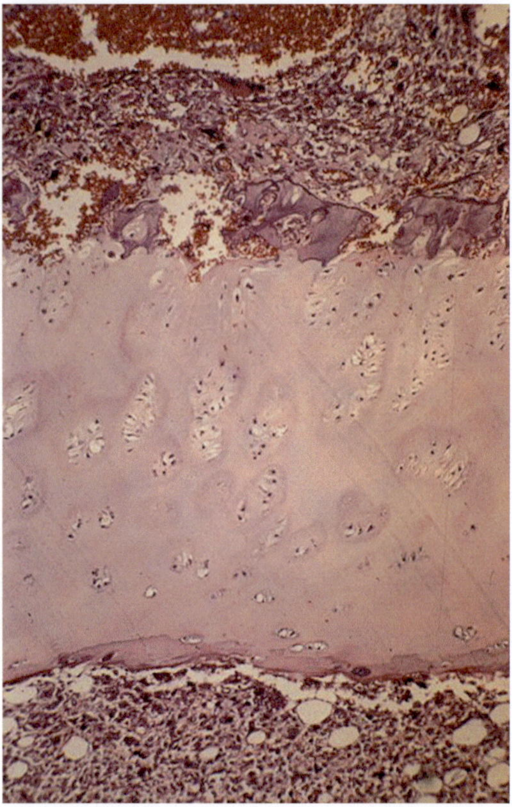

Fig. 6.12 A paradoxical pattern of metaphyseal-epiphyseal infiltration is shown in which there is apparent preservation of the physis, at least on the plane of this section. The case concerns a 15-year-old boy with osteosarcoma (H&E, ×100)

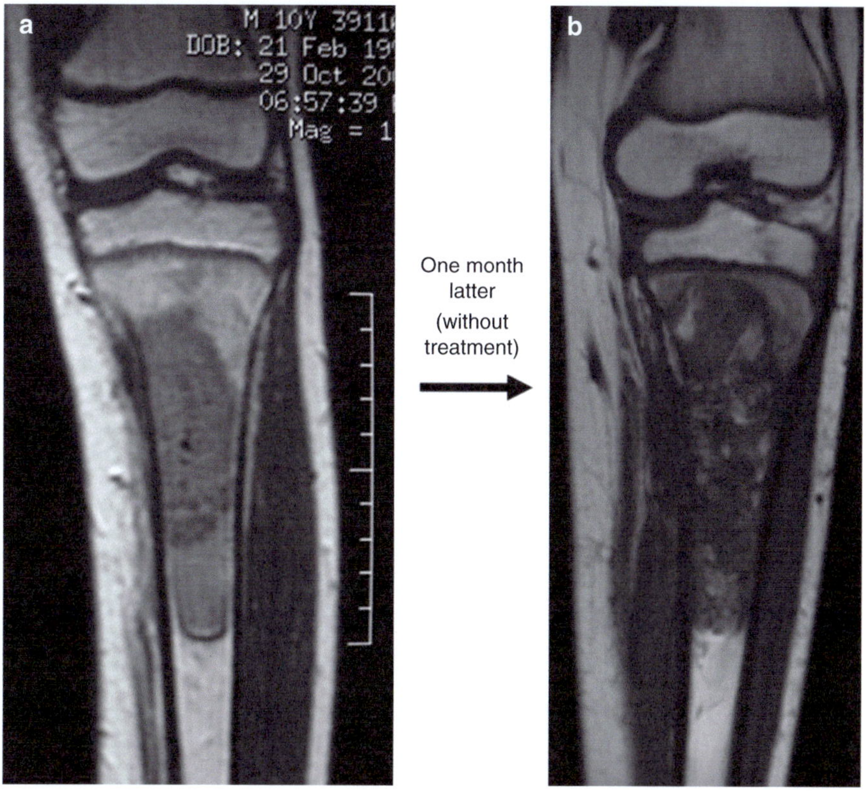

Fig. 6.13 (**a**) The initial MRI scan for this patient with a bone sarcoma was made at a hospital other than our own. Over a month later (**b**), he came to our center, and we took another MRI scan in order to be sure the epiphysis could still be saved. These two consecutive scans and other such sequential scans strongly suggest that invasion of the physis by an osteosarcoma is largely just a matter of time

References

1. Aegerter E, Kirkpatrick J. Orthopaedic diseases. In: Physiology, pathology. Filadelfia: WB Saunders; 1975. p. 519.
2. Brem H, Folkman J. Inhibition of tumour angiogenesis mediated by cartilage. J Exp Med. 1975;141:427.
3. Brighton CT. The growth plate. Orthop Clin North Am. 1984;15:571.
4. Castiella T. El disco fisario frente al osteosarcoma de localización metafisaria. Rev Ortop Traum. 1982;26:301.
5. Chen E, Hermanson S, Ekker SC. Syndecan-2 is essential for angiogenic sprouting during zebrafish development. Blood. 2004;103:1710–9.
6. Dahlin DC. Bone tumours: general aspects and data on 10,165 cases. Philadelphia: Lippincott Williams & Wilkis; 2009.
7. DeChiara TM, Efstratiadis A, Robertson EJ. A growth-deficiency phenotype in heterozygous mice carrying an insulin-like growth factor II gene disrupted by targeting. Nature. 1990;345: 78–80.

8. Ennekingg WF, Kagan A. Skip metastasis in osteosarcoma. Cancer. 1975;36:2192.
9. Ennekingg WF, Kagan A. Transepiphyseal extension of osteosarcoma: incidence, mechanism and implications. Cancer. 1978;41:1526.
10. Folkman J. Tumour angiogenesis: therapeutic implications. N Engl J Med. 1971;285:1182.
11. Ghandur-Mnaymneh L, Mnaymneh WA, Puls S. The incidence and mechanism of transphyseal spread of osteosarcoma of long bones. Clin Orthop Relat Res. 1983;177:210.
12. Iozzo RV, Sanderson RD. Proteoglycans in cancer biology, tumour microenvironment and angiogenesis. J Cell Mol Med. 2011;15:1013.
13. Kuettner KE, Pauli BU, Soble L. Morphological studies on the resistance of cartilage to invasion by osteosarcoma cell "in vitro" and "in vivo.". Cancer Res. 1978;38:277.
14. Kronenberg HM. Developmental regulation of the growth plate. Nature. 2003;423:332–6.
15. Langer R. Isolation of cartilage factor that inhibits tumour neovascularization. Science. 1976;193:70.
16. Missenarg GM. Confrontation anatomoclinique pré et postopératoire: á propos de 30 resections conservatrices pour sarcomes osteogènesis. Rev Chir Orthop. 1986;72:477.
17. Norton KI, Hermann G, Abdelwahab IF, Klein MJ, Granowetter LF, Rabinowitz JG. Epiphyseal involvement in osteosarcoma. Radiology. 1991;180:813–6.
18. Quan GM, Ojaimi J, Nadesapillai AP, Zhou H, Choong PF. Resistance of epiphyseal cartilage to invasion by osteosarcoma is likely to be due to expression of antiangiogenic factors. Pathobiology. 2002–2003;7:361.
19. Simon MA, Bos GD. Epiphyseal extension of metaphyseal osteosarcoma in skeletally immature individuals. J Bone Joint Surg. 1980;62:195.
20. Spira E, Farin I. The vascular supply to the epiphyseal plate under normal and pathological conditions. Acta Orthop Scand. 1967;38:1.
21. Trueta J, Morgan JD. The vascular contribution to osteogenesis. I studies by the injection method. J Bone Joint Surg. 1960;42-B:97.
22. Yamamoto N, Otsuka T, Kondo A, Matsushima-Nishiwaki R, Kuroyanagi G, Kozawa O, Tokuda H. Rac limits TGF-β-induced VEGF synthesis in osteoblasts. Mol Cell Endocrinol. 2015;405:35–41.
23. Zoeller JJ, Whitelock JM, Iozzo RV. Perlecan regulates developmental angiogenesis by modulating the VEGF-VEGFR2 axis. Matrix Biol. 2009;28:284.

Chapter 7
Growth Plate Involvement in Malignant Bone Tumors: Relationship Between Imaging Methods and Histological Findings

Jesús Dámaso Aquerreta, Mikel San-Julián, Alberto Benito, and José Cañadell†

Abstract MRI is a reliable imaging method for detecting physeal and epiphyseal involvement in metaphyseal malignant bone tumors. In our experience, we have had no false negatives.

Keywords Growth plate • Pediatric sarcomas • Physeal involvement • Imaging methods • Sarcoma staging

7.1 Introduction

In the late 1970s and early 1980s, several advances enabled surgeons to broaden the indications for limb salvage: better and more accurate diagnostic imaging techniques became available [2–5, 7–13, 15–17], techniques of bone reconstruction were improved, there was progress in methods for resection of pulmonary metastases, and above all, pre- and post- operative chemotherapy protocols became established. Limb preserving procedures require knowledge of the exact extension of the tumor, and so, in this chapter, we will consider the role of imaging methods and how accurately and specifically they determine the intraosseous extent of tumors. To this end, we carried out a study comparing several imaging methods that are employed in the evaluation of physeal involvement in primary malignant bone tumors.

---

† Author was deceased at the time of publication

J.D. Aquerreta, MD, PhD (✉) • A. Benito, MD, PhD
Department of Radiology, Clínica Universidad de Navarra, Pamplona, Navarra, Spain
e-mail: jdaquerret@unav.es

M. San-Julián, MD, PhD • J. Cañadell†, MD, PhD
Department of Orthopaedic Surgery, University of Navarra, Pamplona, Navarra, Spain

M. San-Julian (ed.), *Cañadell's Pediatric Bone Sarcomas: Epiphysiolysis before Excision*, DOI 10.1007/978-3-319-24220-0_7

7.2 Patients and Methods

We analyzed metaphyseal malignant bone tumors in children who were treated in our department between 1982 and 1995. Of the 65 tumors studied, 47 were osteosarcomas and 18 were Ewing's sarcomas. The mean age of the patients was 11 (3–16) years.

Standard radiographs were available for all patients. Computed tomography (CT) scans were available for 51 patients, digital angiography (Fig. 7.1) images for 48, and magnetic resonance imaging (MRI) T1- and T2-weighted sequences for 31. All methods were evaluated by the same radiologist.

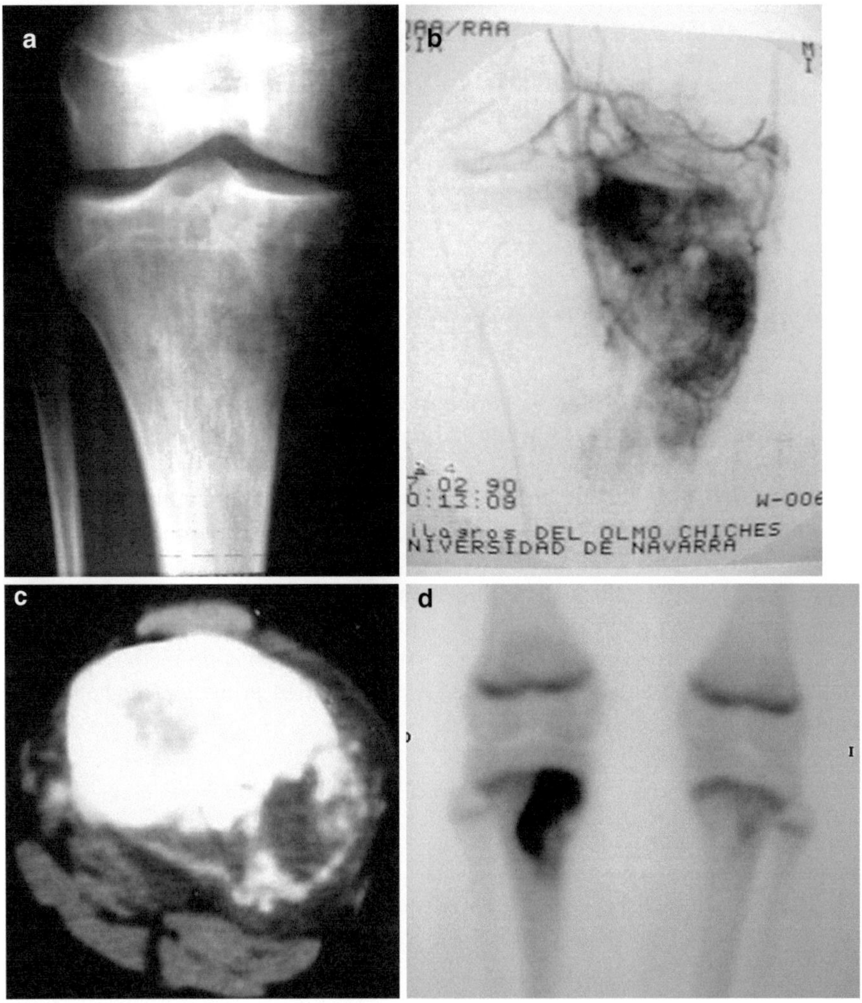

Fig. 7.1 X-ray (**a**), angiography (**b**), and CT (**c**) images used for assessing tumor involvement of the epiphysis. (**d**) A bone scan of a different case showing an epiphysis free of tumor

Careful histological examination of all the resected pieces was performed, especially of the metaphyseal margin in cases in which the epiphysis was preserved.

The proximity of the tumor to the growth plate was evaluated with as many of the different methods as possible. A tumor was considered to be at *distance zero* if it was in contact or had crossed the growth plate. On the basis of the histological findings, we studied the following statistical parameters of the four imaging methods: sensitivity, specificity, accuracy, and positive and negative predictive values.

7.3 Results

The physis was affected in 53 % of cases (Figs. 7.2 and 7.3). Table 7.1 presents the relationship between histological findings and the evaluation of growth plate involvement based on the different imaging methods.

The sensitivity with CT and MRI was 100 %, with X-ray and angiography, over 90 %. The specificity with MRI was 78.5 %.

Predictive value and accuracy data is given in Table 7.2. The positive predictive value (the probability of actual involvement of the growth plate given that with the imaging method it was *seen* to be involved) was more than 80 % for all the methods studied. The negative predictive value (the probability that the imaging method correctly indicated that the growth plate was not involved) was 100 % in CT and

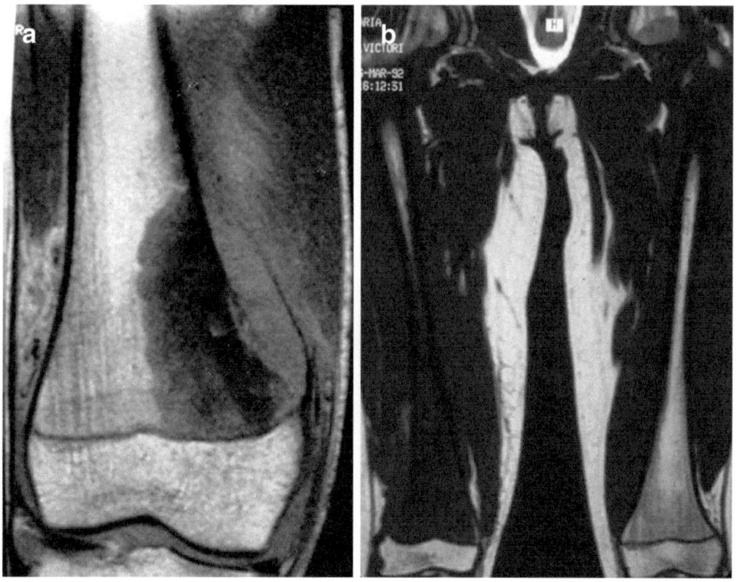

Fig. 7.2 MRI was the best imaging method for assessing tumoral involvement of the growth plate. T1 weighted images of patients with metaphyseal osteosarcoma showing extensive contact with the physis, but without epiphyseal involvement

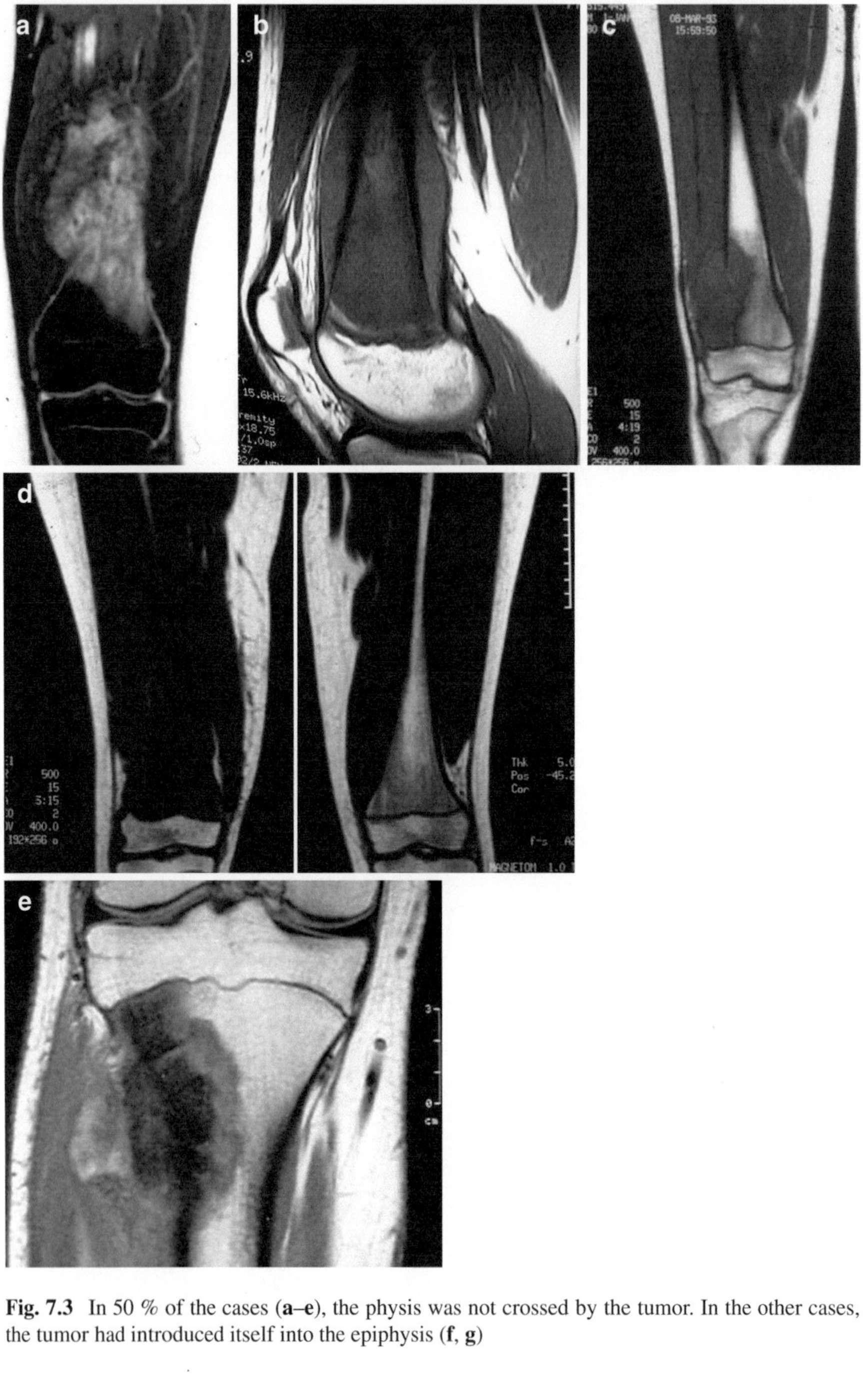

Fig. 7.3 In 50 % of the cases (**a–e**), the physis was not crossed by the tumor. In the other cases, the tumor had introduced itself into the epiphysis (**f**, **g**)

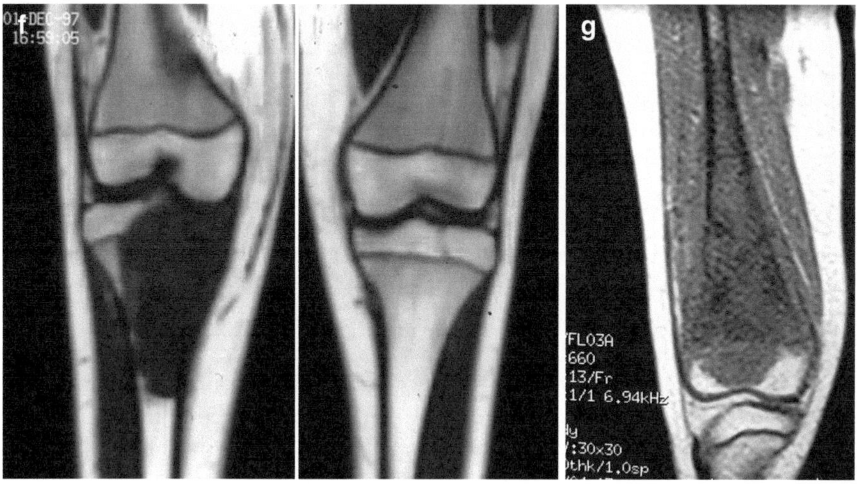

Fig. 7.3 (continued)

Table 7.1 Relationship between imaging and histological findings

No of cases studied with every imaging method	False (–)	False (+)	Total
X-ray (65)	1	6	7 (10.7 %)
CT (43)	0	6	6 (13.9 %)
Angiography (30)	1	3	4 (13.3 %)
MRI (31)	0	3	3 (9.6 %)

f cases studied with every imaging method False (–) False (+) Total

Table 7.2 Accuracy of the imaging methods

Imaging method	PPV	NPV	Accuracy
X-ray	82.7	94.7	87.5
CT	81.5	100	86.5
Angiography	85.1	80	84
MRI	87.1	100	90.3

MRI. The greatest accuracy (the average of the positive and negative predictive values) was obtained with MRI (90.3 %). With MRI, we found that it was possible to distinguish three types of lesion:

- The tumor was not in contact with the growth plate. In some cases, the radiologist could discern edema between the tumoral lesion and the growth plate, and this was an important feature in determining the surgical approach.
- The tumor was in contact with part or all of the growth plate. In some of these cases, it was possible to resect the tumor while preserving the epiphysis (*see* Chap. 9).
- The tumor transgressed the physis.

7.4 Discussion

Despite the general low specificity of X-rays, over a century of experience with X-ray imaging make it the primary and indispensable methodology for visualization of bone pathologies. CT can be regarded as a complementary technique to X-ray because it provides better imaging of complex zones such as pelvic bones. Currently, CT can provide high-quality multi-plane reconstructions. However, this requires acquisition of images with fine slices, which in turn requires higher radiation doses. Although CT enables detection of injury to the edge of the physis, it does not enable evaluation of physeal invasion as reliably as magnetic resonance imaging (MRI).

A technique not included in our study is scintigraphy, which, due to its very high sensitivity, is more generally used in cancer patients to determine whether or not there is multiple bone involvement. For the purpose of evaluating involvement of the growth plate, the low specificity of scintigraphy means it is not particularly useful: in most cases, both the lesion and the growth plate show increased up-take of the radiopharmaceutical (Fig. 7.1d).

Angiography shows the vascular supply to tumors and facilitates staging a tumor. Angiography is also helpful for evaluating the likely effectiveness of intra-arterial chemotherapy, which is useful in the treatment of bone tumors, above all in osteosarcoma.

Pre-operative chemotherapy, which initially confirmed the action in vivo of drugs on tumor tissue, can improve limb preservation. Angiography may also facilitate evaluation of whether or not a tumor has involved the epiphysis, since neovascularization can be observed in this area. With digital subtraction angiography, however, it is more difficult to distinguish bone structures, and thus this method is less useful for the purposes of evaluating growth plate involvement.

In our study, there were more false positive results than false negative ones. With CT and MRI, there were no false negatives. We conclude that, for our purposes, CT and MRI are safe and reliable diagnostic techniques [2–5, 7–13, 15–17], (Figs. 7.4 and 7.5).

Although diagnosis should never be based solely on MRI, it is the best available technique for staging a bone tumor because of its high sensitivity and the possibility of multi-planar imaging. MRI provides a clear delineation of tumor extension and shows the association between the tumor and the growth plate. We prefer the T1-weighted image in coronal sections because it enables the use of thin slides with which high contrast between fat and tumor signal intensity can be achieved. The accuracy of this technique in determining physeal involvement was better than that of the other techniques [11, 14] (Figs. 7.1, 7.2, and 7.3).

The application of contrast media does not improve the specificity and accuracy of the sequences without contrast to differentiate between tumor and edema [6].

PET is now a well-developed imaging technique of considerable importance in the study of tumors. PET enables assessment of the degree of metabolic activity of a tumoral lesion and can be used to determine the level of response to treatment (chemotherapy) based on the quantification of the SUV (standard uptake value).

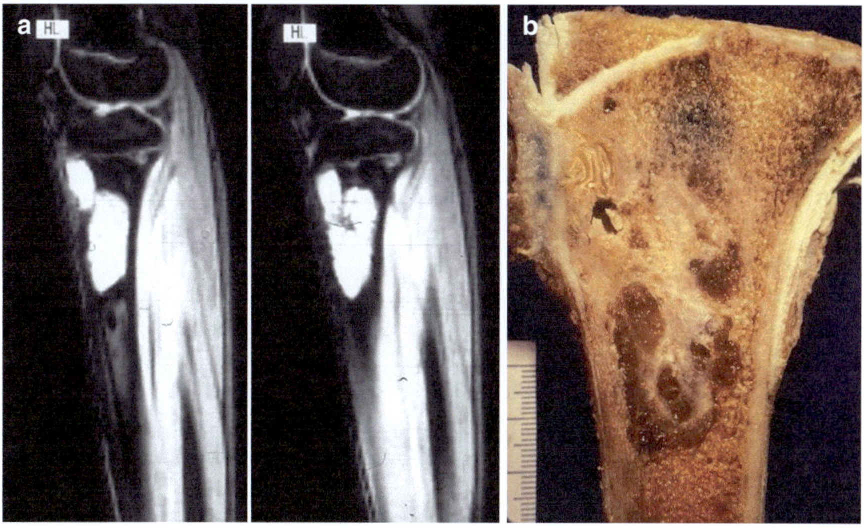

Fig. 7.4 (**a**) Sagittal T2-weighted images showing contact between the metaphyseal injury and physeal cartilage in the anterior region. (**b**) Sagittal section of the surgical specimen showing integrity of the physis

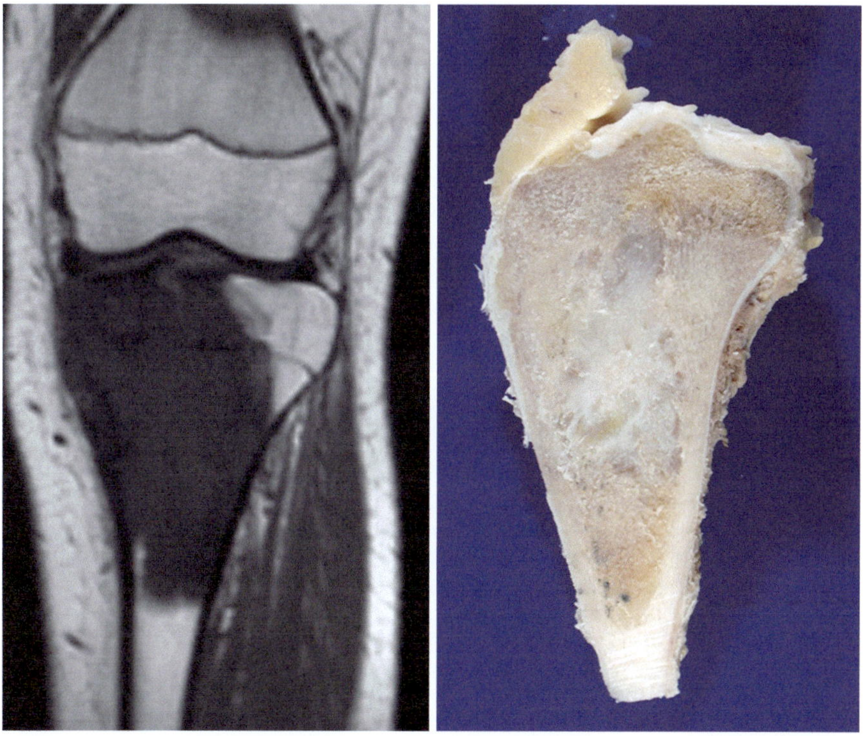

Fig. 7.5 An example of metaphyseal osteosarcoma extending across the growth plate

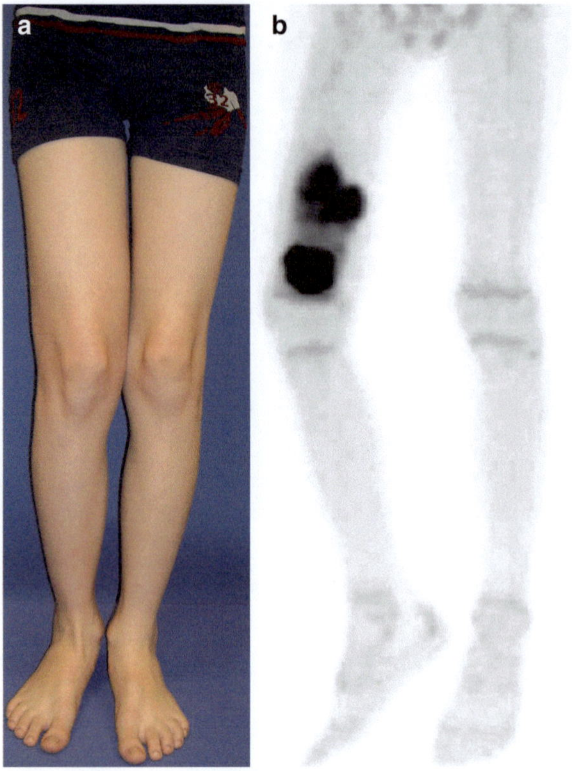

Fig. 7.6 Clinical aspect (**a**) and PET image (**b**) of a metaphyseal bone sarcoma that is not crossing the physis. The metabolism of FDG is increased in the metaphysis, but not in the epiphysis. Note the up-take in every growth plate

The spatial resolution of PET is not always sufficient to make it a reliable technique for assessing the involvement of physeal cartilage, although the involvement of the epiphysis and the presence of bone metastases can be determined [1] (Fig. 7.6).

References

1. Byun BH, Kong CB, Lim I, et al. Comparison of (18)F-FDG PET/CT and (99 m)Tc-MDP bone scintigraphy for detection of bone metastasis in osteosarcoma. Skeletal Radiol. 2013;42(12):1673–81.
2. Estes DN, Magill HL, Thompson EL, Hayes FA. Primary Ewing's sarcoma: follow up with Ga-67 scintigraphy. Radiology. 1990;177:449.
3. Exner GU, Von Hochstetter AR, Augustiny N, Von Schulthess G. Magnetic resonance imaging in malignant bone tumors. Int Orthop. 1990;14:49.
4. Frank JA, Ling A, Patronas NJ, et al. Detection of malignant bone tumors: MR imaging vs scintigraphy. AJR Am J Roentgenol. 1990;155:1043.
5. Golfieri R, Baddeley H, Pringle JS, Souhami R. The role of the STIR sequence in magnetic resonance imaging examination of bone tumors. Br J Radiol. 1990;63:251.
6. Hoffer FA, Nikanorov AY, Reddick WE, et al. Accuracy of MR imaging for detecting epiphyseal extension of osteosarcoma. Pediatr Radiol. 2000;30(5):289–98.
7. Hudson TM, Hamlin DS, Enneking WF, Peterson H. Magnetic resonance imaging of bone and soft tissue tumors. Skeletal Radiol. 1985;13:134.

8. Kattapuram SV. Imaging of musculoskeletal tumors. Curr Opin Orthop. 1991;2:781.
9. Knop J, Delling G, Heise U, Winkler K. Scintigraphic of tumor regression during preoperative chemotherapy of osteosarcoma: correlation of Tc-99m-methylene diphosphonate parametric imaging with surgical histopathology. Skeletal Radiol. 1990;19:165.
10. Lemmi MA, Fletcher RB, Marina NM, et al. Use of L MR imaging to assess results of chemotherapy for Ewing sarcoma. AJR Am J Roentgenol. 1990;155:343.
11. Muscolo DL, Ayerza MA, Aponte-tinao LA, Ranalletta M. Epiphyseal preservation and intercalary allograft reconstruction in osteosarcoma of the knee. J Bone Joint Surg. 2004;86-a(12): 2686–93.
12. O'Flanagan SJ, Stack JP, Mccee HM, Dervan P, Hurson B. Imaging of intramedullary tumor spread in osteosarcoma: a comparison of techniques. J Bone Joint Surg Am. 1991;73-A:998–1001.
13. San Julian M, Aquerreta JD, Benito A, Cañadell J. Indications for epiphyseal preservation in metaphyseal malignant bone tumors of children. Relationship between image methods and anatomopathological findings. Am J Pediatr Orthop. 1999;19:543–8.
14. Saifuddin A. The accuracy of imaging in the local staging of appendicular osteosarcoma. Skeletal Radiol. 2002;31:191–201.
15. Sundaram M, McLeod RA. MR imaging of tumor and tumor-like lesions of bone and soft tissue. AJR Am J Roentgenol. 1990;155:817.
16. Vander Griend RA, Eenneking WF. Radiologic imaging techniques in the diagnosis and treatment of osteogenic sarcoma. Semin Orthop. 1988;3:59.
17. Zimmer WD, Berquist TH, McLeod RA, et al. Bone tumors: magnetic resonance imaging versus computer tomography. Radiology. 1985;155:709.

Chapter 8
Consequences of Delayed Diagnosis

Blanca L. Vazquez-García, Mikel San-Julian, Ana Patiño-García, Luis Sierrasesúmaga, Antonie H.M. Taminiau, and P.D. Sander Dijkstra

Abstract Background: To determine for pediatric patients with high grade metaphyseal osteosarcoma whether there are any correlations between delay in diagnosis (time between appearance of symptoms and start of treatment), tumoral spread across physis and outcome.

Procedure: The clinical records, imaging methods and histology reports of 157 patients with high grade metaphyseal pediatric osteosarcoma of a long bone were reviewed. The mean follow-up time was 102 months. Location, histological subtype, time from initial symptoms to start of treatment, major diameter, percentage of necrosis, whether the physis was crossed by the tumor, and outcome (recurrence, metastasis and status) were collated and statistically analyzed with SPSS v15.0.

Results: Compared to the group of patients with unbreached physis, the group with tumors that had crossed the physis (58 % of patients) was older (13.4 vs 11.9 years; $p=0.05$), had longer diagnostic delay (4 vs 2 months; $p<0.0001$), had almost twice the incidence of metastasis at diagnosis (38 % vs 22 %, $p=0.043$) and had poorer outcome (overall survival 49 % vs 67 %). Statistical analysis demonstrated an age-independent correlation between diagnostic delay and tumoral spread across the physis ($p<0.0001$).

Conclusion: Breach of the physis by a metaphyseal pediatric osteosarcoma is a matter of time. Outcomes for patients with tumors that had crossed the physis were worse than for patients with tumors that had not. Diagnostic delay of over 2 months

B.L. Vazquez-García, MD (✉)
Department of Orthopaedic Surgery, Complejo Hospitalario de Navarra, Pamplona, Navarra, Spain
e-mail: blanca.vazquezgarcia82@gmail.com

M. San-Julian, MD, PhD
Department of Orthopaedic Surgery, University of Navarra, Pamplona, Navarra, Spain

A. Patiño-García, MD, PhD
Department of Pediatrics, University Clinic of Navarra, IdiSNA, Navarra Institute for Health Research, Pamplona, Navarra, Spain

L. Sierrasesúmaga, MD PhD
Department of Pediatrics, University Clinic of Navarra, Pamplona, Navarra, Spain

A.H.M. Taminiau, MD, PhD • P.D.S. Dijkstra, MD, PhD
Department of Orthopaedic Surgery, Leiden University Medical Center, Leiden, The Netherlands

M. San-Julian (ed.), *Cañadell's Pediatric Bone Sarcomas: Epiphysiolysis before Excision*, DOI 10.1007/978-3-319-24220-0_8

was associated with poor prognosis. We urge that a major effort be undertaken to facilitate early diagnosis of all patients who might be suffering from this lesion.

Keywords Delay diagnosis • Osteosarcoma • Physis

8.1 Introduction

Pediatric osteosarcoma usually arises on the metaphysis of long bones, the most common site being around the knee (in the distal femur or proximal tibia). The standard treatment includes wide surgery and chemotherapy. The type of surgery differs according to such considerations as the age, extension of the tumor, the involvement of the joint, and the need for growth plate removal [1].

Tumors arising on the metaphysis sometimes proceed to invade the epiphysis by crossing the growth plate, which can be regarded as representing a temporary and somewhat imperfect barrier to tumoral spread. According to previous studies [1–7] such breaching of the growth plate and spread into the epiphysis occurs in between 50 and 70 % of cases. The large difference in these percentages can be explained in several ways: by variation in aggressiveness of tumors, by the age of patients (the younger the patient the thicker the growth plate), or by delay in starting treatment (the longer the tumor is allowed to develop the greater its chances of breaching the temporary barrier that the growth plate implies). In this respect it would be useful to establish whether tumors that cross the physis are qualitatively different from those that do not. The question arises: are tumors that invade the epiphysis more aggressive? Alternatively, do the cases with invasive tumors tend to be the cases that were diagnosed later? The outcomes for patients with tumors confined to the metaphysis are better than those for patients with epiphyseal involvement, is this attributable to differences in tumor aggressiveness or to earlier diagnosis?

The diagnostic and staging process for an osteosarcoma case includes obtaining the clinical history, imaging (x-ray, CT, MRI, bone scan) and a biopsy study. In the centers at which the authors work, all diagnostic tests, can be performed within 1 or 2 days. In non-reference centers, however, the diagnostic process can take up to several months.

The aim of this study of pediatric patients with high grade metaphyseal osteosarcoma is to determine whether there are any correlations between delay in diagnosis, tumoral spread across the physis, and final outcome. We define delay in diagnosis as the interval between appearance of initial symptoms and the beginning of treatment.

8.2 Patients and Methods

We reviewed the clinical data by patient records, imaging methods and histology reports for the pediatric osteosarcoma patients treated at two large tumor reference centers in two different countries (referred to here as hospitals A and B) between 1980 and 2009. For inclusion, patients had to be of pediatric age (under 15 years old for girls and under 17 years old for boys), to have a diagnosis of classic high grade osteosarcoma with a metaphyseal location in a long bone, and to have been treated in standard manner, that is, with neoadjuvant chemotherapy, surgery and adjuvant chemotherapy. Patients with metastasis at diagnosis were included. Patients of adult age were excluded as were patients with tumors affecting flat bones, of low grade or located in the diaphysis. Data for location, histological subtype, time from initial symptoms to start of treatment, major diameter, percentage necrosis, whether the physis had been crossed by the tumor or not, and outcome (recurrence, metastases and status) were collated. Statistical analysis was by SPSS v15.0.

The study included 157 patients, with a mean follow-up of 102 months. The characteristics of these patients are given in Table 8.1.

8.3 Results

The tumor crossed the physis in 56 % (89/157) of patients. Comparison of patients in whom tumors crossed the physis and patients in whom tumors did not revealed statistically significant differences in age, time from initial symptoms to start of treatment, presence of metastases at diagnosis and outcome (Table 8.2).

Patients in whom tumors did not cross the physis were younger than those in whom the epiphysis was involved. The mean age at diagnosis was slightly lower in patients from hospital A (12.5 years vs 13.2 years), and the percentage of patients with tumors crossing the physis was correspondingly lower for hospital A than for hospital B (54 % compared to 61 %, respectively).

For the group of patients with epiphyseal involvement, the median time between initial symptoms and start of treatment was 4 months (range 1–16 months). For the group in which the physis was not crossed, the median diagnostic delay was 2 months (range 1–7 months). The difference is statistically significant ($p < 0.0001$).

In order to control for confounding factors, a regression analysis with age stratification was performed (Table 8.3 and Table 8.4). Regardless of the age at diagnosis, there was a statistically significant correlation ($p < 0.0001$) between delay in starting treatment and tumoral spread across the physis.

Clinical outcome in terms of survival, local recurrence and metastasis was impaired when the physis was crossed by the tumor ($p = 0.04$, 0.07 and 0.04, respectively). In the group of patients with tumors that crossed the physis, the number of cases with metastasis at diagnosis was almost twice that in the group with unbreached physis (42 % vs 22 %) (Table 8.2).

Metastasis at diagnosis was the prognostic factor ($p < 0.0001$) most indicative of poor survival (Figs. 8.1 and 8.2). Local recurrence was almost three times higher in patients with tumors that crossed the physis (14 % vs 5 %). Overall long-term survival in the group of patients with tumors that crossed the physis was almost 20 % worse than that in the group with unbreached physis.

Table 8.1 Clinical characteristics of the patients included in the study

	Osteosarcomas (n = 157)	
	No.	%
Age at diagnosis (years)		
Median	13.3	
Range	(0–44)	
Sex		
Female	68	43.3
Male	89	56.7
Location		
Proximal femur	9	5.7
Distal femur	79	50.3
Proximal tibia	39	24.8
Distal tibia	11	7
Proximal fibula	5	3.2
Proximal humerus	11	7
Distal humerus	2	1.3
Distal radio	1	0.6
Necrosis		
Good (>90 %)	59	37.6
Poor (<90 %)	86	54.8
Not available	12	7.6
Histologic subtype		
Osteoblastic	132	84.1
Chondroblastic	16	10.2
Fibroblastic	3	1.9
Telangiectasic	6	3.8
Metastasis at diagnosis		
No	105	66.9
Yes	52	33.1
Status		
Alive	101	64.3
Dead	48	30.6
Not available	8	5.1
Follow-up (months)		
Mean	102	
Median	69.5	
Range	(2.6–363.7)	

8.4 Discussion

We have studied the relationships between breach of the physis by metaphyseal pediatric osteosarcoma, delay in diagnosis and clinical outcome. Our main finding, that outcomes for patients with tumors that had crossed the physis were worse than for patients with tumors that had not, is, to the best of our knowledge, the first

Table 8.2 Differences between patients grouped according to whether the tumor crossed the physis or not. (Contingency tables)

	Physis crossed (%)	Physis not crossed (%)	
Number	89 (56 %)	68 (44 %)	
Mean age	13.4	11.9	p=0.05
Diagnostic delay[a]	4 months	2 months	p<0.0001
Metastasis at diagnosis	37 (42 %)	15 (22 %)	p=0.04
Local recurrence	12 (14 %)	3 (5 %)	p=0.07
Overall survival	44 (49 %)	46 (67 %)	p=0.04

[a]Mean time in months between initial symptoms and start of treatment

Table 8.3 Regression analysis with age stratification

	Diagnostic delay (months)	
	Crude mean (95 % CI)	Age-adjusted mean[a]
With physis-crossing	2.21 (1.90–2.53)	2.20 (1.58–2.82)
Without physis-crossing	4.05 (3.40–4.69)	4.06 (3.53–4.58)

Analysis of covariance (ANCOVA)
Model: the dependent variable is time; independent variables are physis-crossing (dichotomous) and age (continuous)
[a]Analysis of Covariance ANCOVA (equivalent to linear ordinary least-squares regression). p<0.0001

Table 8.4 Regression analysis with age stratification

Time	N	OR (95 % CI)	Age-adjusted OR* (95 % CI)
≤1	31	1 (ref)	1 (ref)
1.5–2	37	1.99 (0.71–5.53)	1.88 (0.67–5.29)
2.5–3	31	4.04 (1.38–11.86)	4.67 (1.54–14.14)
4–16	49	9.14 (3.13–26.69)	9.36 (3.16–27.7)

* Odds ratio (95 % CI) for physis-crossing according to time between initial symptoms and start of treatment

demonstration of the veracity of the supposition, based on experience with other pediatric cancers, that the earlier a pediatric osteosarcoma is diagnosed and treated, the better the oncological outcome.

The current study confirms the suggestion present in other published reports that invasion of the physis by a metaphyseal osteosarcoma is likely to be a matter of time [1, 3] osteosarcoma usually arises in the metaphysis of long bones, and the growth plate is thought to represent a temporary barrier to tumoral spread across the physis and into the epiphysisis. We found that for tumors that had crossed the physis, the mean time between initial symptoms and start of treatment was approximately twice the mean for tumors constrained in the metaphysis.

The physis can be regarded as representing a temporary barrier to tumoral spread from metaphysis to epiphysis. Because the thickness of the physis decreases with age, it is reasonable to hypothesize that breaching of the physis by a metaphyseal

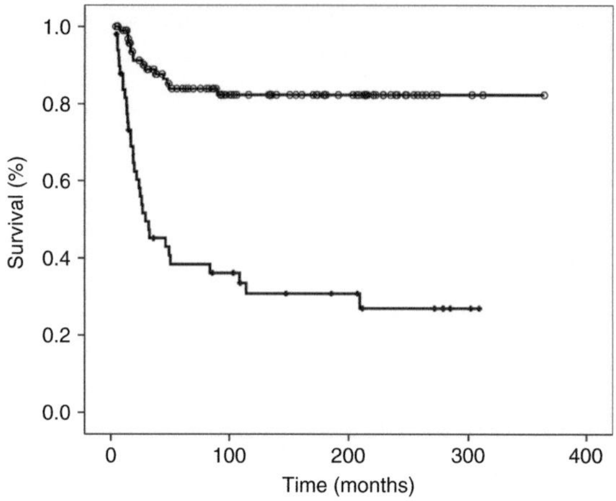

Fig. 8.1 Kaplan-Meier survival plot comparing patients in whom the tumor crossed the physis with patients in whom the tumor did not. The graph includes patients who were metastatic at diagnosis

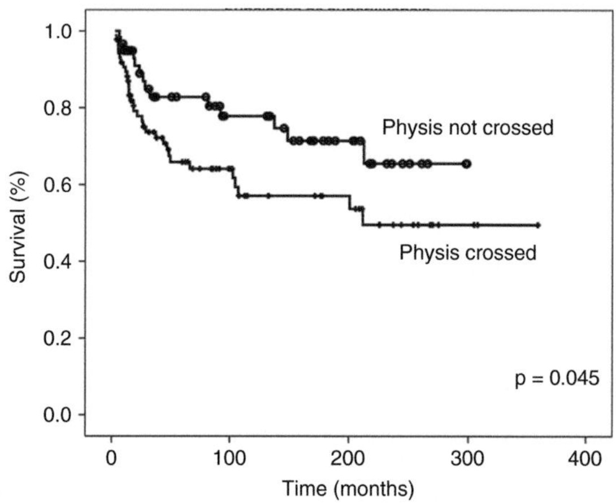

Fig. 8.2 Kaplan-Meier survival plot comparing patients with metastasis at diagnosis and those without ($p<0.0001$)

osteosarcoma may depend to some degree on a patient's age. One would expect that the younger the patient, the better the barrier to epiphyseal invasion posed by the physis. In view of the fact that diagnostic delay increases correspondingly a patient's age, could this putative age effect confound our results? After taking into account patient age by applying regression analysis with age stratification to our data, we found that patients in whom the tumor had crossed the physis were still associated with significantly longer diagnostic delay than patients in whom the tumor remained constrained in the metaphysis.

Patients with tumor crossing the physis had worse outcomes than those with a tumor that had not crossed the physis: the percentages with metastases at diagnosis and with local recurrence were higher, and overall survival was impaired (49 % vs 67 %).

From the point of view of surgical technique, surgery is simpler when the epiphysis is free of tumor. There is no need for joint resection, reconstruction is simpler, and clinical results are usually better in terms of function [7–9]. Preserving the joint and, when possible, the potential for growth is the best way to avoid further complications and further surgery, especially in young children.

In children, tumor breaching of the physis is not only bad news in terms of post-treatment joint function, it is also a strong indicator of poor prognosis. As demonstrated by this study, whether a tumor breaches the physis depends on the speed with which treatment is started. It is of paramount importance to minimize the time interval between appearance of symptoms and start of treatment, because the consequences of a diagnostic delay of 2 months are, quite frankly, terrible.

It may not be possible to change the behavior and other characteristics of a tumor, but we can improve time intervals of the diagnostic procedures and avoid delays. The use of screening protocols in oncological centers is mandatory. In addition, we suggest implementation of educational measures so that general physicians and general orthopedic surgeons become the sufficiently aware of this pathology to send possible patients immediately to reference centers. This will improve prognosis and functional outcome in pediatric osteosarcoma.

8.5 Conclusion

Breaching of the physis by a metaphyseal pediatric osteosarcoma is a matter of time. Outcomes with tumors that have crossed the physis are worse than outcomes with tumors that have not. Regardless of age, a delay of 2 months between the appearance of symptoms and the start of treatment worsens the clinical outcome drastically. For this reason, we urge implementation of measures to guarantee early diagnosis of all patients who might be suffering from metaphyseal pediatric osteosarcoma.

References

1. Cañadell J, San-Julian M, editors. Pediatric bone sarcomas: epiphysiolysis before excision. Heidelberg/London/NewYork: Springer; 2009.
2. Cañadell J, San-Julian M. Growth plate involvement by malignant bone tumours. Seminar book of the meeting Update in Malignant bone tumors in children and adolescents. CL meeting Mapfre-EPOS-POSNA (European Pediatric Orthopaedic Society and Pediatric Orthopaedic Society of North America), Madrid; 1997.
3. De-Pablos J, Idoate M, Gil J, Vázquez J, Cañadell J. Estudio clínico sobre el efecto barrera de las fisis ante el osteosarcoma metafisario. Rev Ortop Traum. 1990; 34IB(5):472–81.
4. Enneking WF, Kagan 2nd A. Transepiphyseal extension of osteosarcoma: incidence, mechanism, and implications. Cancer. 1978;41(4):1526–37.
5. Panuel M, Gentet JC, Scheiner C, Jouve JL, Bollini G, Petit P, Bourliere-Najean B, Devred P. Physeal and epiphyseal extent of primary malignant bone tumors in childhood. Correlation of preoperative MRI and the pathologic examination. Pediatr Radiol. 1993;23:421–4.
6. Spina V, Torricelli P, Montanari N, Manfrini M, Picci P, Sangiorgi L, Romagnoli R. The epiphyseal involvement of metaphyseal bone sarcomas in patients with fertile growth plates. A magnetic resonance assessment. Radiol Med. 1994;88(3):190–7.

7. Muscolo DL, Ayerza MA, Aponte-Tinao LA, Ranalletta M. Partial epiphyseal preservation and intercalary allograft reconstruction in high-grade metaphyseal osteosarcoma of the knee. J Bone Joint Surg Am. 2005;87 Suppl 1(Pt 2):226–36.
8. San-Julian M, Aquerreta JD, Benito A, Cañadell J. Indications for epiphyseal preservation in metaphyseal malignant bone tumors of children. Relationship between image methods and anatomopathological findings. Am J Pediatr Orthop. 1999;19:543–8.
9. San-Julian M, Dölz R, Garcia-Barrecheguren E, Noain E, Sierrasesúmaga L, Cañadell J. Limb salvage in bone sarcomas in patients younger than age 10. A 20-year experience. J Pediatr Orthop. 2003;23(6):753–62.

Chapter 9
Imaging-Based Indications for Resection with Epiphyseal Preservation

Mikel San-Julian and José Cañadell†

Abstract The findings of imaging methods can be used to select cases in which we can try to preserve the epiphysis during tumor resection. In the 1980s, we were more cautious; with time and experience we have enlarged the indications for the technique.

Keywords Epiphyseal distraction • Limb salvage • Bone sarcomas • Growth plate • Epiphysis preservation • Indications • Imaging methods

9.1 Introduction

On the basis of the findings of the various imaging methods considered in Chap. 7, we can identify cases in which the tumor does not involve the epiphysis and in these cases adopt an approach to tumor resection which attempts to preserve the epiphysis. Such an approach involves a carefully coordinated chemotherapy program before resection, with the aim of minimizing the risk of local recurrence.

We carried out a study comparing several imaging methods that are employed in the evaluation of physeal involvement in primary malignant bone tumors. By correlating our findings with the histological features of each case, we were able to establish indications for our technique of epiphyseal preservation through physeal distraction (epiphysiolysis) before excision of metaphyseal bone tumors in children [1].

In our imaging study (Chap. 7), there were more false positive than false negative results; in the CT and MRI studies, there were no false negatives which confirms that MRI and CT scan are safe and reliable diagnostic techniques that allow us to

† Author was deceased at the time of publication

M. San-Julian, MD, PhD (✉) • J. Cañadell†, MD, PhD
Department of Orthopaedic Surgery, University of Navarra, Pamplona, Navarra, Spain
e-mail: msjulian@unav.es

M. San-Julian (ed.), *Cañadell's Pediatric Bone Sarcomas: Epiphysiolysis before Excision*, DOI 10.1007/978-3-319-24220-0_9

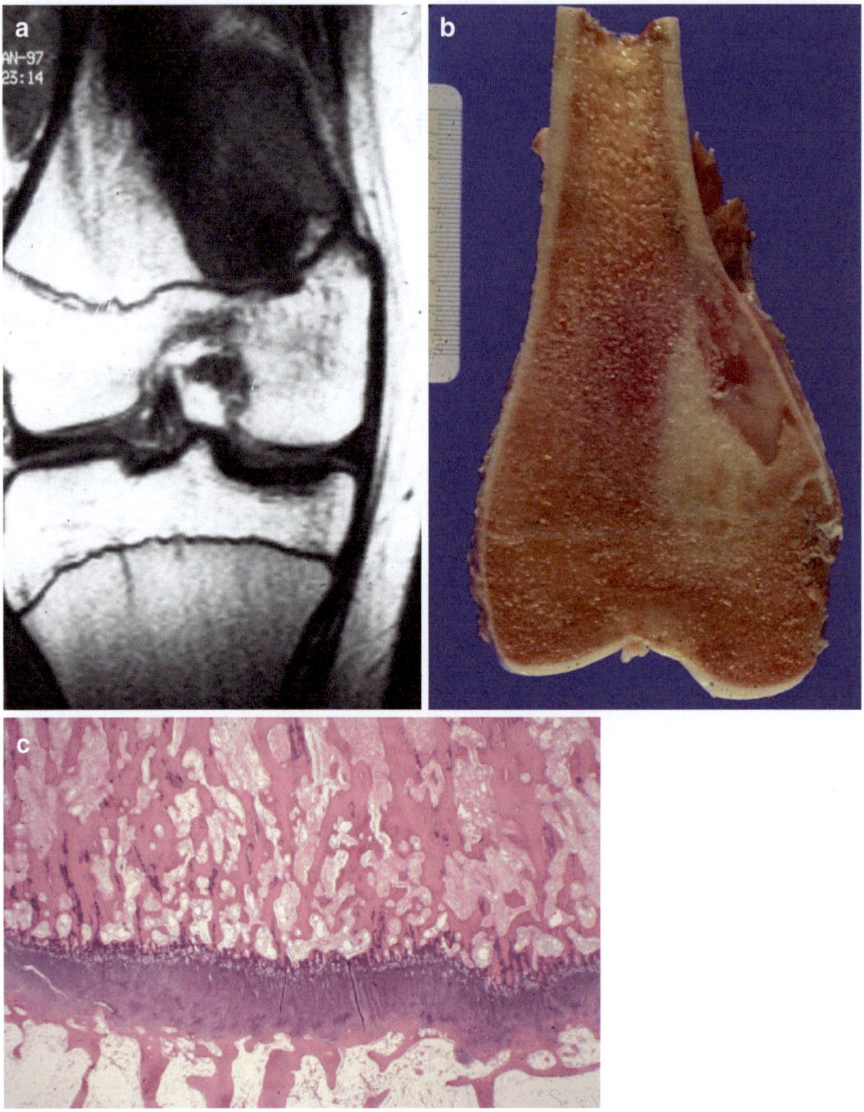

Fig. 9.1 (**a**) Osteosarcoma in the distal metaphysis of the femur of a 15-year-old boy. The tumor seems to have crossed the physis in the MRI image. (**b**, **c**) However, the histological study found no tumor cells in the physis

predict the location and extent of a tumor and, where oncologically appropriate, reduce the amount of bone resected [3–14]. The problem of false positives with CT and MRI (Fig. 9.1), however, could lead us to a sub-optimal treatment of certain tumors in terms of limb function preservation.

9.2 Stages of Invasion of the Epiphysis

Several years ago, in our department, we carried out a retrospective histological study of a series of malignant bone tumors in children [2] (*see* Chap. 6). The proportion of cases in which the tumor infringed the physis, about 50 %, was similar to that found with our subsequent study of imaging methods (*see* Chap. 7). In the histological study, we found that morphological lesions at the physis could be categorized into three types:

- The growth plate was not in contact with tumoral tissue.
- Areas of the growth plate were in contact with tumor tissue but were not penetrated by the tumor. Voluminous capillary sinusoids had introduced themselves between the columns of the matrix of the cartilage. The remainder of the physis appeared to be free of alterations.
- The physis was clearly invaded by the tumor. The areas crossed by tumor were surrounded by zones of thinned cartilage, similar to what was observed in the second type of lesion.

The implication of these observations is that invasion of the epiphysis by the tumor progresses in a predictable manner: first there is a hypervascularization reaction which leads to an early ossification of the growth plate, and after that the tumor crosses the physis.

9.3 Surgical Treatments

The surgical treatment we recommend for these tumors depends on the stage of invasion of the epiphysis as revealed by MRI. The three possibilities are presented below.

1. *The tumor has crossed the physis.*
   In such cases, preservation of the epiphysis is not possible (Fig. 9.2).
2. *The tumor is in contact with the physis.*
   There are three scenarios:

   - If all of the physis is affected (Fig. 9.3), the probability that tumor cells have crossed over the physis is high (*see* Chap. 5). However, most Ewing sarcomas and many osteosarcomas respond well to neoadjuvant chemotherapy, and if this response is particularly strong, preservation of the epiphysis should not be ruled out.
   - If the tumor is only in contact with part of the growth plate, tumor cells are less likely to have crossed over the physis and consequently we can try to preserve the epiphysis. After resection, external fixation can be maintained until intraoperative histological studies determine whether tumor cells are present in the physeal margin of the resection (Fig. 9.4). Then, on the basis of

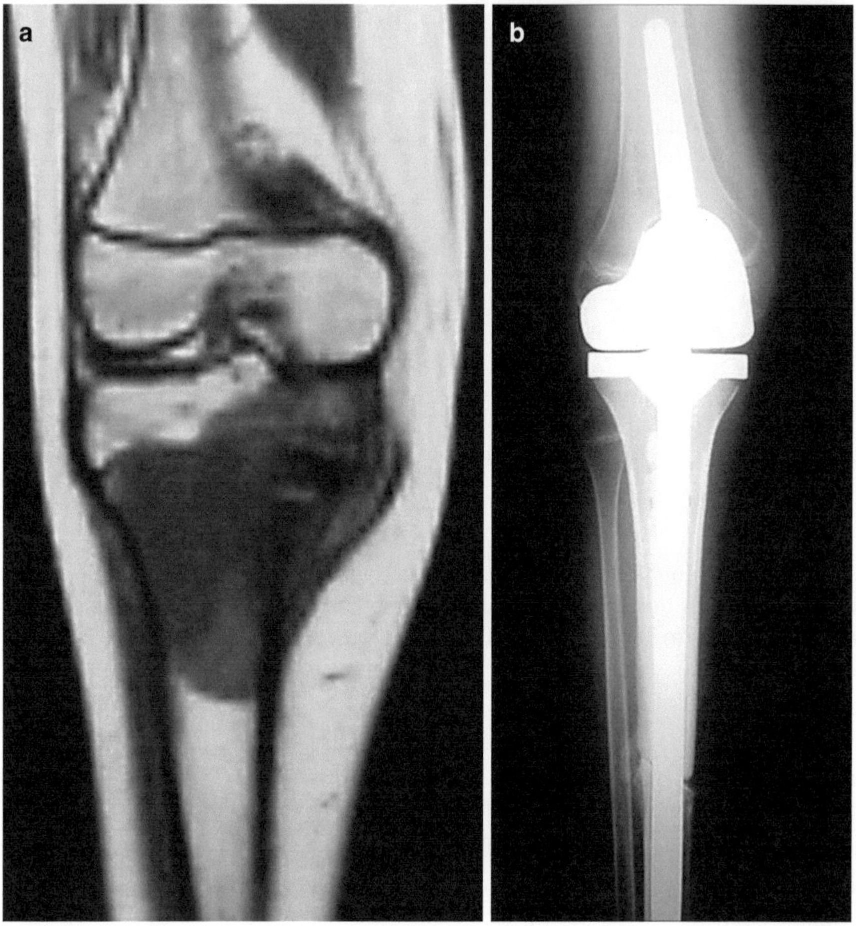

Fig. 9.2 (**a**) The growth plate has been crossed by this osteosarcoma in the proximal metaphysis of the tibia. (**b**) Reconstruction with a composite allograft-prosthesis

the histology, the appropriate manner in which to complete the surgical treatment (*see* Chap. 10) can decided. Before the advent of MRI, due to the lower accuracy of the other imaging methods employed, we used this methodology more frequently.

- An alternative method for preserving the epiphysis in cases when a tumor is in contact with only a part of the physis but does not cross it is intra-epiphyseal osteotomy, which may be useful especially in certain cases in children who are nearing the end of growth.

3. *The tumor is near to but not in contact with the physis.*
Physeal distraction before excision is, in our experience, the best technique in such cases (Fig. 9.5). The safety of physeal distraction and the fact that it can preserve the whole epiphysis and most of the growth plate make it superior to other techniques such as epiphyseal osteotomy.

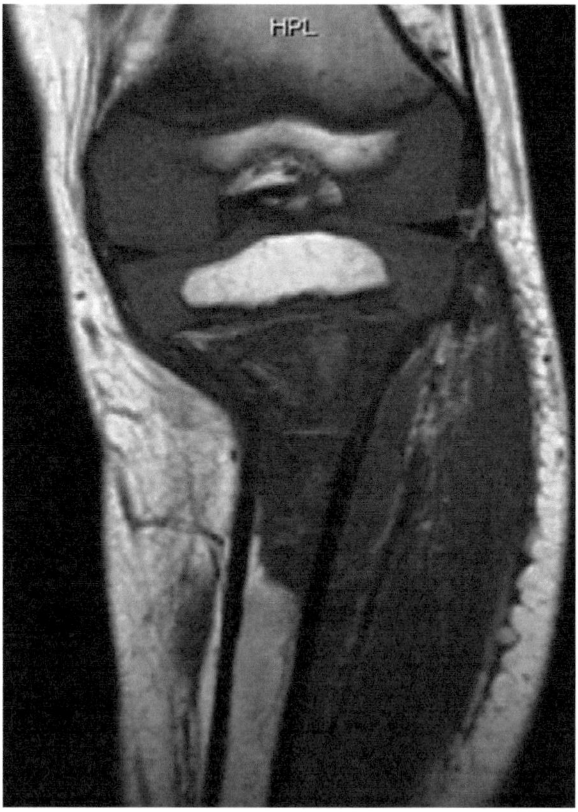

Fig. 9.3 Osteosarcoma in contact with the whole of the physis

9.4 Other Considerations

The fact that there are no anastomoses between epiphyseal and metaphyseal vessels, the possibility of using imaging methods to determine whether or not the tumor has involved the epiphysis, and the Cañadell technique for resection through physeal distraction [1, 11] together make it feasible, in selected cases, to preserve the epiphysis and the joint during tumor resection.

Physeal distraction is used in tumors of the distal femur, proximal tibia, proximal humerus, distal radius, distal tibia, and distal fibula. In locations such as the proximal fibula or proximal femur, physeal distraction is not used for obvious reasons (Fig. 9.6). In tumors involving the proximal metaphysis of the humerus, the particular morphology of the growth plate makes it possible to employ physeal distraction (Fig. 9.7).

The presence of a pathological fracture (Fig. 9.8) contraindicates physeal distraction because the distraction will occur through the fracture instead of through the growth plate. In such cases, intra-epiphyseal osteotomy could be used to conserve the epiphysis. However, if a fracture heals during the period of neo-adjuvant chemotherapy, it is still possible to perform physeal distraction (Fig. 9.9).

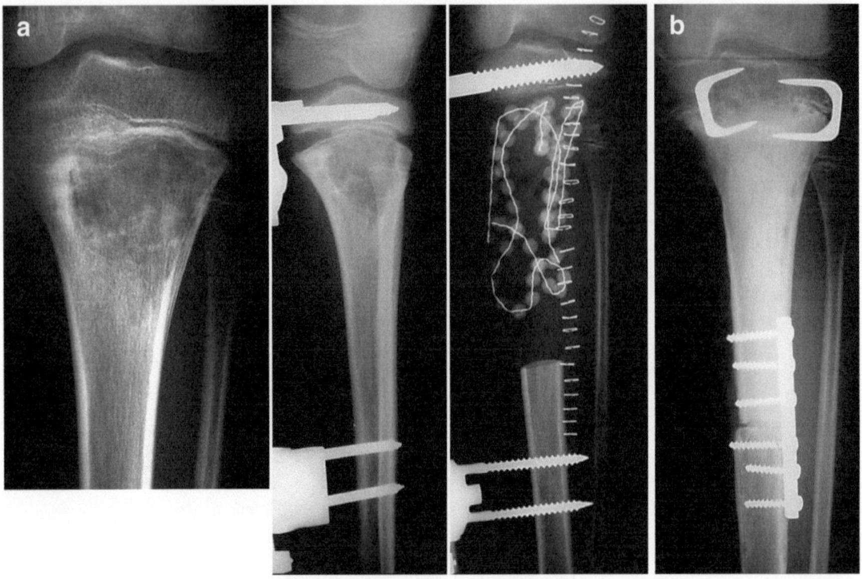

Fig. 9.4 Physeal distraction according to Cañadell's technique in a case in which involvement of the physis was uncertain, before the MRI era. (**a**) External fixation was kept in place after resection until histological study of the resection margins had been carried out. (**b**) After histological confirmation of the absence of tumor cells in the metaphyseal margin of the resection, the reconstruction was carried out with an intercalary allograft

Finally, note that physeal distraction serves no purpose in cases of diaphyseal tumors with a safe margin between the tumor and the physis [5] (Fig. 9.10).

Figure 9.11 provides a summary of the MRI-based indications and contraindications for tumor resection with physeal distraction in order to preserve the epiphysis. Of the patients we have operated on in accordance with the prescriptions of the Cañadell technique, none have suffered a local recurrence of the tumor in the retained epiphysis.

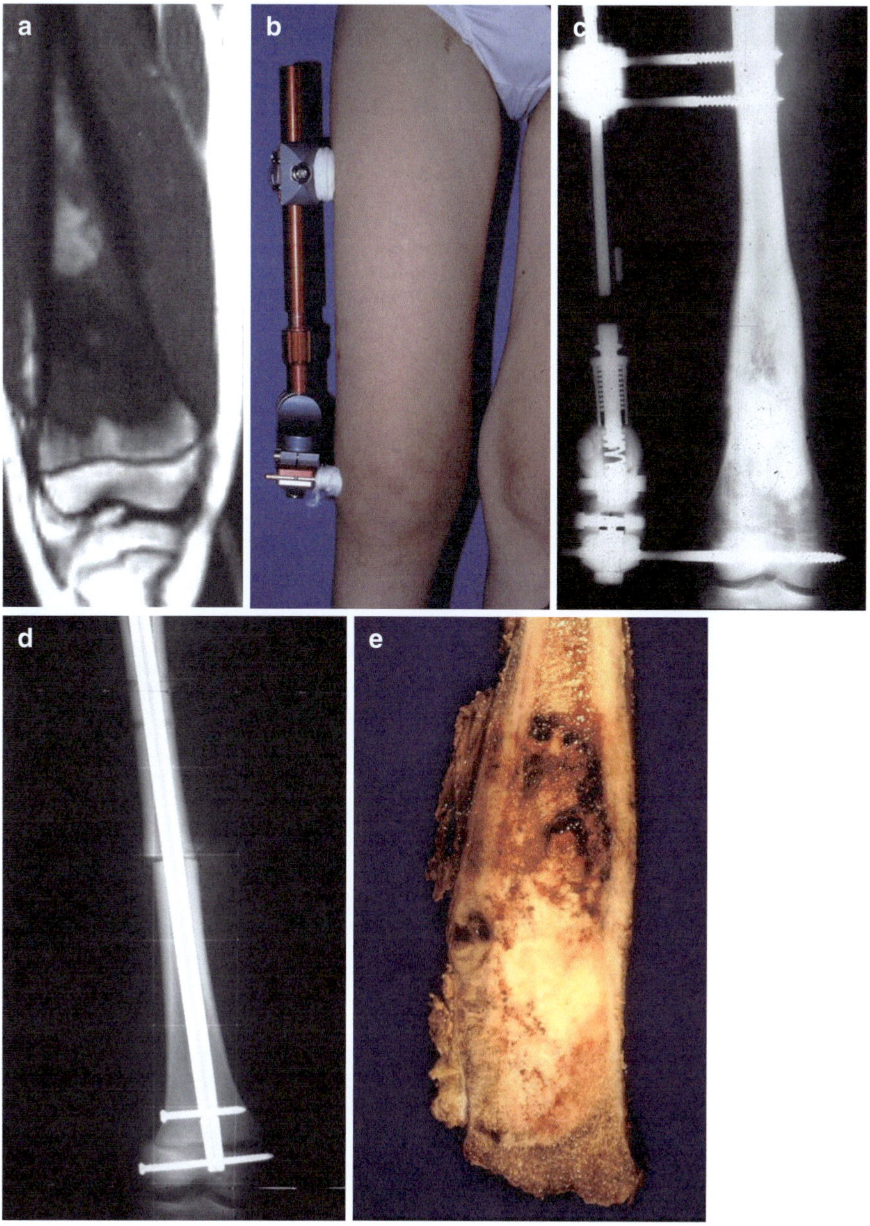

Fig. 9.5 (**a**) Osteosarcoma in the distal femur. The tumor is not in contact with the growth plate. There are some areas of edema between the tumor and the physis. (**b**, **c**) Physeal distraction was performed. (**d**) Reconstruction was by intercalary allograft. (**e**) Macroscopic appearance

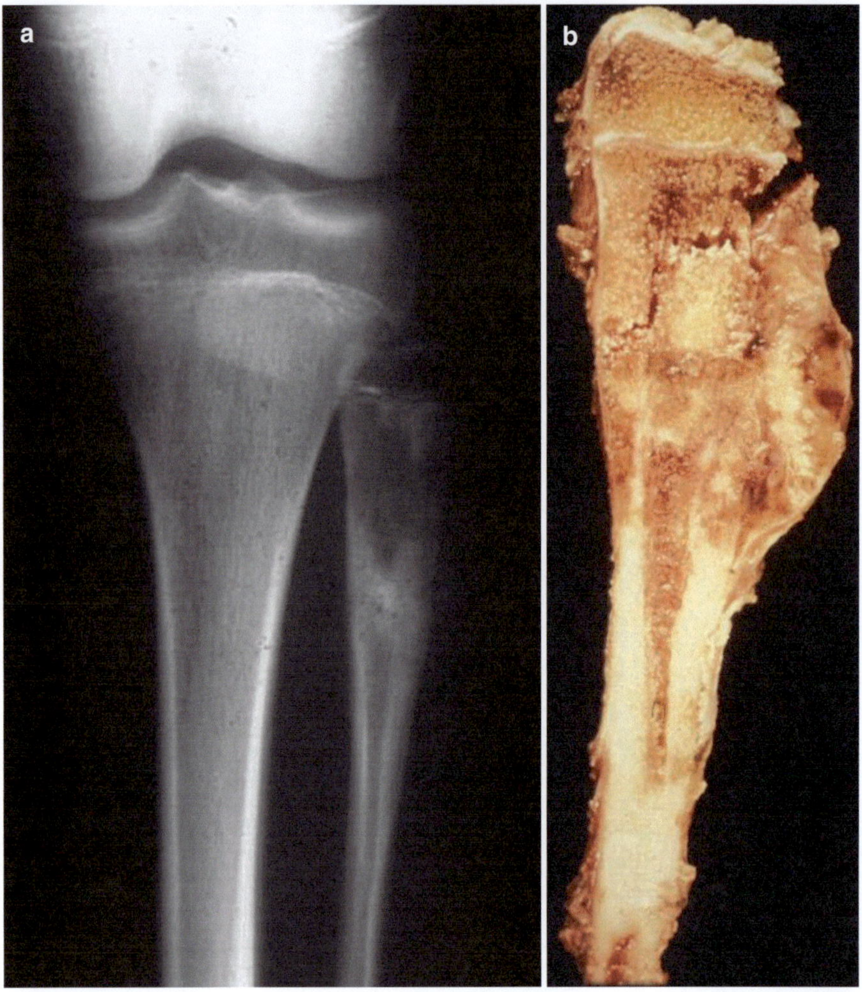

Fig. 9.6 X-Ray (**a**) and macroscopic view (**b**) of an osteosarcoma in the proximal metaphysis of the fibula of a 15-year-old girl. In such cases, it would not be appropriate to attempt to use physeal distraction and to preserve the epiphysis because of the risk of lesion to the peroneal nerve when placing the pins. Aside from this consideration, in this patient, the loss of the epiphysis does not imply any impairment in knee function

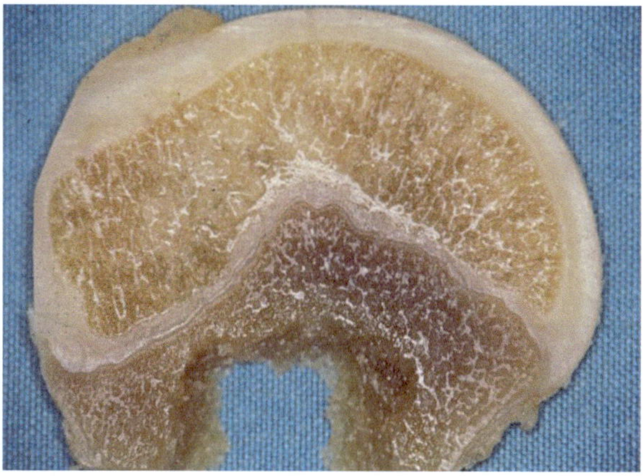

Fig. 9.7 The particular morphology of the growth plate of the proximal humerus allows placement of pins for physeal distraction

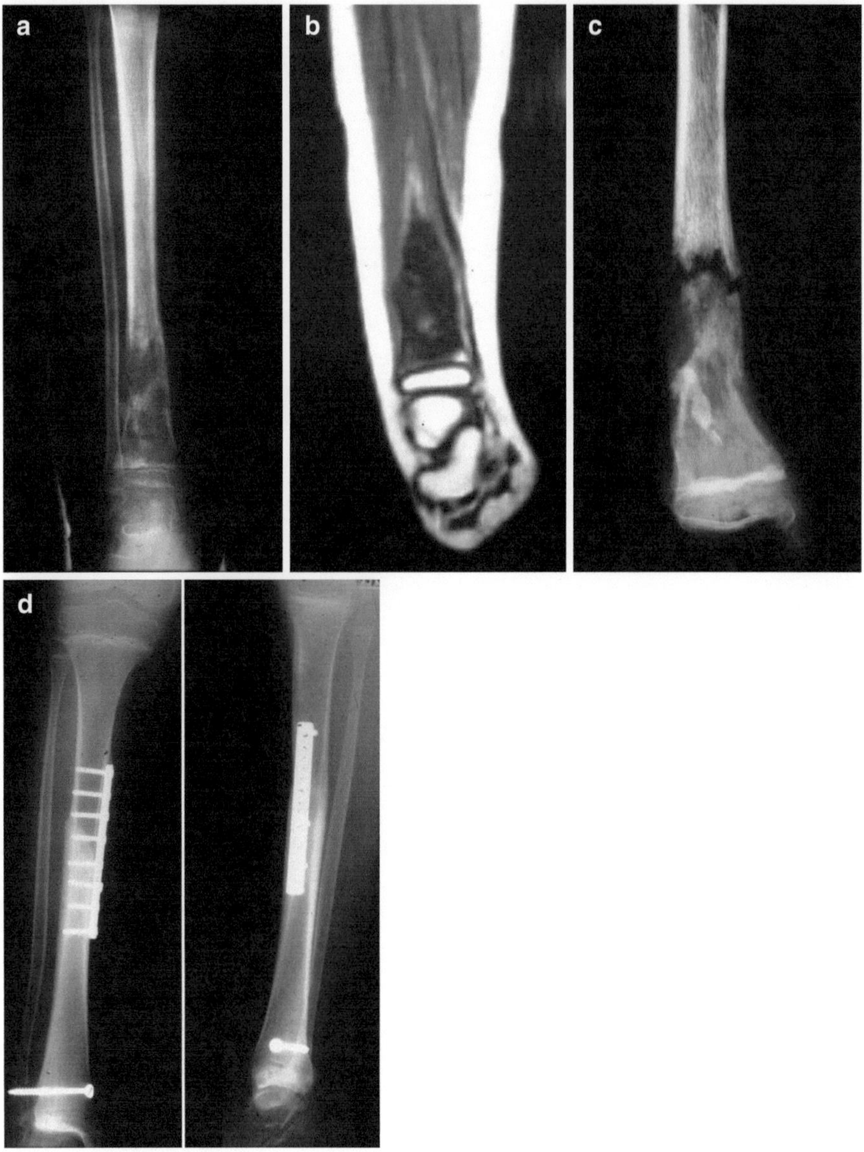

Fig. 9.8 (**a**) Pathological fracture in the distal tibia of a 9-year-old boy with an osteosarcoma. (**b**) The tumor did not transgress the physis. (**c**) X-ray of the resected piece. (**d**) Reconstruction was done by osteoarticular allograft

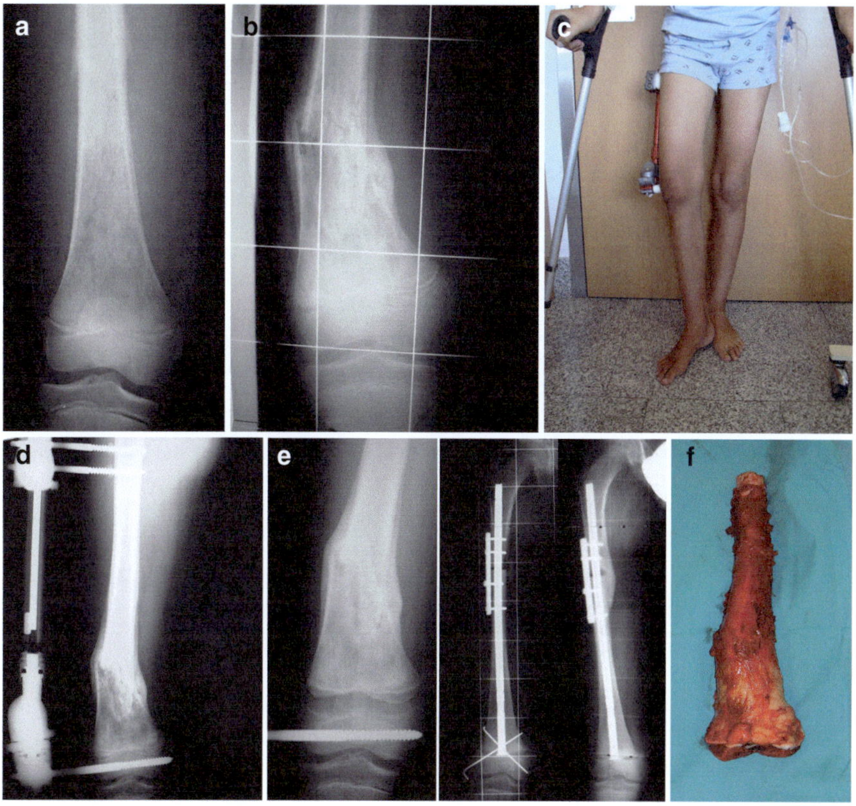

Fig. 9.9 (**a**) Ewing's sarcoma in the distal femur of a 10-year-old boy. Note the osteolysis in the metaphysis and the Codman triangle in the middle shaft. (**b**) A few days after diagnosis, this patient suffered a pathological fracture which healed after a few weeks. (**c**) The external fixation was placed. (**d**) Note the varus and shortening due to the fracture. (**e**) Epiphysiolysis was successful. The tumor was resected and the limb was reconstructed. The allograft healed. (**f**) The resected piece; note a fine layer of growth plate tissue covering the distal margin of resection

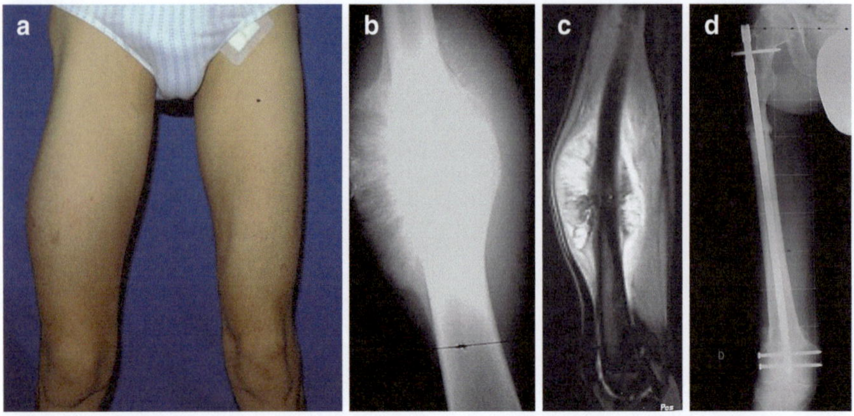

Fig. 9.10 Clinical picture (**a**) and X-ray (**b**) of an osteosarcoma in a 15-year-old boy. There was a safe margin between the tumor and the growth plate (**c**). The tumor was resected and reconstruction was carried out with an intercalary allograft (**d**)

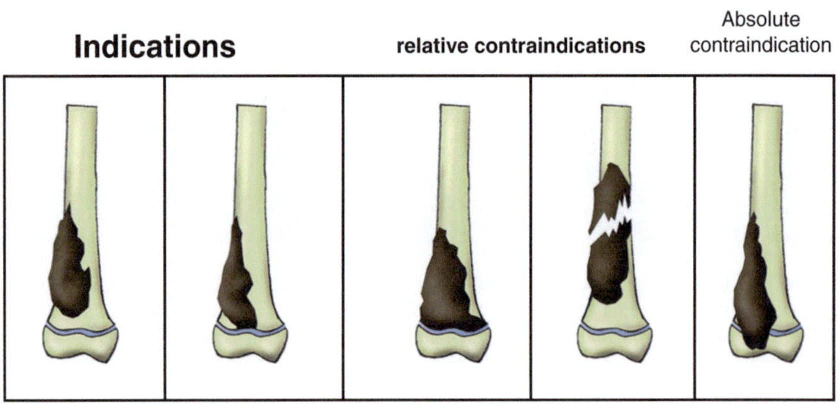

Fig. 9.11 MRI-based indications and contraindications for physeal distraction before resection of metaphyseal tumors

References

1. Cañadell J, Forriol F, Cara JA, San-Julian M. Removal of metaphyseal bone tumors with preservation of the epiphysis. Physeal distraction before excision. In: Cañadell J, San-Julian M, Cara JA, editors. Surgical treatment of malignant bone tumors. Pamplona: Ediciones Universidad de Navarra; 1995. p. 153–60.
2. De Pablos J, Cañadell J, Vazquez J, Idoate M. Clinical study on the barrier effect of the physis in metaphyseal osteosarcoma. In: Cañadell J, Sierrasesúmaga L, Calvo F, Ganoza C, editors. Treatment of malignant bone tumors in children and adolescents. Pamplona: Ediciones Universidad de Navarra; 1991. p. 221–45.
3. Exner GU, Von Hochstetter AR, Augustiny N, Von Schulthess G. Magnetic resonance imaging in malignant bone tumors. Int Orthop. 1990;14:49.

4. Golfieri R, Baddeley H, Pringle JS, Souhami R. The role of the STIR sequence in magnetic resonance imaging examination of bone tumors. Br J Radiol. 1990;63:251.
5. Grimer RJ, Bielack S, Flege S, et al. and from The European Musculo Skeletal Oncology Society (EMSOS) Periosteal osteosarcoma. A European review of outcome. Eur J Cancer. 2005; 41(18):2806–11.
6. Hudson TM, Hamlin DS, Ennekingg WF, Peterson H. Magnetic resonance imaging of bone and soft tissue tumors. Skeletal Radiol. 1985;13:134.
7. Kattapuram SV. Imaging of musculoskeletal tumors. Curr Opin Orthop. 1991;2:781.
8. Knop J, Delling G, Heise U, Winkler K. Scintigraphic of tumor regression during preoperative chemotherapy of osteosarcoma: correlation of Tc-99m-methylene diphosphonate parametric imaging with surgical histopathology. Skeletal Radiol. 1990;19:165.
9. Lemmi MA, Fletcher RB, Marina NM, et al. Use of LMR imaging to assess results of chemotherapy for Ewing sarcoma. AJR Am J Roentgenol. 1990;155:343.
10. O'Flanagan SJ, Stack JP, Mccee HM, Dervan P, Hurson B. Imaging of intramedullary tumor spread in osteosarcoma: a comparison of techniques. J Bone Joint Surg Am. 1991;73-A: 998–1001.
11. San Julian M, Aquerreta JD, Benito A, Cañadell J. Indications for epiphyseal preservation in metaphyseal malignant bone tumors of children. Relationship between image methods and anatomopathological findings. Am J Pediatr Orthop. 1999;19:543–8.
12. Sundaram M, McLeod RA. MR imaging of tumor and tumor-like lesions of bone and soft tissue. AJR Am J Roentgenol. 1990;155:817.
13. Vander Griend RA, Ennekingg WF. Radiologic imaging techniques in the diagnosis and treatment of osteogenic sarcoma. Semin Orthop. 1988;3:59.
14. Zimmer WD, Berquist TH, Mcleod RA, et al. Bone tumors: magnetic resonance imaging versus computer tomography. Radiology. 1985;155:709.

Chapter 10
Conservation of the Epiphysis While Removing Metaphyseal Bone Tumors: Epiphysiolysis Before Excision

José Cañadell†, Mikel San-Julian, Jose A. Cara, and Francisco Forriol

Abstract Physeal distraction – when used for epiphysiolysis rather than for lengthening – provides a safe margin of resection in appropriate patients. The technique does not delay tumor treatment. Placement of the external fixator requires only 15 min and should be done a fortnight before the date established for surgery. We include in this chapter a video tutorial of the placement technique.

10.1 Introduction

Physeal distraction has been extensively used for bone lengthening [4–6] and for correcting angular deformities [1, 2, 8]. We now describe its use in facilitating the excision of malignant bone tumors of the metaphysis. Such use can enable preservation of the epiphysis.

The absence of anastomoses between epiphyseal and metaphyseal vessels means that in those cases where imaging methods determine that the epiphysis has not been affected by the tumor, it is possible to conserve the epiphysis and the joint

---

Electronic supplementary material The online version of this chapter (doi:10.1007/978-3-319-24220-0_10) contains supplementary material, which is available to authorized users.

† Author was deceased at the time of publication

J. Cañadell†, MD, PhD • M. San-Julian, MD, PhD (✉)
Department of Orthopaedic Surgery, University of Navarra, Pamplona, Navarra, Spain
e-mail: msjulian@unav.es

J.A. Cara, MD, PhD
Servicio Médico San Pedro, Department of Orthopaedic Surgery, San Pedro de Alcántara, Málaga, Spain

F. Forriol, MD, PhD
School of Medicine, Department of Clinical Sciences, University San Pablo – CEU, Campus de Monteprincipe, Madrid, Spain

M. San-Julian (ed.), *Cañadell's Pediatric Bone Sarcomas: Epiphysiolysis before Excision*, DOI 10.1007/978-3-319-24220-0_10

while resecting the tumor. This is made possible by physeal distraction according to Cañadell's technique.

10.2 Patients and Methods

Between March 1980 and December 2014, we operated on more than 1000 patients with pediatric bone sarcomas. Intercalary reconstructions were carried out in 168 patients, and many of these reconstructions were made possible by means of physeal distraction. Of these 168 patients, the mean age was 9.4 years; there were similar numbers of males and females. The histological diagnosis was osteosarcoma in two-thirds of the patients (n: 109) and Ewing's sarcoma in the remaining one-third (n: 59).

10.3 Indications Conservation of the Epiphysis While Removing

The indications for Cañadell's technique were:

1. *Location of the tumor in the metaphyseal region.*
2. *The physeal cartilage had to be open.* A patient's age is an important consideration here. In about half of our pediatric patients, the tumor had not involved the physis; the mean age of this group was 11 years. In patients who have nearly finished growing, the probability of tumoral cells having crossed the physis is higher, and it is more difficult to achieve physeal distraction. Other authors [7] have reported a similar incidence of micro- or gross- extension to the epiphysis from metaphyseal bone tumors.
3. *The tumor must not have transgressed the physis.* Radiography, arteriography, CT, and particularly MRI were used to demonstrate this pre-operatively, and histological examination was then used to corroborate the findings of such imaging studies [3].

10.4 Operative Technique (Video 10.1)

The surgical technique usually consists of two phases:

Phase one (Fig. 10.1). Two pins are inserted into the epiphysis and another two into the diaphysis at a distance from the tumor (8–10 cm away if possible). An external monolateral fixator with a T-shaped piece (Fig. 10.2) for the epiphyseal pins is attached (Fig. 10.3). We usually use Schanz pins of 5 or 6 mm diameter. In very young children, 4 mm pins could be strong enough for epiphysiolysis.

Fig. 10.1 Diagram showing the first surgical step

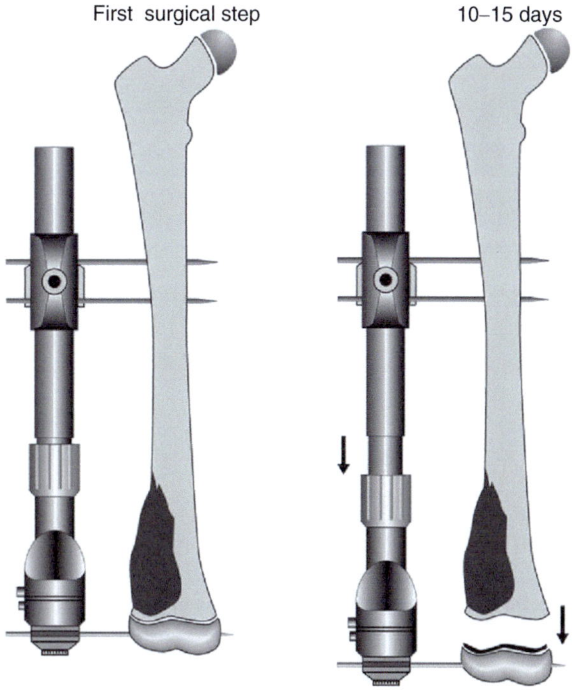

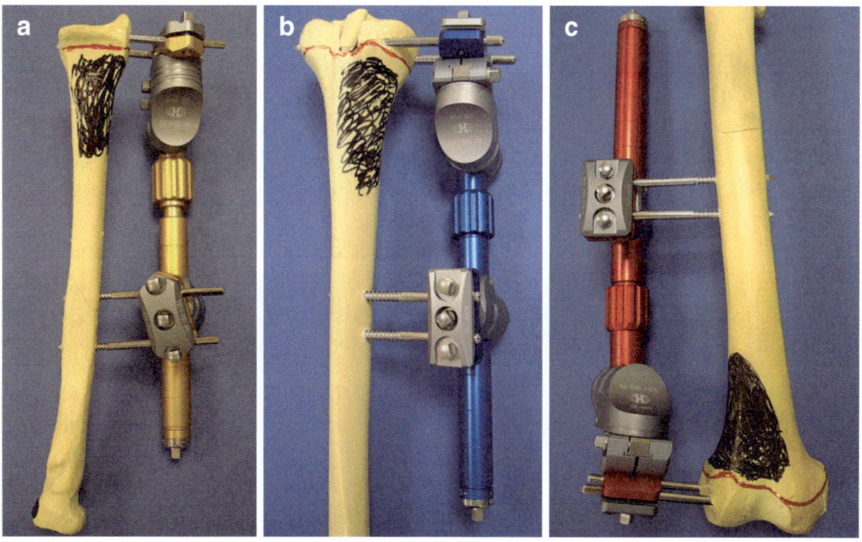

Fig. 10.2 (**a–c**) Devices used in young children for distal tibia, distal fibula, and distal radius (*yellow*) and in adolescents for proximal tibia and humerus (*blue*) and distal femur (*red*). All devices have a T-shaped piece in order to put the two epiphyseal pins perpendicular to the diaphysis

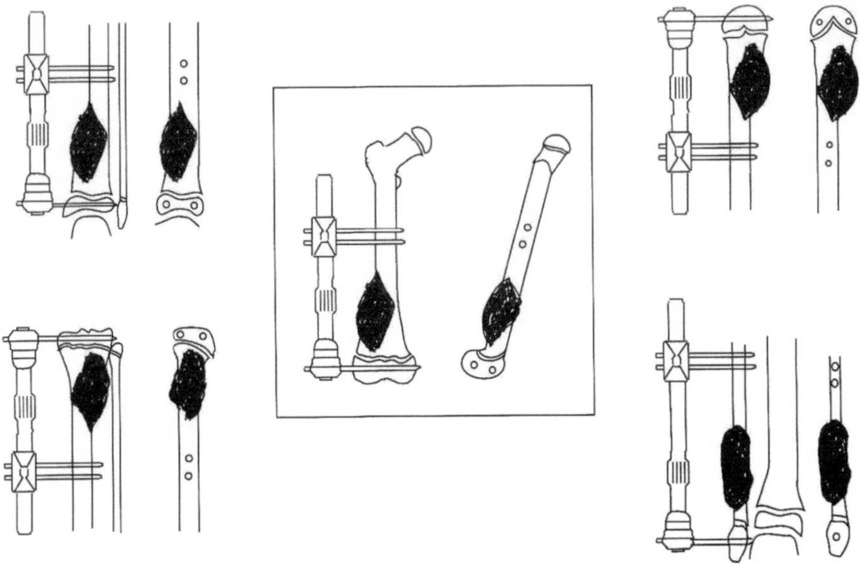

Fig. 10.3 Diagrams showing the placement of the pins in distal femur, proximal and distal tibia, proximal humerus, and distal fibula

Distraction is begun in the operating room and continues at the rate of 1–1.5 mm/day until 1 or 2 cm of distraction is achieved. During the first few days nothing happens, but after between 7 and 14 days of distraction the patient usually reports pain, and this indicates rupture of the growth plate: radiography will show disruption of the physis. In our series, the mean time over which distraction was applied was 10 days. This first phase can be carried out while the patient is finishing the course of neoadjuvant chemotherapy; despite the external fixator being in place, even intra-arterial procedures can be used without problems [9] (Fig. 10.4). We usually operate on a patient the day after the final intraarterial neoadjuvant procedure.

Phase two. En-bloc resection of the tumor is performed by diaphyseal osteotomy, leaving a wide margin. The metaphyseal end of the resection is already effected by the distraction. If the prior imaging methods clearly indicated an absence of tumor in the epiphysis, the operation is completed, in this second surgical step, by reconstruction with an intercalary graft (Fig. 10.5).

In the past, before the advent of MRI, with cases for which we could not be sure that the tumor had not involved the epiphysis, the resected tumor was sent immediately for histological examination, and chains of PMMA containing gentamicin were inserted into the space held open by the fixator. If the pathologist reported absence of tumor at the edges of the resected segment, the chains of beads were withdrawn and a bone graft was inserted (Fig. 10.4). If, on the other hand, the pathologist were to find tumor cells, the procedure would be to resect the epiphysis and reconstruct the limb by other means: prosthesis, osteoarticular allograft, or arthrodesis. In our series the latter scenario was only necessary in

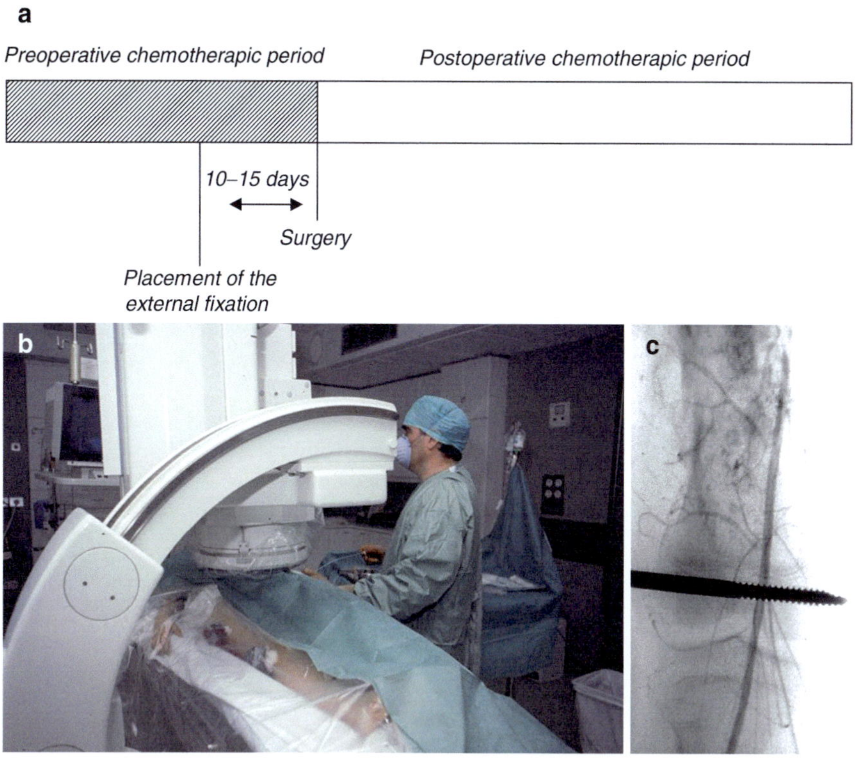

Fig. 10.4 (**a**) It not necessary to delay the protocol of treatment. The first surgical step is carried out during the pre-operative chemotherapy period. (**b**, **c**) In osteosarcoma patients, we use intra-arterial cisplatin as a part of the neo-adjuvant chemotherapy protocol. The angiogram also clearly shows that vascularization of the epiphysis is not connected with that of the metaphyseal tumor. We usually carry out resection of the tumor the day after the last intra-arterial neoadjuvant procedure

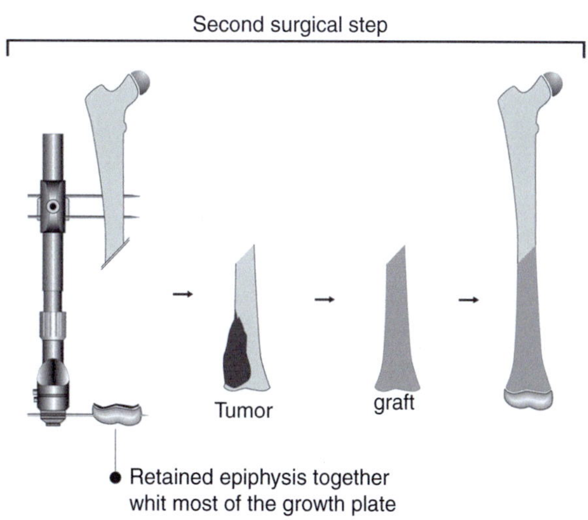

Fig. 10.5 Diagram showing resection and reconstruction

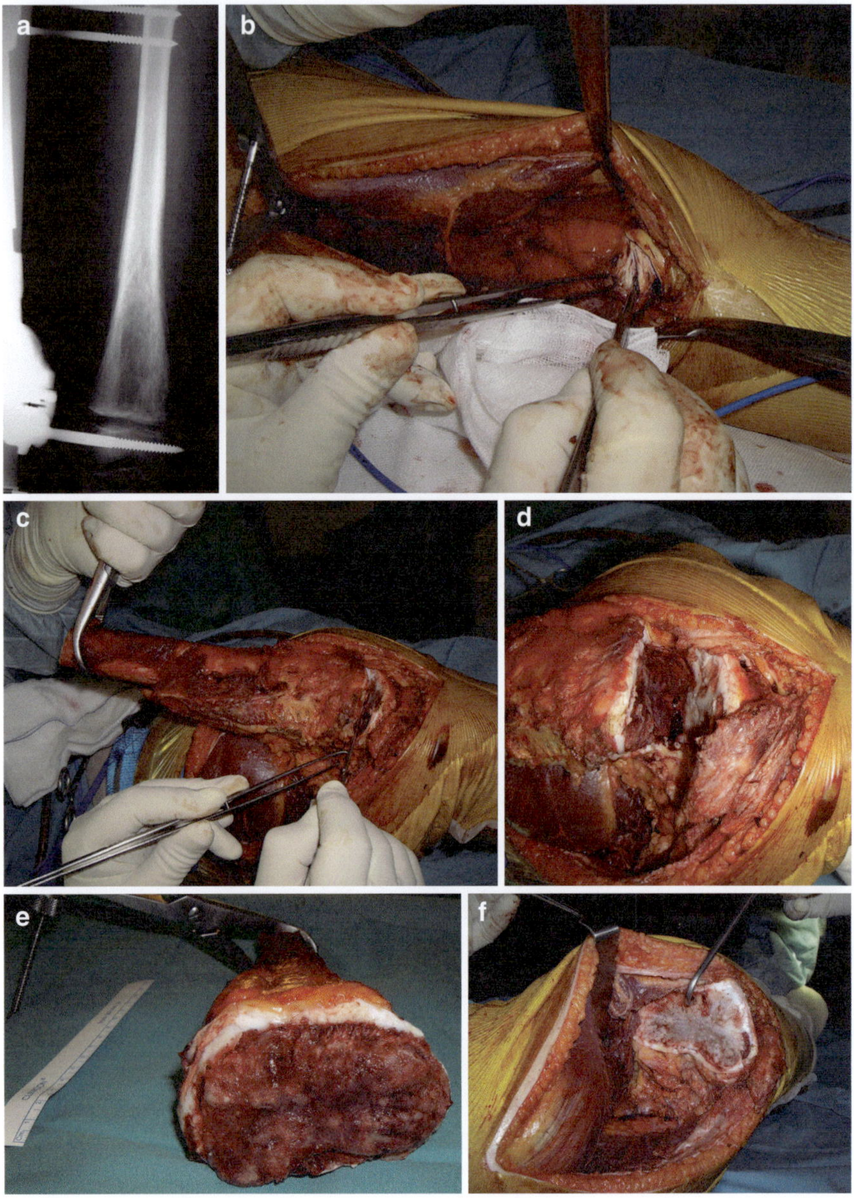

Fig. 10.6 After distraction (**a**), surgery is easier. The perichondrium is cut (**b–d**). Only diaphyseal osteotomy is required (**c**), because the metaphyseal "osteotomy" is already done. The resected piece is covered by a thin layer of growth plate which constitutes a safe margin (**e**), while most of the growth plate remains attached to the epiphysis in the patient (**f**)

one patient, whose prosthetic reconstruction proceeded without problem, and who suffered no local recurrence. MRI has removed the uncertainty over epiphysis involvement, and the so the three-step technique described in this paragraph is no longer generally required (Figs. 10.6 and 10.7).

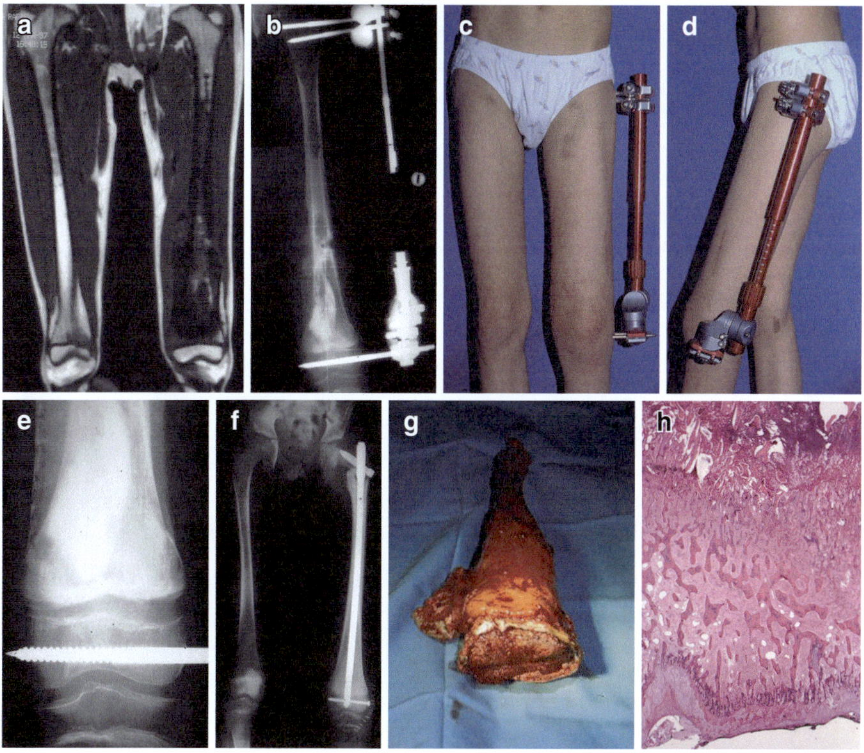

Fig. 10.7 Osteosarcoma involving two-thirds of the femur in a 13-year-old boy. MRI (**a**) shows some edema between the tumor and the growth plate. In this particular case, the proximal pins were placed in the femoral neck due to the tumoral extension (**b–d**). Physeal distraction was achieved (**e**). Reconstruction was carried out with an intercalary allograft in the second surgical step (**f**). The allograft used was 2 cm longer than the resected piece (**g**, **h**). The resected piece (**g**) together with the biopsy scar. Staining of the distal margin with Indian ink (**h**) shows that the margin is free of tumor, because there is a thin layer of growth plate cells covering the resected bone

In cases of large femoral tumors, sometimes the proximal pins have to be inserted in the femoral neck (Figs. 10.7 and 10.8).

The choice of the kind of osteosynthesis device in the graft and in the remaining physis and epiphysis can play an important role in the final leg-length discrepancy (*see* Chap. 12). In this respect, for children near the end of growth, it may be appropriate to insert an allograft longer than the resected piece.

10.5 Discussion

When resecting a tumor, the surgeon must be certain that no malignant tissue is left behind. Many authors agree that a 2–3 cm margin is safe in bone sarcomas. This means that, when the tumor is in the metaphysis close to the growth plate, resection with such a margin implies loss of the adjacent joint.

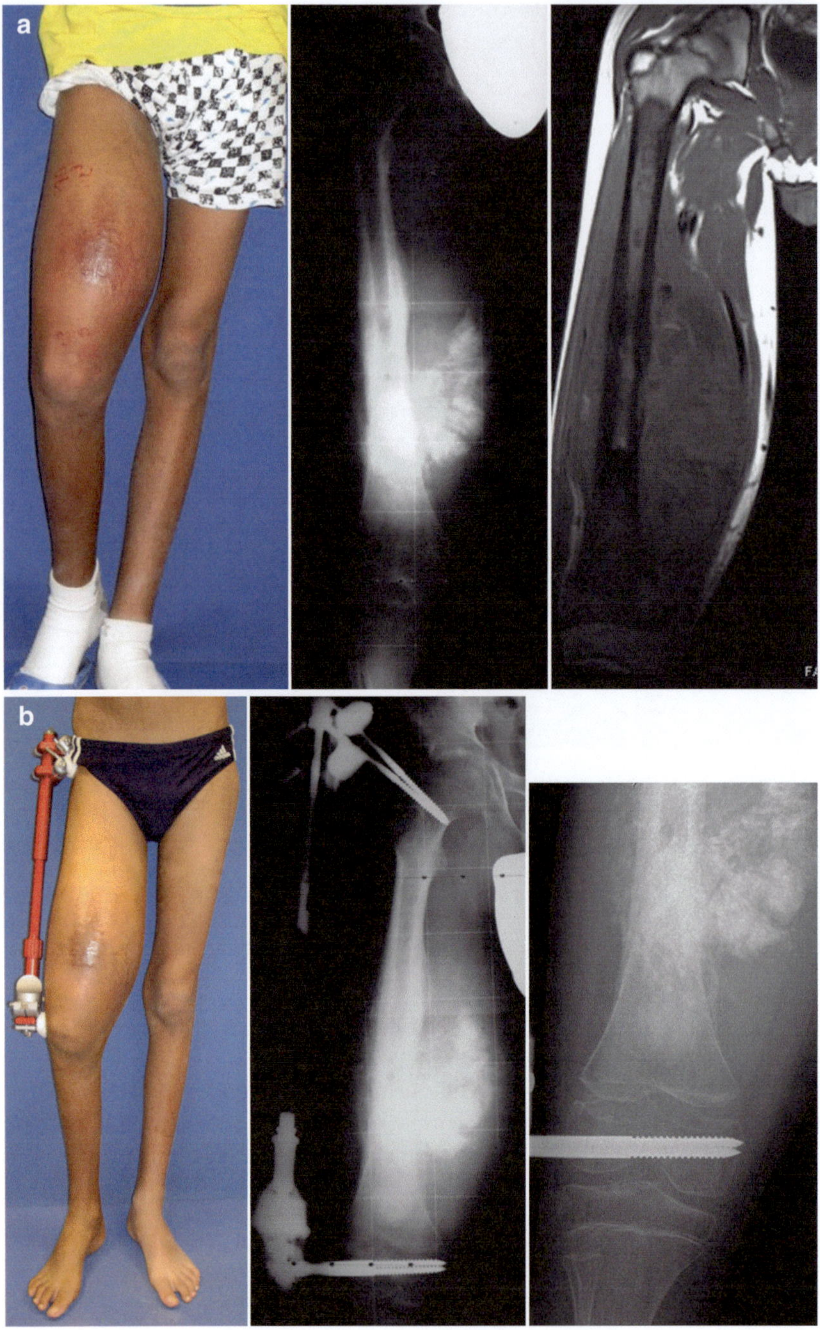

Fig. 10.8 (**a**) A huge osteosarcoma in the right femur of a 12 year-old boy. A large transquadricipital open biopsy was performed elsewhere, and amputation was advised. MRI shows extension of the tumor near the distal epiphysis. (**b**) After neoadjuvant chemotherapy an external fixator was placed. Note the location of the proximal pins. Epiphysiolysis was achieved. (**c**) An intra-operative picture showing dissection of the vessels. (**d**) Postoperative x-ray. (**e**) The patient's leg function 7 years later was acceptable

Fig. 10.8 (continued)

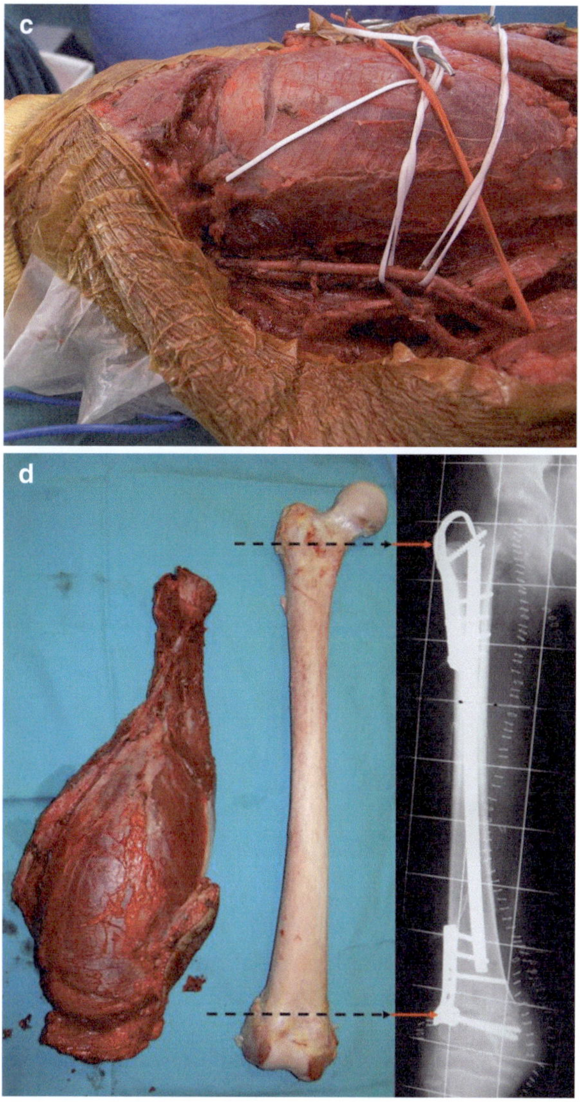

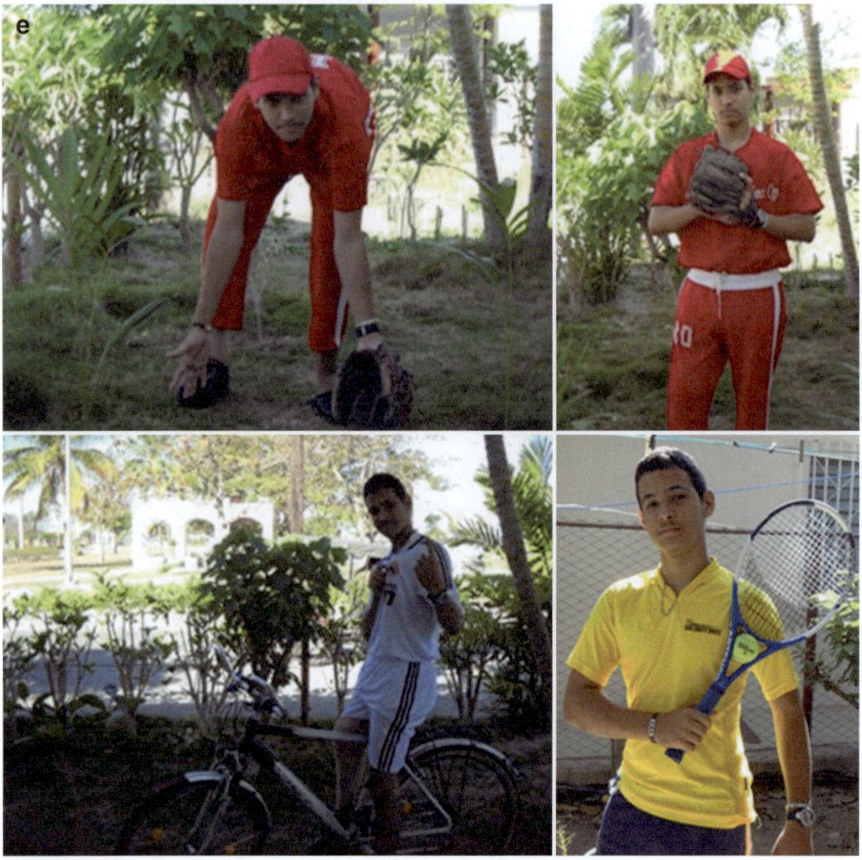

Fig. 10.8 (continued)

However, by definition, the wide margin is assumed to refer to a layer of normal tissue, as opposed to reactive or inflammatory tissue surrounding the tumor.

In tumors that do not cross the growth plate, our technique based on previous physeal distraction, provides a safe margin while averting loss of the epiphysis. When present, the growth cartilage itself provides a dependable margin of safety: the 2–3 cm margin suggested by most authors is unnecessary in this specific context. This view is supported by the fact that in our series as well as in other series (see Chap. 14) no tumor has been observed to recur locally in epiphysis that has been conserved in accordance with the procedure we describe.

References

1. Cañadell J, De Pablos J. Breaking bone bridges by physeal distraction: a new approach. Int Orthop. 1985;9:223–9.
2. Cañadell J, De Pablos J. Correction of angular deformities by physeal distraction. Clin Orthop. 1992;283:98.

3. Daffner RH, Lupetin AR, Dash N, et al. MRI in the detection of malignant infiltration of bone marrow. AJR Am J Roentgenol. 1986;146:353–8.
4. De Bastiani G, Aldegheri R, Renzi Brivio L, Triviella G. Limb lengthening by distraction of the epiphyseal plate. A comparison of two techniques in the rabbit. J Bone Joint Surg (Br). 1986;68-B:545–9.
5. De Pablos J, Villas C, Cañadell J. Bone lengthening by physeal distraction: an experimental study. Int Orthop. 1986;10:163–70.
6. Monticelli G, Spinelli R. Distraction epiphysiolysis as a method of limb lengthening. III clinical applications. Clin Orthop. 1991;154:274–85.
7. Neel M, Bush C, Scarborough M, Enneking W. Transepiphyseal extension of osteosarcoma. Abstract book of the 8th ISOLS international symposium on limb salvage, Florence, 10th–12th May 1995, p. 107.
8. Peltonen JI, Karaharku EO, Alitalo I. Experimental epiphysiolysis distraction producing and correcting angular deformities. J Bone Joint Surg (Br). 1984;66-B:598–602.
9. Sierrasesúmaga L, Antillon F, Patiño A, San Julian M. Oncología pediátrica. Madrid: Pearson; 2005.
10. San Julian M, Vazquez-García BL, Sierrasesúmaga L. Limb salvage in children. In: Bentley G. (ed): European Surgical Orthopaedics and Traumatology. The EFORT textbook. Springer-Verlag Berlin Heidelberg, London, 2014, p. 4251–80.

Chapter 11
Complications of the Technique and Solutions

Blanca L. Vázquez-García and Mikel San-Julián

Abstract Limb salvage in children with bone tumors consists in a long surgical intervention divided in two-steps. The first step is to resect the tumor; the second step is to reconstruct the limb. In appropriate cases, Cañadell's technique has been demonstrated to be a safe and effective technique that facilitates resection of the tumor whilst providing a safe margin. Reconstruction after the use of Cañadell's technique has similar rates of complications as reconstructions after other surgical procedures.

With distraction of the growth plate at a rate of 1 mm per day, the physis usually breaks through the layer of degenerative cells. This chapter will focus on an unusual complication of the Cañadell technique: rupture in the wrong site. The solution should this occur is intra-epiphyseal osteotomy, which can be undertaken without sacrificing the articulation.

Keywords Complications • Epiphysiolysis distraction • Intra-epiphyseal osteotomy

11.1 Introduction

Bone sarcoma surgery consists of two steps: resection and reconstruction San-Julian et al. [5]. Complications in the reconstruction step are the same as with reconstruction after other surgical procedures or pathological conditions, such as, fractures, pseudoarthrosis, and infections. For more information see Chap. 12: "Clinical Results".

As a tumor resection technique, epiphysiolysis before excision has, over time, proved to be a safe and effective technique. It has, however, had critics, who have expressed concern about the possibility of higher rates of complications (infection,

B.L. Vázquez-García, MD (✉)
Department of Orthopaedic Surgery, Complejo Hospitalario de Navarra, Pamplona, Navarra, Spain
e-mail: blanca.vazquezgarcia82@gmail.com; blankita290@hotmail.com

M. San-Julián, MD, PhD
Department of Orthopaedic Surgery, University of Navarra, Pamplona, Navarra, Spain
e-mail: msjulian@unav.es

M. San-Julian (ed.), *Cañadell's Pediatric Bone Sarcomas: Epiphysiolysis before Excision*, DOI 10.1007/978-3-319-24220-0_11

for example) that might result from placing an external fixator so close to the tumor. Another concern has been the possibility that tumor cells might be left in the joint area. These considerations have been cautiously investigated over the years and the security and efficacy of the technique has been established (Cañadell and San Julian 2009) [2]. There is no increased risk of local recurrence or infection as a result of the use of an external fixator before resection (Xu et al. 2014) [6]. In this chapter we take a look at a different complication of the Cañadell technique: distraction through an unexpected plane.

When distraction is through the physis at a rate of 1 mm/day, the break usually occurs through the calcified layer in the metaphyseal zone of the growing plate (de Pablos 1986) [1]. This is the desired site of rupture. On some occasions (about 2–3 % of cases), however, the break occurs in a different place. In this chapter we analyze this unusual scenario, and explain how to detect it and what to do in response.

11.2 Material and Methods

We have reviewed our series of more than 160 cases during the last 30 years.

11.3 Results

In our series, there were only two cases of complications related to epiphysiolysis before excision, and both of these cases were distraction in an unexpected site: through the tumor. Our colleagues in Switzerland have reported a third case of such distraction (Betz et al. 2012) [1].

There were no complications related to the external fixator, which was in position for only 10–12 days. The infection rate was 9 %/low, comparable to that for the cases in which epiphysiolysis was not used

11.3.1 Case 1

Case 1 was a 10-year-old boy who presented with pain in his left knee and a limp, which had been ongoing for 2 months. Initially, the patient attended a hospital other than ours. An X-ray was taken and a cortical defect observed (Fig. 11.1).

Suspecting a bone tumor, an MRI scan was taken. Subsequently, the boy underwent open biopsy (of 6 cm of length) with curettage. After this procedure the patient was not able to walk with that leg due to the pain. The tumor was diagnosed as osteosarcoma.

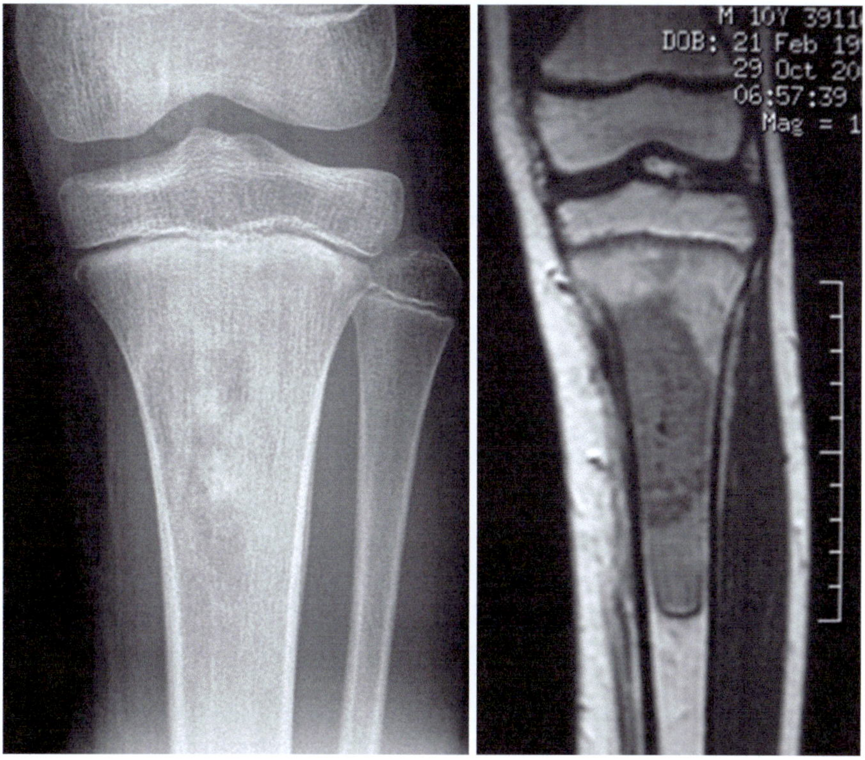

Fig. 11.1 XR and MRI of a 10 y-o male who complains of knee pain. Bone alteration is seen on the XR. MRI shows no affectation of the physis. So limb salvage is the indication in this cases

At this point, the boy was brought to our center to receive treatment. After evaluation of the case (Fig. 11.2), we decided that limb salvage was possible by means of the Cañadell technique and posterior reconstruction. The patient started chemotherapy and received three sessions of intra-arterial chemotherapy. We placed the external fixator and distraction was carried out at a rate of 1 mm per day.

After between 7 and 10 days of distraction or if the patient reports pain, we typically request an X-ray to confirm rupture through the growth plate. In this case, the X-ray revealed that separation had occurred through the biopsy tract (Fig. 11.3).

The external fixation was removed and intra-epiphyseal osteotomy undertaken. We were able to preserve the proximal tibiae epiphysis and the knee joint. We reconstructed with an intercalary allograft with an intramedullary nail (Fig. 11.4 and 11.5).

Postoperatively, the patient recovered in a normal way. He continued with chemotherapy treatment. The excised tumor had 100 % necrosis. The patient started walking with crutches and then with full weight-bearing and demonstrated complete range of motion of the knee.

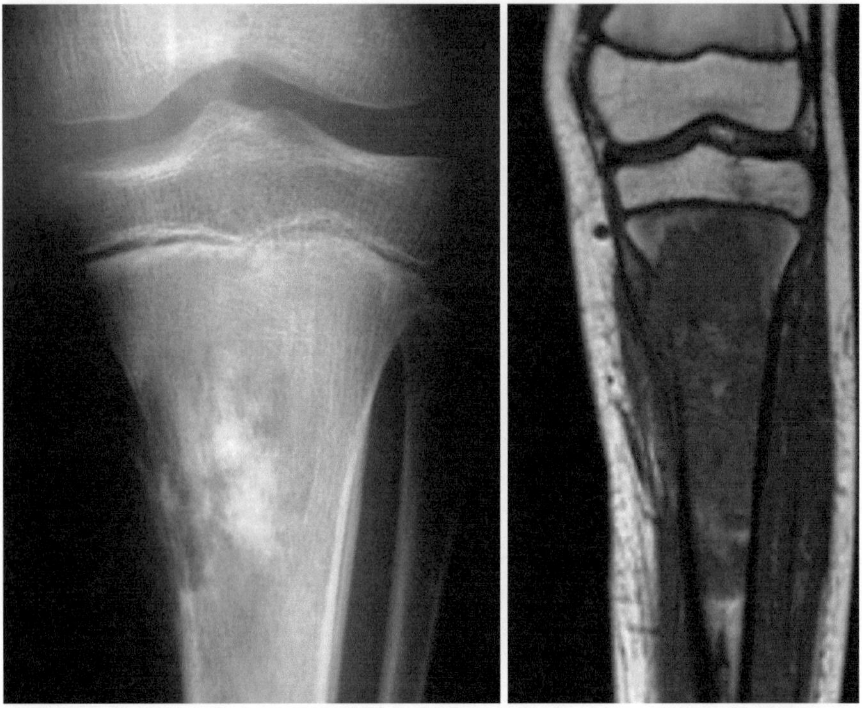

Fig. 11.2 XR and MRI after open biopsy elsewhere. The tumor has grown without the treatment

Nine months after completion of chemotherapy (one and a half years after surgery) the patient reported a pain in the contralateral knee (Fig. 11.6). This turned out to be a single bone metastasis without lung affectation. We decided to treat the metastasis as if it were a primary tumor. Intra-venous and intra-arterial chemotherapy was initiated. As the tumor was in contact with all of the physis, we performed intra-epiphyseal osteotomy rather than the Cañadell technique. Then we proceeded with reconstruction (Fig. 11.7)

The tumor was 90 % necrotic. The patient continued to receive chemotherapy, but 3 months later developed lung metastases and further bone metastases. He died 4 months later.

11.3.2 Case 2

This concerns a 9 year-old boy who presented with pain and a limp, without any trauma, in his right leg. At that time, the symptoms had persisted for 4 months. He was taken to hospital (not initially our hospital) because of an increase in the intensity of pain and the fact that pain continued even during the night (Fig. 11.8a). By means of closed biopsy, the diagnosis of osteosarcoma was established. There was

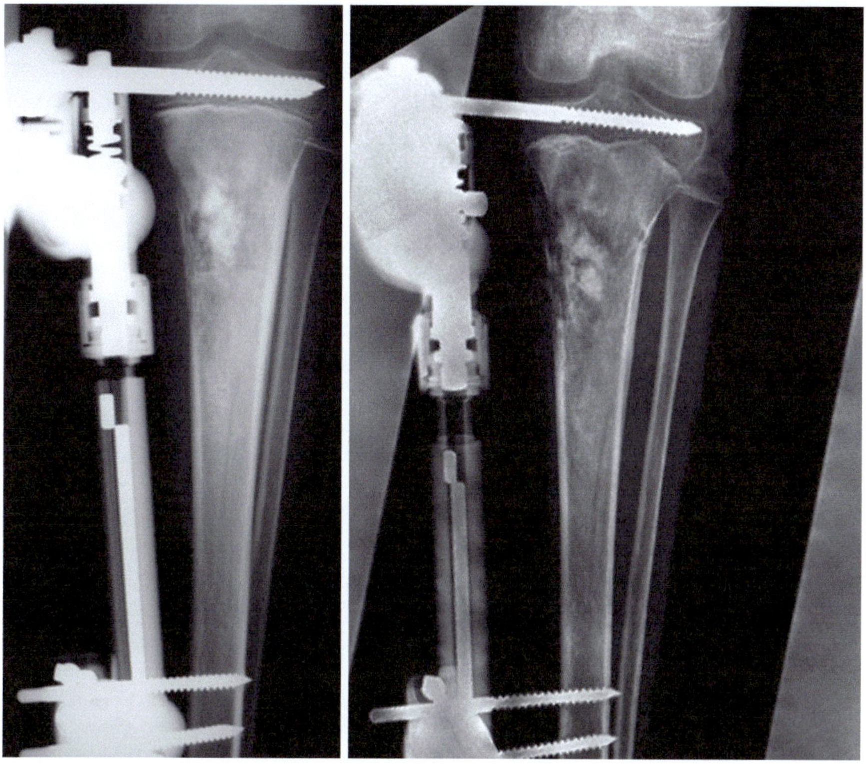

Fig. 11.3 Control XR of the external Fixator. We observed that the distraction has not been done through the physis, is been done through the biopsy tract. At this point we remove the EF

no lung metastasis. He started chemotherapy, and with two courses of intravenous chemotherapy there was a clear decrease in the pain. His referral center proposed amputation as surgical treatment, and it was in search of other possibilities that he came to our hospital.

After evaluation of the case (Fig. 11.8b, c), we decided that limb salvage was achievable by means of epiphysiolysis (Fig. 11.9) before excision (Cañadell's technique). We gave just one session of intra-arterial chemotherapy before placing the external fixation, because, as mentioned above, he had already started neoadjuvant chemotherapy elsewhere, with an apparently good response.

During the preoperative planning session, we saw the possibility that the distraction had not occurred in the expected place, and that the rupture was through the tumor; a CT scan confirmed our suspicion (Fig. 11.10).

To save the articulation we performed intra-epiphyseal osteotomy. As the growth plate is not tibial plateau, for surgeons with less experience in intra-epiphyseal osteotomy we recommend the use of a k-wire under fluoroscopy control to be more accurate with the saw when performing the osteotomy (Fig. 11.11). In the case of this patient, we had to sacrifice the patellar tendon insertion. For reconstruction we

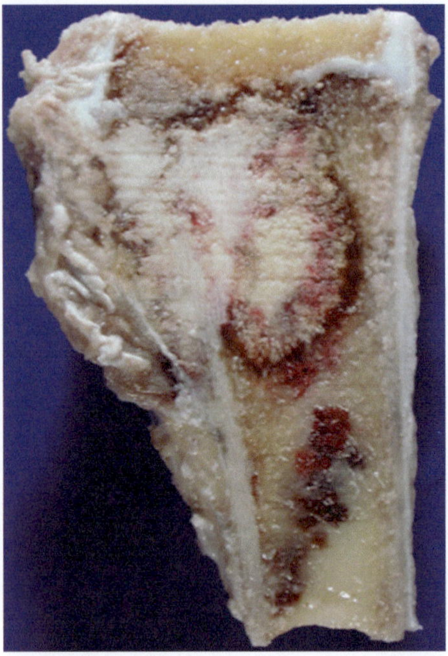

Fig. 11.4 Specimen. We performed an intra-epiphyseal osteotomy. See how we get a secure margin above the physis. Histology showed complete necrosis of the tumor

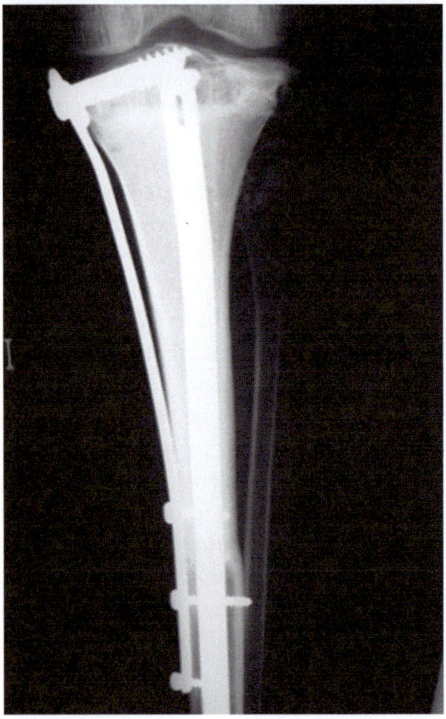

Fig. 11.5 Postoperative RX of the reconstruction with allograft and intramedullary nail and scaffolding with a plate fixing the rest of the epyphisis. We conserve the articular surface

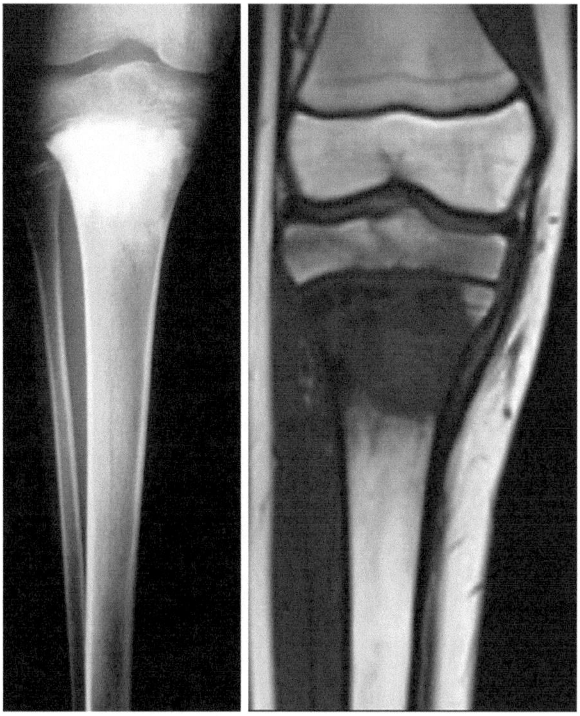

Fig. 11.6 Xr and MRI of the right tibiae. The patient presented a bone metastasis in contact with the whole physis without lung mets. We decided to do an intra-epiphyseal osteotomy as he has before in the other leg

used a humerus intercalary allograft, as this was the most suitable for this patient. Because we had not been able to preserve the growth plate, we used a slightly larger allograft in order to compensate for future dissymmetry (Fig. 11.12).

The tumor was 99 % necrotic. The patient continued with standard chemotherapy and follow up. He had complete articular range of motion and walked without crutches. He had slightly instability in varus-valgus angulation of the knee. After 3 years the patient developed lung metastasis. He underwent thoracotomy of the left lung and then, 4 months later, video-thoracoscopy of the right lung. One year later he developed bone metastasis. Currently, 4 years after the initial surgery, the patient is alive but with disease that is still under treatment with chemotherapy and radiotherapy.

11.4 Discussion

The two complications that we have observed with epiphysiolysis were by no means catastrophic and had an easy work-around.

The two cases described are surprising in that we would not expect metastatic disease when the rates of necrosis of the tumor in response to chemotherapy were so high (99 % and 100 %). In this sense these two cases are exceptional.

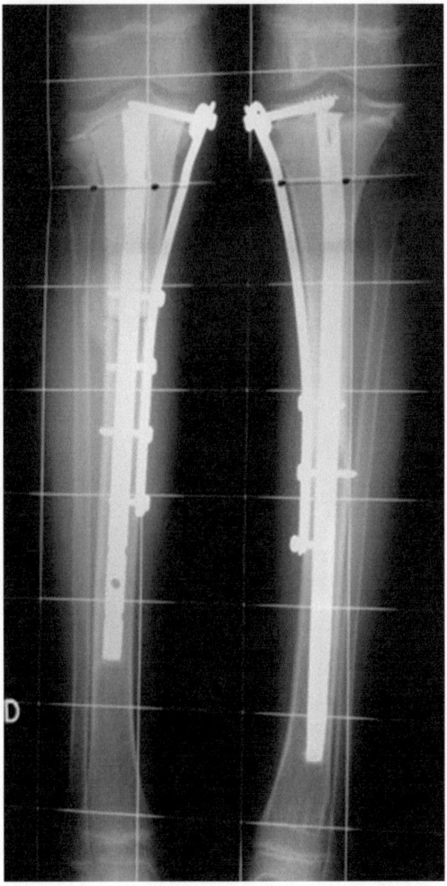

Fig. 11.7 XR control of both legs

Both patients had complete range of motion of the knee, could walk, and returned to their normal way of life. In view of the short follow-up, we were not able to evaluate residual dissymmetry due to loss of the growth plate.

11.5 Conclusions

Epiphysiolysis before excision has been shown to be a safe technique (Eralp and Enar 2013) [4] (Zhang et al. 2014) [7]. Distraction at an unexpected site occurred in only 2–3 % of cases. Should this happen, treatment can proceed with intra-epiphyseal osteotomy, and so there is still a chance to preserve the joint, without increasing the local recurrence rate. In case of doubt about the location of the distraction, we recommend taking a CT scan.

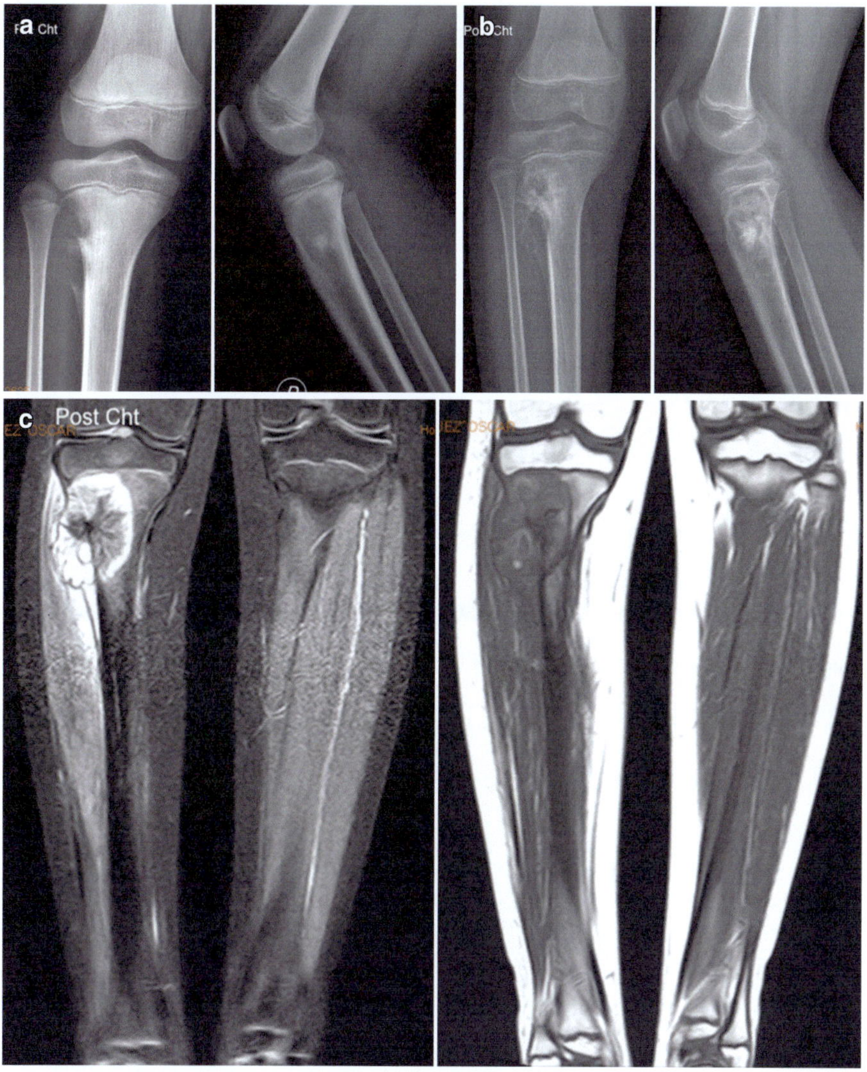

Fig. 11.8 (**a**) 9 yo boy who complains of knee pain. A simple XR showed a cortical bone defect and soft tissue mass. Diagnosed of osteosarcoma. (**b**) XR post chemotherapy. We observed how the tumor has not grown and is delimitate. (**c**) T1 and T2 sequences of the tumor which is in contact to 50 % of the physis

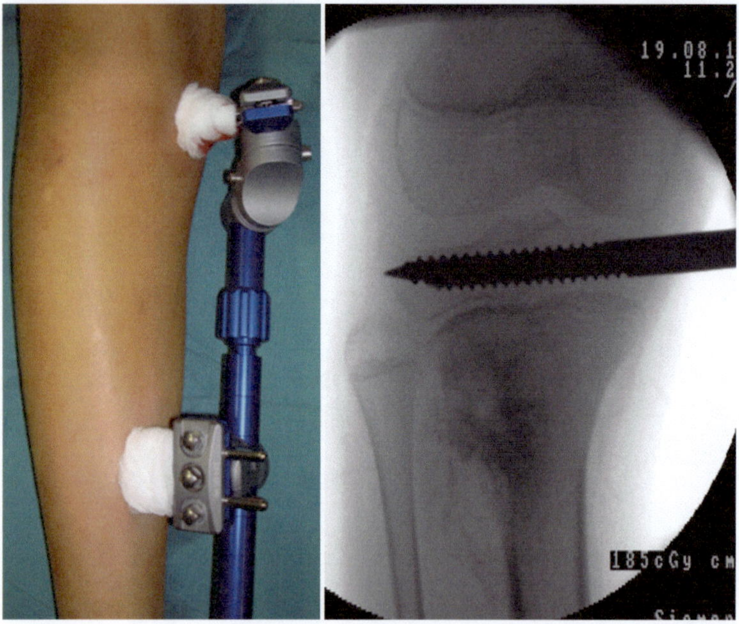

Fig. 11.9 We decided to do limb salvage with epiphysiolysis. We place the external fixation

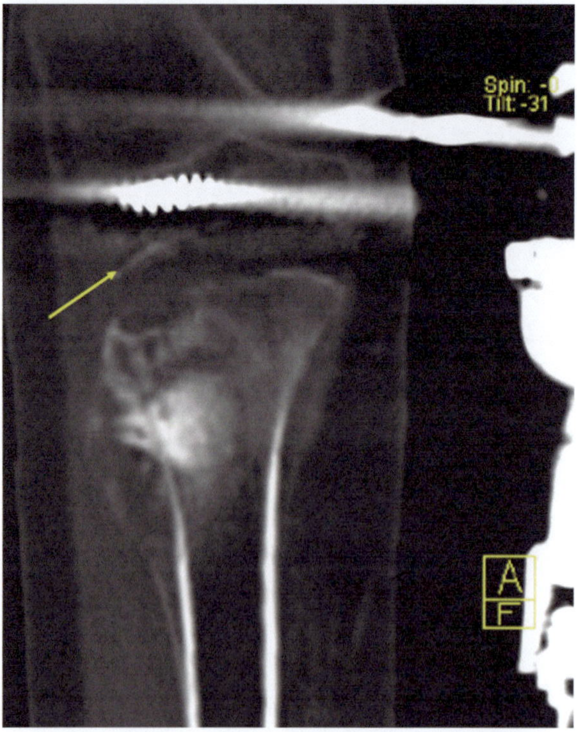

Fig. 11.10 CT were we observe the Fracture line

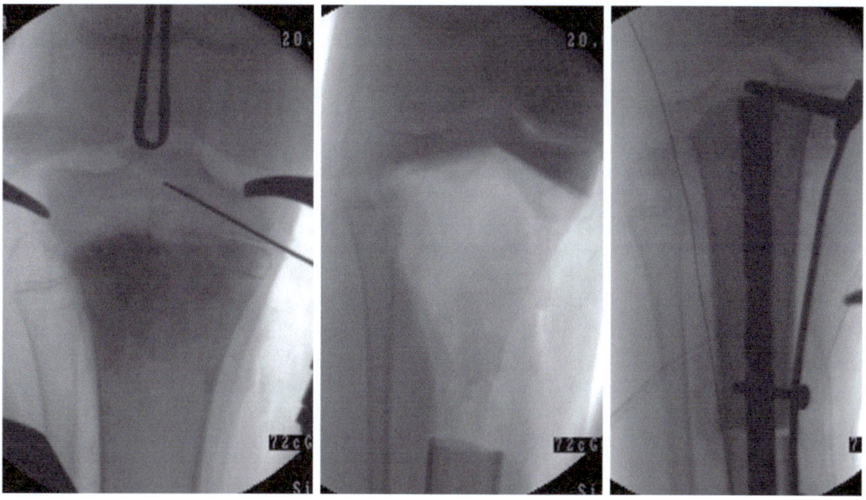

Fig. 11.11 (*1*) K-wire helps us to do the osteotomy, (*2*) Removal of the tumor, (*3*) Reconstruction with allograft with intramedullary nail and plate

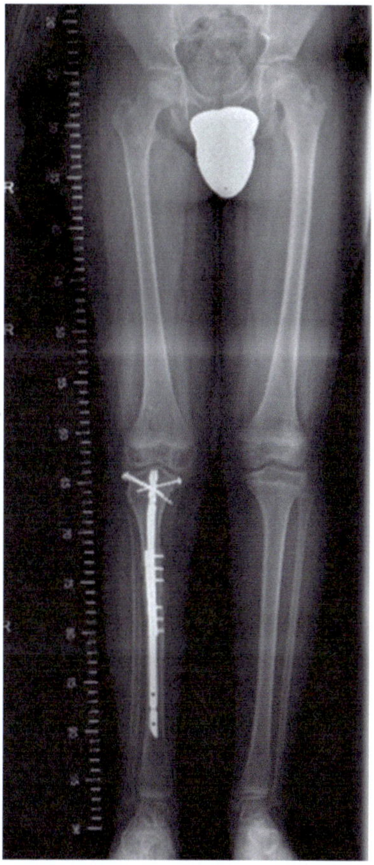

Fig. 11.12 Postop XR

Bibliography

1. Betz M, Dumont CE, Fuchs B, Exner GU. Physeal distraction for joint preservation in malignant metaphyseal bone tumors in children. Clin Orthop Relat Res. 2012;470(6):1749–54.
2. Cañadell J, San-Julian M. Pediatric bone sarcomas. Springer-Verlag London; 2009.
3. de Pablos J. Bone lengthening by means of physeal distraction. An experimental study. Int Orthop (SICOT). 1986;10:163–70.
4. Eralp L, Eran I. Distraction epiphysiolysis prior to resection of malignant bone tumour (Osteosarcoma). In: Limb lengthting and reconstruction surgery case atlas. Springer International Publishing; 2015.
5. San-Julian M, Vázquez-García B, Sierrasesúmaga L. Limb salvage in children. In: European surgical orthopaedics and traumatology. Springer Berlin Heidelberg; 2014. p. 4251–80. ISBN: 978-3-642-34745-0.
6. Xu S, Yu X, Xu M, Fu Z, Chen Y, Sun Y, Su Q. Limb function and quality of life after various reconstruction methods according to tumor location following resection of osteosarcoma in distal femur. BMC Musculoskelet Disord. 2014;15(1):453. doi:10.1186/1471-2474-15-453.
7. Zhang P, Feng F, Cai Q, Yao W, Gao S, Wang J, Wang X. Effects of metaphyseal bone tumor removal with preservation of the epiphysis and knee arthroplasty. Exp Ther Med. 2014;8(2): 567–72. Epub 2014 May 28.

Chapter 12
Clinical Results

Mikel San-Julian and Jose Canadell†

Abstract There were no cases of local recurrence in the retained epiphysis. The rate of complications was similar to that with other reconstruction procedures. The retained growth plate can continue growing. Functional results are excellent.

Keywords Overal survival • Local control • Recurrence rate • Functional results • Complications • Infection • Fracture • Non-union • Subsequent growth • Limb length discrepanvies

12.1 Control of Disease

In this chapter, we present a review of the clinical results obtained with the Cañadell technique for patients who were treated according to the protocol of treatment for osteosarcoma and Ewing's sarcoma at the Clínica Universidad de Navarra [28, 36, 37]. Mean follow up was 146 months (ranging from 12 to 366 months), and most patients were followed up for at least 2 years. There were no cases of local recurrence in the epiphyseal region, and only three cases of recurrence in the diaphysis, which occurred 18, 22 and 36 months after the operation. (A colleague working in Brazil has reported a case of local recurrence in the metaphysis; this occurred after reconstruction with recycled/sterilized tumoral bone [see Chap. 14].) The rate of local recurrence is actually lower than that for our complete series of osteosarcomas. This low rate might be explained under the hypothesis that tumors not crossing the physis are less aggressive than those that do. Another possible explanation is that these tumors contained within the metaphysis, without invasion of the physis, were diagnosed earlier (see Chap. 8). Aponte et al. [1] published similar results, but in their series they only included

Electronic supplementary material The online version of this chapter (doi:10.1007/978-3-319-24220-0_12) contains supplementary material, which is available to authorized users.

† Author was deceased at the time of publication

M. San-Julian, MD, PhD (✉) • J. Canadell†, MD, PhD
Department of Orthopaedic Surgery, University of Navarra, Pamplona, Navarra, Spain
e-mail: msjulian@unav.es

M. San-Julian (ed.), *Cañadell's Pediatric Bone Sarcomas: Epiphysiolysis before Excision*, DOI 10.1007/978-3-319-24220-0_12

osteosarcomas that responded well to chemotherapy, a finding that could be interpreted to support the hypothesis that tumors that do not cross the physis are less aggressive.

At present (2015), the disease-free survival rate is 85 %. This rate is slightly better than that for the overall series of osteosarcoma and Ewing's sarcoma patients treated in our hospital (Fig. 12.1); tumors that did not cross the physis may have been less aggressive than those that did. Other authors, reporting on surgery without preservation of the epiphysis in tumors that did not cross the physis, present similar results (85 % of survival) [21].

12.2 Histological Study of Margins

Previous studies by our team indicate that invasion of the epiphysis by a tumor seems to be a question of time: there is a hypervascularization reaction which leads to an early ossification of the growth plate, and after that the tumor transgresses the physis. However, for epiphysiolysis to be indicated, the tumor must not have crossed the physis. For the series of patients reported here, imaging methods accurately revealed whether or not the physis had been involved by the tumor.

Histological examination of resected pieces confirmed in all cases that the tumor had not involved the growth plate. We used Indian ink staining to study the physeal margin of resection, where – because at the rate of distraction employed (1 mm/day) the growth plate is disrupted at the degenerative layer of cells – there is a thin layer of growth plate cells covering the bone (Fig. 12.2). Note that the 1 mm/day rate of distraction results in most of the growth plate being retained with the epiphysis.

12.3 Limb Function (Videos 12.1 and 12.2)

In most patients, preservation of the epiphysis has resulted in an excellent functional outcome. In addition, the long-term complications of joint substitution are avoided [3–5, 29–31] (Figs. 12.2, 12.3, 12.4, 12.5, and 12.6). The rates and natures of complications due to reconstruction procedures are similar to those encountered with other limb salvage techniques.

12.4 Complications

12.4.1 Infection

This occurred in 7 % of patients, and therefore we conclude that the risk of infection is the same as in other limb salvage procedures. The risk is not higher because the external fixator is placed for only 10–15 days (Fig. 12.7). Most infections occurred

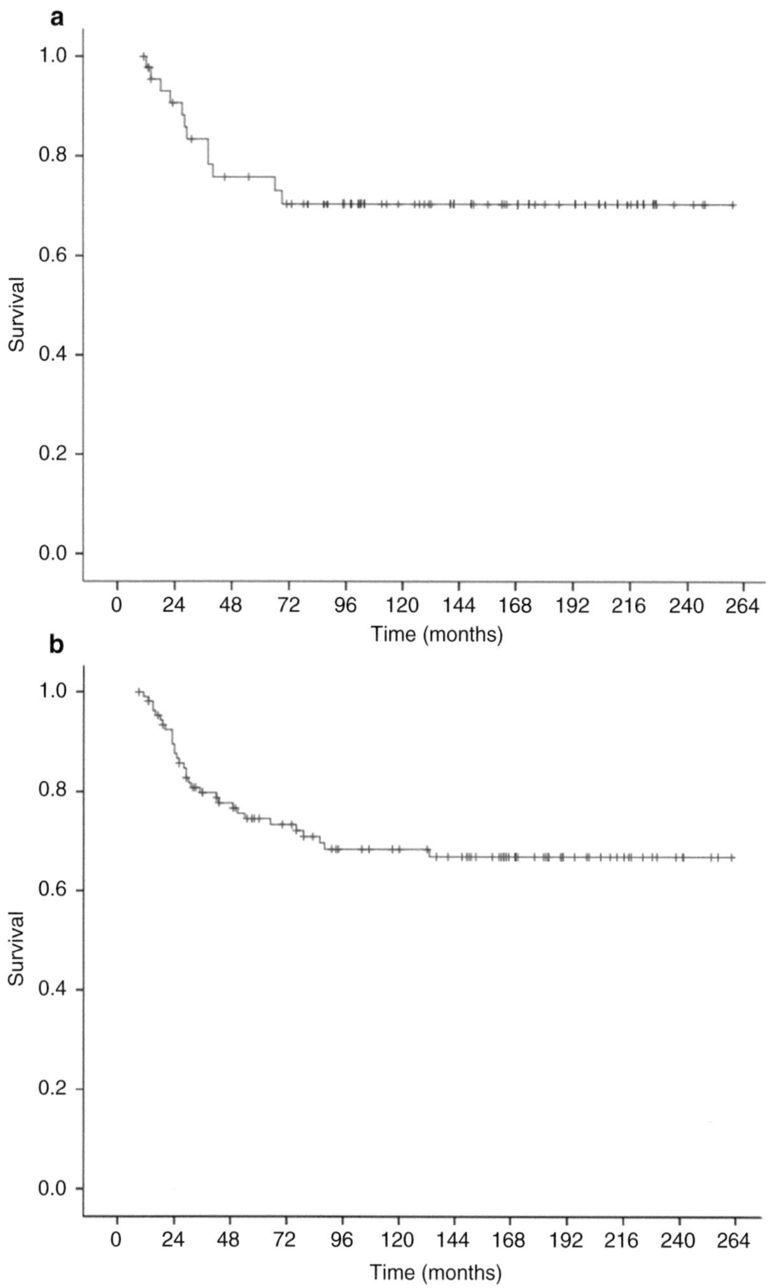

Fig. 12.1 Long term survival of osteosarcoma (**a**) and Ewing's sarcoma patients (**b**) treated at our institution. Percentage of DFS at 15 years is 72 % for osteosarcoma patients and 68 % for Ewing's sarcoma patients

after secondary operations performed in response to some other complication, such as, non-union or fracture of the graft. Therefore, in our series, infections were not related to the external fixator.

Of the cases with infection, some were cured by systemic antibiotic therapy, but most required removal of an allograft, reattachment of the external fixator, insertion of gentamicin-impregnated cement, systemic antibiotic therapy [8], and, after elimination of the infection, implantation of a new allograft. The risk of infection is higher in allografts in comparison to autografts. This is another reason

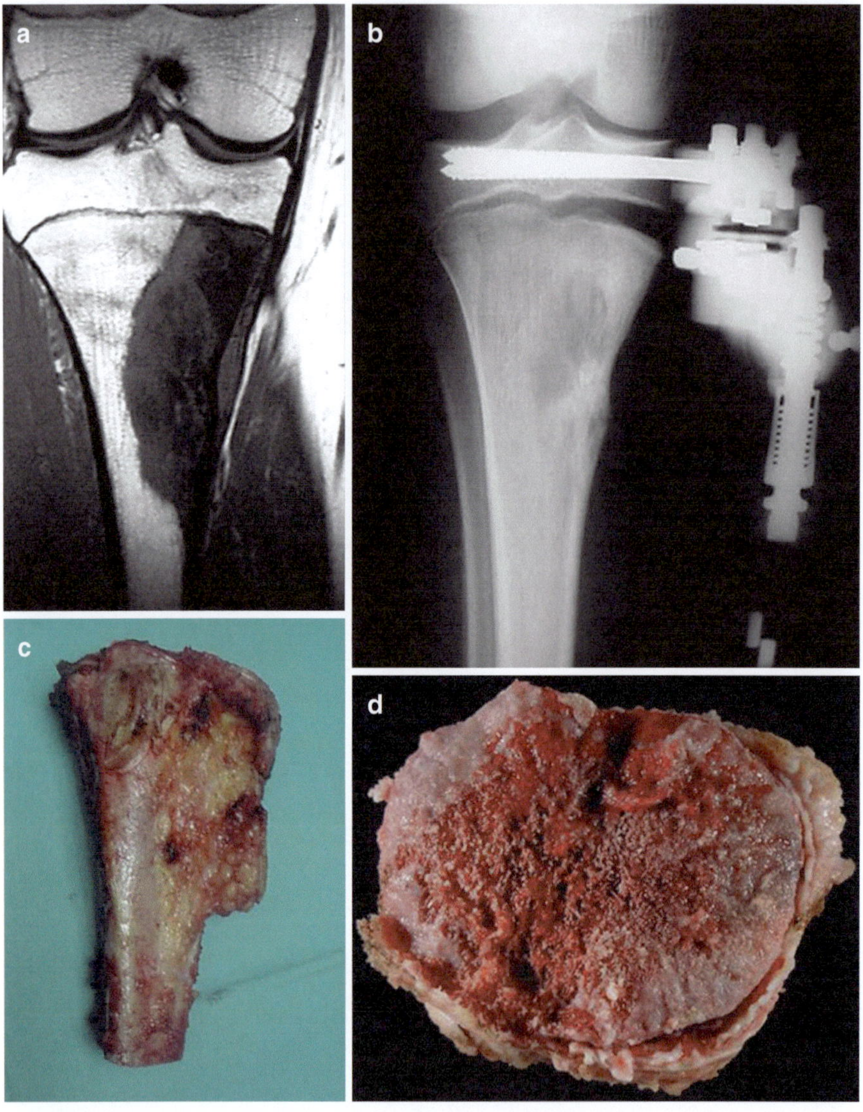

Fig. 12.2 Proximal tibia osteosarcoma apparently in contact with the growth plate. (**a**) After epiphysiolysis (**b**). This is, by definition, a wide margin (that is, there is no reactive tissue) (**c–f**)

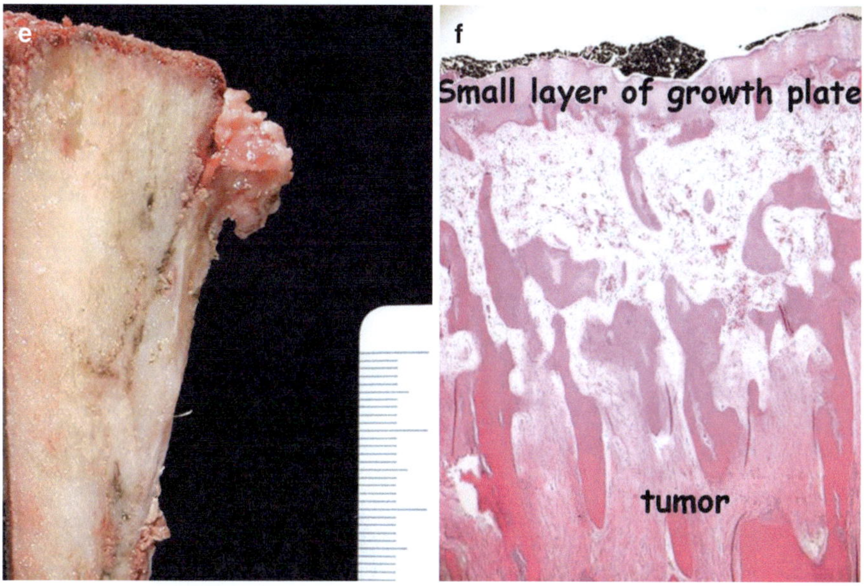

Fig. 12.2 (continued)

for choosing autografts for reconstruction in young children or after resection of small tumors.

12.4.2 Non-union of the Graft

About 14 % of patients required a further operation, with the addition of autologous grafts, to achieve union between the allograft and the host bone. Healing was achieved in all but one case.

12.4.3 Other Complications

As with other tumoral resection procedures, peroneal nerve palsy can occur; the neurotoxicity of chemotherapy is also involved in this palsy. Another complication is fracture of the united allograft, which can usually be successfully treated by osteosynthesis with a plate and screws and autologous graft.

Despite the number of complications, the results of intercalary reconstructions are better than those from other kinds of limb salvage surgery in growing children. The results published for old models of expandable prosthesis are generally poor. For example, recently, Manfrini et al. [15] reported that nine out of ten expandable prostheses required revision surgery (in some cases even twice) before the end of growth. The high price of expandable prostheses is another important factor to take into account. Nowadays, however, results are improving as new models are developed (see Chap. 3).

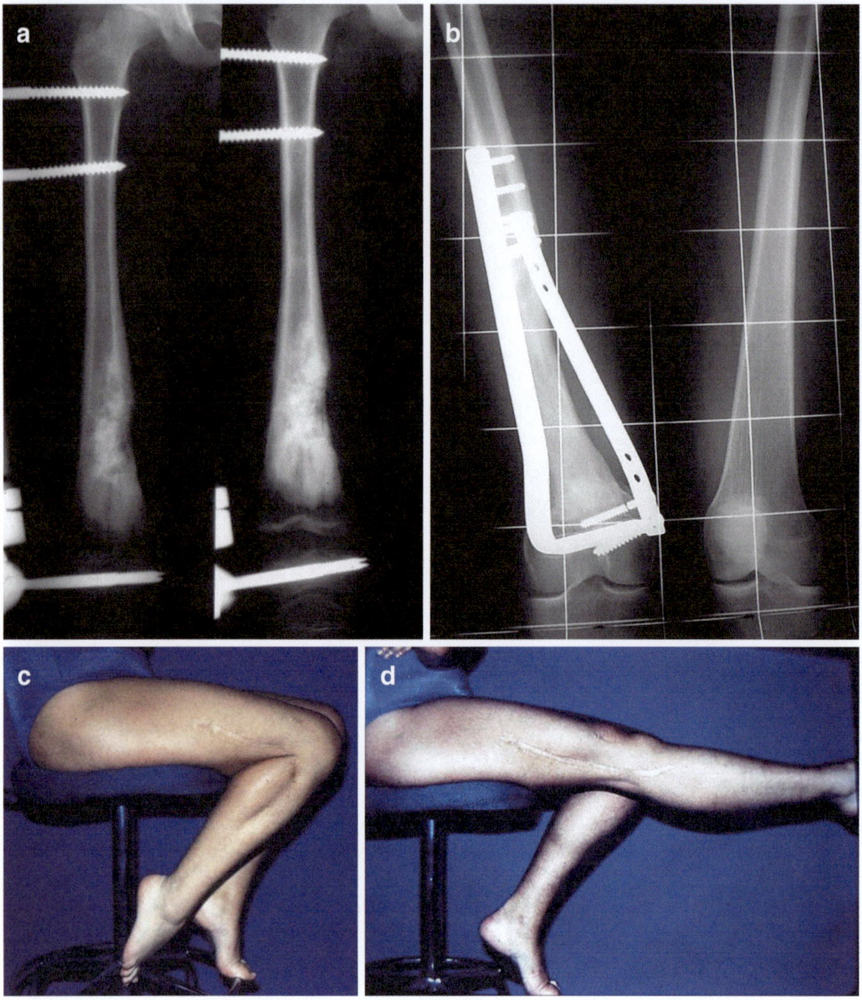

Fig. 12.3 (**a**) Physeal distraction in a metaphyseal osteosarcoma of the femur. (**b**) The reconstruction was carried out with autografts from the tibia and iliac crests. Twenty-three years after operation, the joint (**b**) and the functional results (**c**, **d**) remain excellent

12.5 Incorporation of Graft

Before 1986, as we did not have a bone bank, we used autografts from the ipsilateral or contralateral tibia, and iliac crests (Fig. 12.8). Since 1986, for most patients with big tumors [32–34], we have used allografts [25].

The use of autografts resulted in an average of 2.8 operations per patient before graft consolidation [6, 40]. With allografts this average was reduced to 0.74, but it should be noted that patients were affected by other complications.

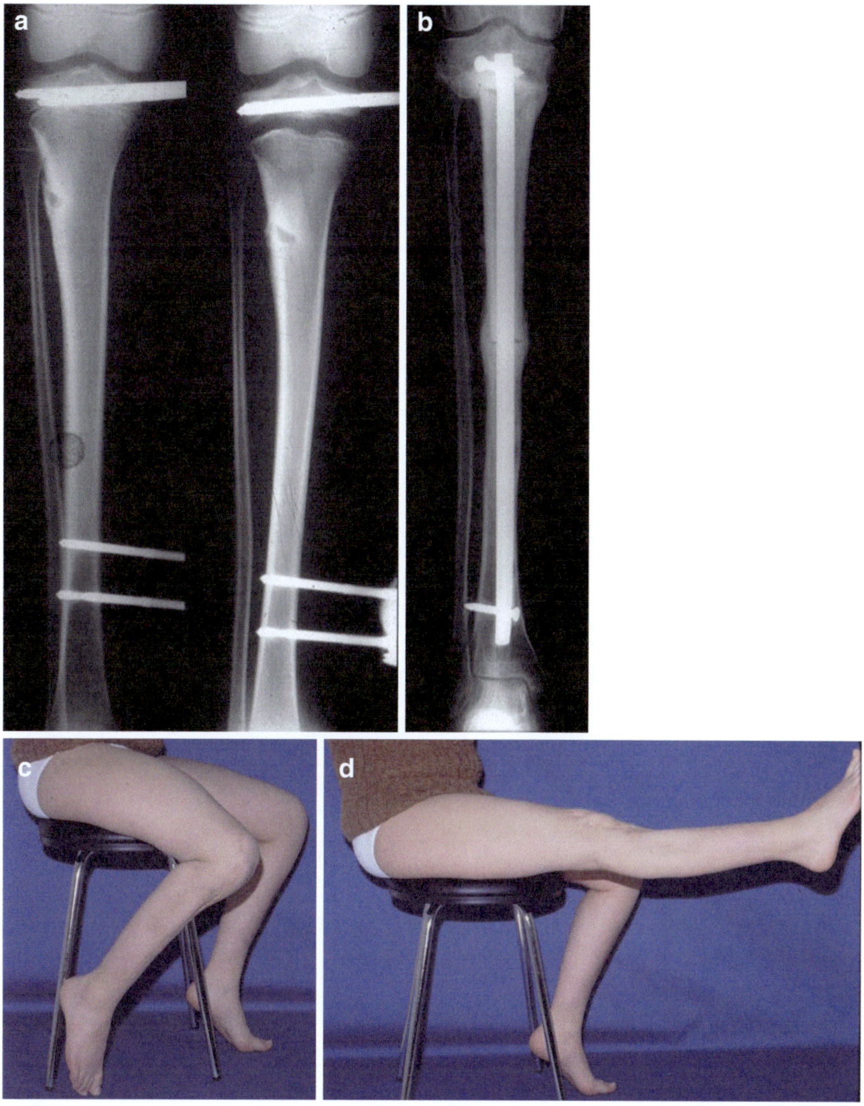

Fig. 12.4 (**a**) Ewing's sarcoma in the proximal metaphysis of the tibia. Physeal distraction was performed. (**b**) The reconstruction was carried out with an intercalary allograft. (**c**, **d**) Functional result

Consolidation at the metaphysis generally occurred before 6 months had elapsed, but at the diaphyseal end it often took longer than a year. In metaphyseal unions we used several types of osteosynthesis devices, such as, Kirschner wires, Enders, screws, and staples. Diaphyseal osteotomy and osteosynthesis devices are discussed at the end of this chapter.

Since 1987, at the Clínica Universidad de Navarra, we have used more than 1000 massive bone allografts in the conservative treatment of malignant bone tumors.

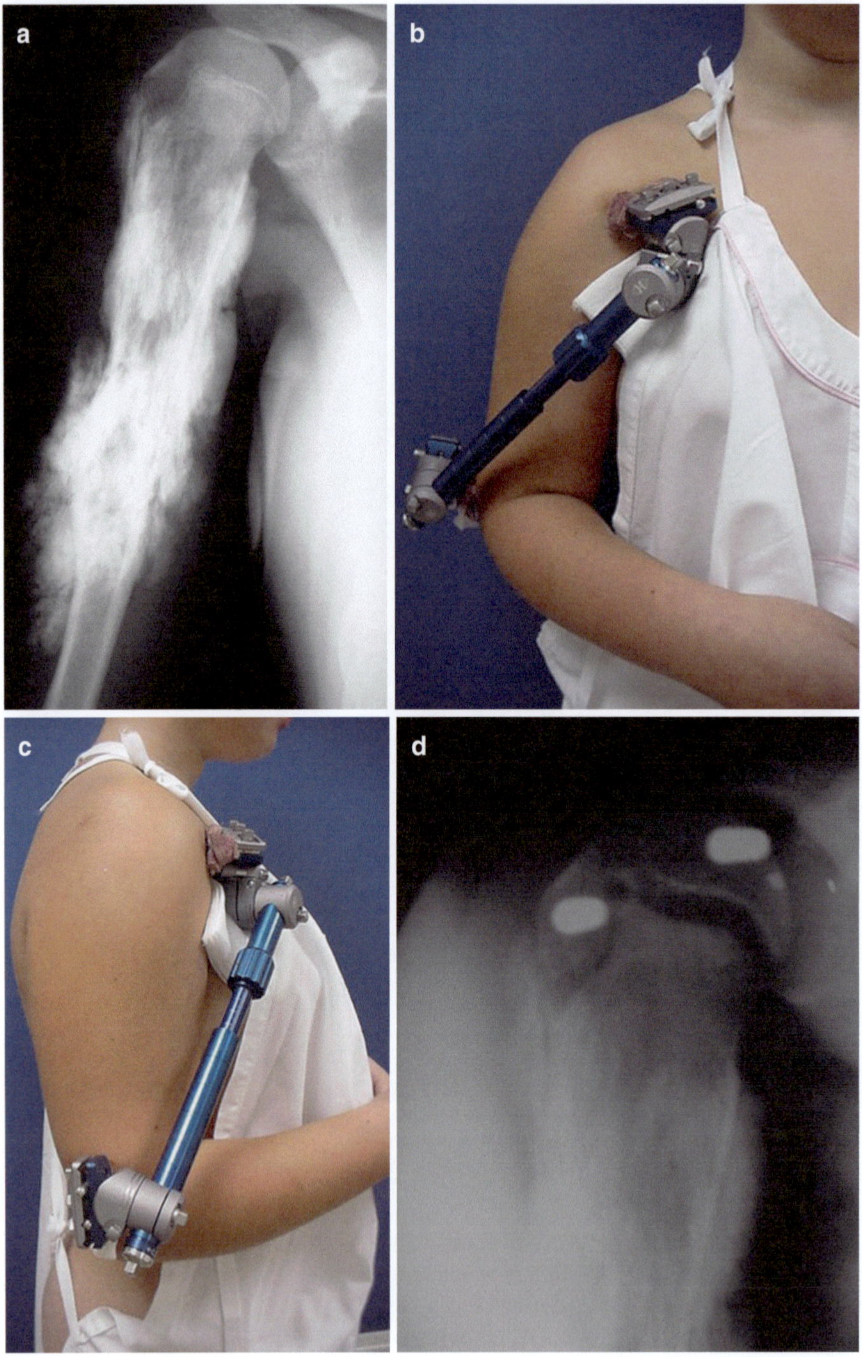

Fig. 12.5 (**a–c**) In the proximal humerus, due to the particular morphology of this growth plate, the pins should be placed anteriorly in the humeral head (see also Fig. 7.7), and posteriolaterally in the distal part, in order to avoid radial nerve damage. (**d**) After distraction, reconstruction was carried out (**e**) with an allograft. (**f**) Because it was possible to preserve the joint, the attachment of the rotator cuff and the axillary nerve, abduction of the shoulder is almost complete

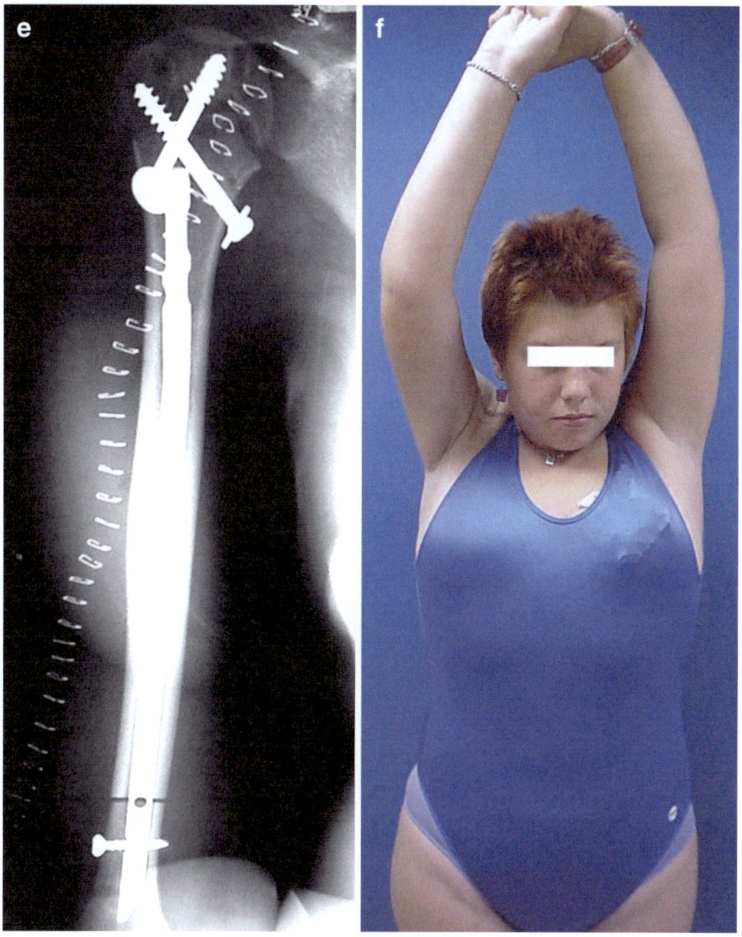

Fig. 12.5 (continued)

The allograft type used depended on how the cartilage growth plate was affected and on the possibilities of preserving the joint near the tumor.

Monthly radiological follow-ups were carried out during the first year of systemic chemotherapy, with diagnostic studies to assess the local and systemic control of disease. Afterwards, follow-ups were every 3 months for another year, and subsequently every 6 months. In all cases, chemotherapy and radiotherapy were in accordance with the hospital's cancer protocol [36] for the type of tumor.

12.5.1 Radiological Study

We used the ISOLS criteria (Table 12.1) to evaluate consolidation results [20] and analyzed the following factors which can influence consolidation: host and donor age, allograft length and location, osteotomy and osteosynthesis type, intra-arterial

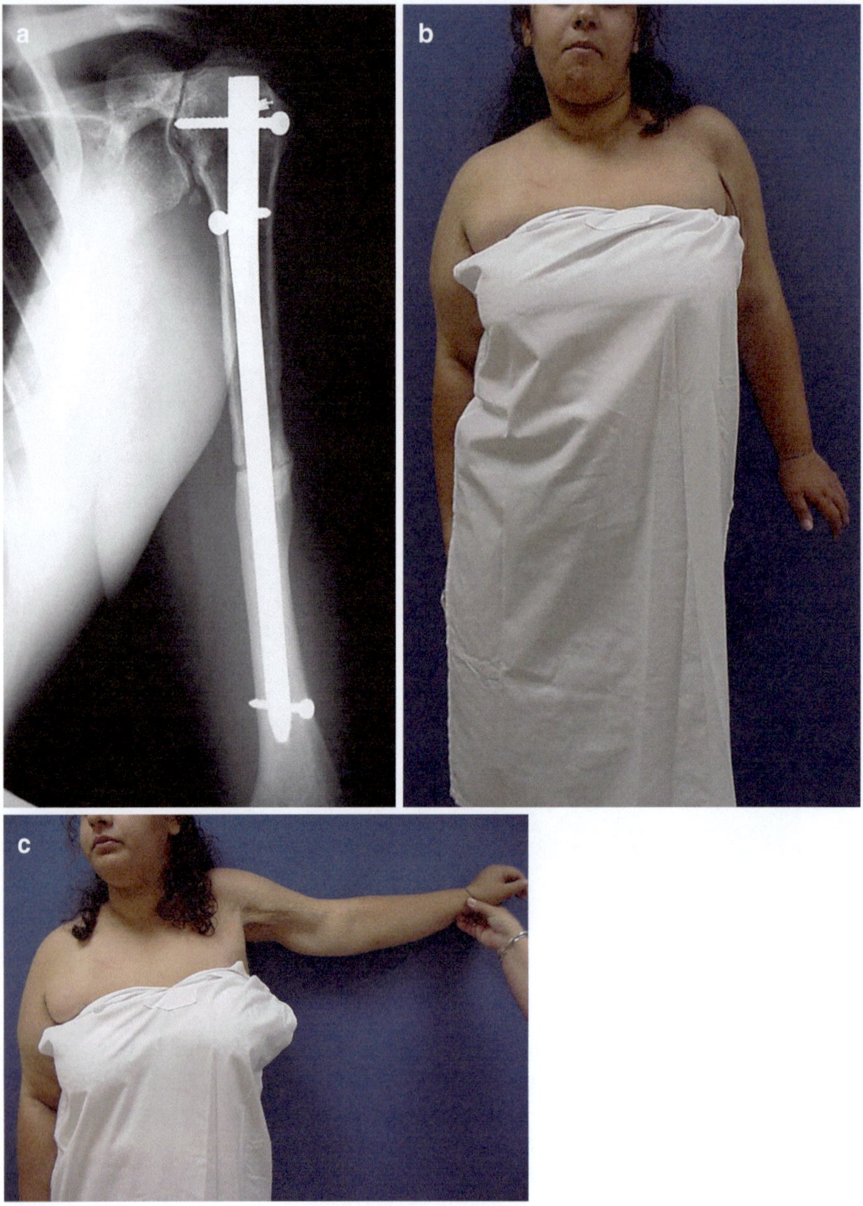

Fig. 12.6 (**a**) Osteoarticular allograft for reconstruction of the shoulder after resection of a Ewing's sarcoma in the proximal humerus. When the joint cannot be preserved, abduction of the shoulder, both active (**b**) and passive (**c**), is poor

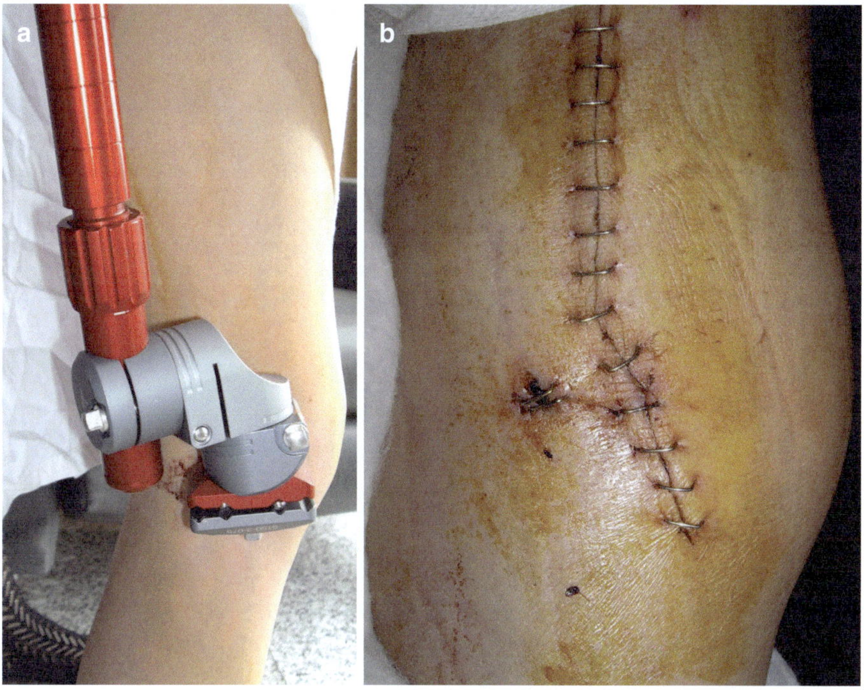

Fig. 12.7 (**a**) The risk of infection is not higher because the external fixator is only in place for 10–15 days. (**b**) In this case, one pin tract was removed in the surgical approach

and systemic chemotherapy, and intraoperative and external radiotherapy. We performed a multi-variant statistical analysis with StatView software.

The mean consolidation time of metaphyseal osteotomies (including those cases in which physeal distraction was used before excision of the tumor) was 6.5 months; none of the factors studied had a statistically significant influence on consolidation. In metaphyseal osteotomies consolidation was achieved with minimal osteosynthesis (Fig. 12.9).

The mean consolidation time of diaphyseal osteotomies was 16 months (Fig. 12.10). We found no statistically significant differences in consolidation with the use of intra-arterial chemotherapy, intraoperative radiotherapy, donor age, osteosynthesis type (plates vs. intramedullary devices), osteotomy type (horizontal vs. oblique), type of tumor, or location of the tumor.

The mean consolidation time of metaphyseal osteotomies (6.5 months) is similar to that reported by others [16, 39]. Systemic chemotherapy delayed consolidation and this finding is supported by clinical data from other series [9–11, 17, 37, 38]. Experimental studies [14, 42] have also demonstrated that chemotherapeutic agents impair bone healing, and that allogeneic cortical bone grafts incorporate more slowly when chemotherapy is administered. External radiation also delayed consolidation. Radiation damages small and medium-sized blood vessels that supply nutrients to the bone, making it more difficult for the irradiated bone to heal [12].

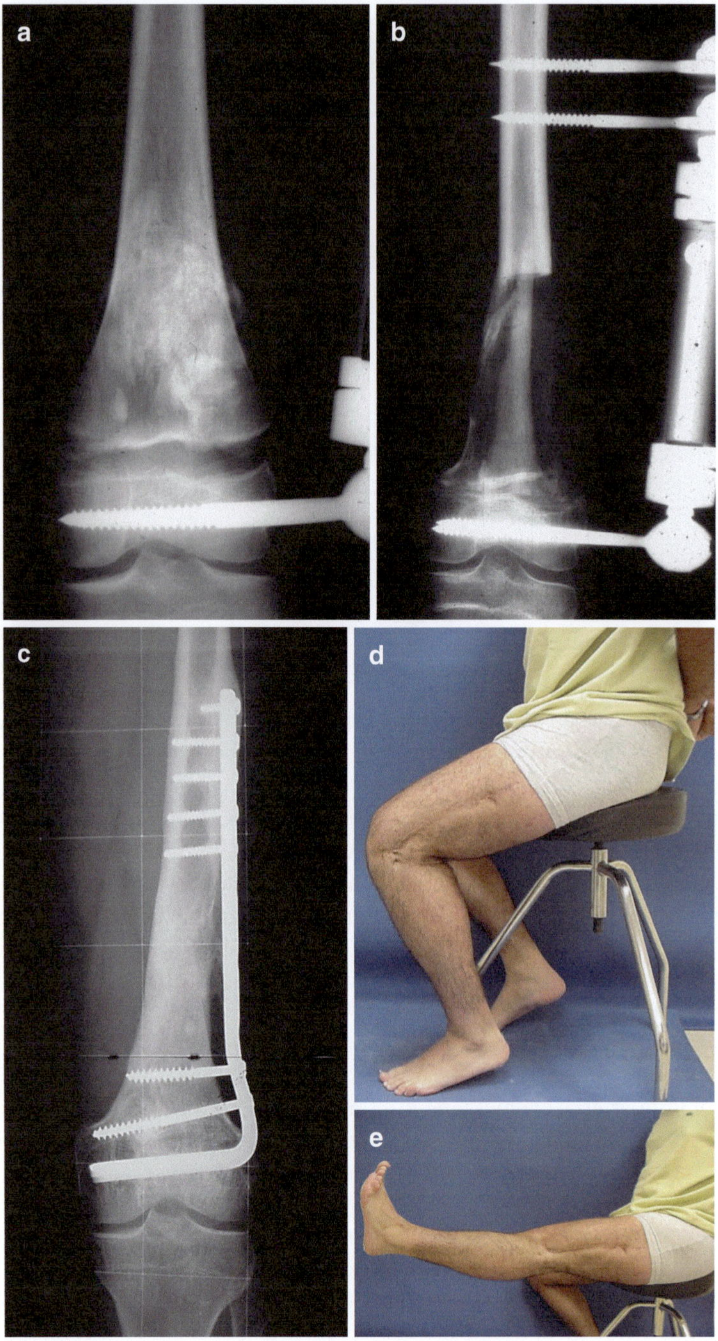

Fig. 12.8 (**a**) Radiograph showing an osteosarcoma of the femur in a 14-year-old boy after physeal distraction. (**b**) After resection of the tumor and autografting from the left tibia. The same frame was used for stabilizing the graft. (**c**) Twenty-two years later, the knee joint has an excellent aspect. (**d, e**) The function of the knee remains excellent. This patient plays sports without restrictions

Table 12.1 ISOLS criteria regarding fusion of allografts

Excellent: Fusion complete. Osteotomy line not visible
Good: Fusion >75 %. Osteotomy line still visible
Fair: Fusion 25–75 %
Poor: Fusion <25 %. No evidence of callus

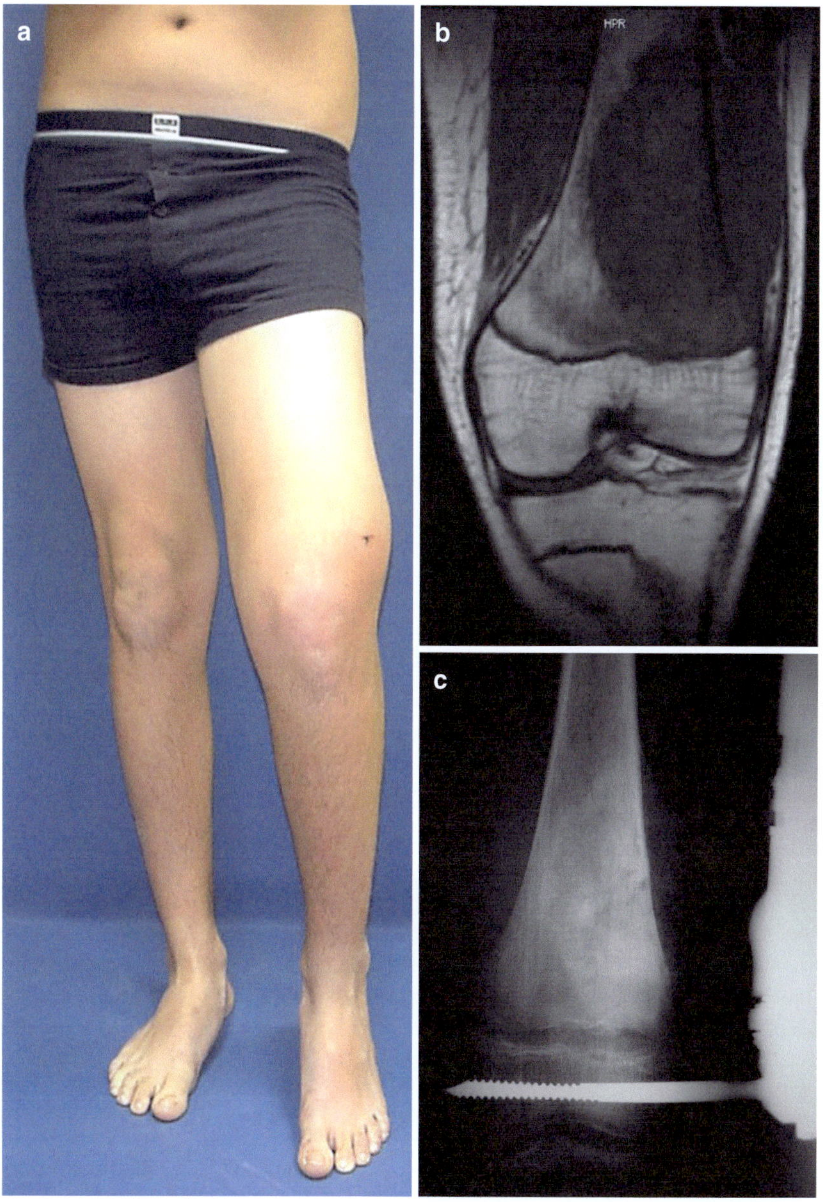

Fig. 12.9 (**a**, **b**) Osteosarcoma in the distal metaphysis of the femur of a 14-year-old boy. (**c**) Physeal distraction was performed and (**d**) an intercalary allograft was used for reconstruction. The healing at the distal junction was achieved with two Kirschner wires, while the diaphyseal junction required stronger osteosynthesis. (**e**) The same patient surfing

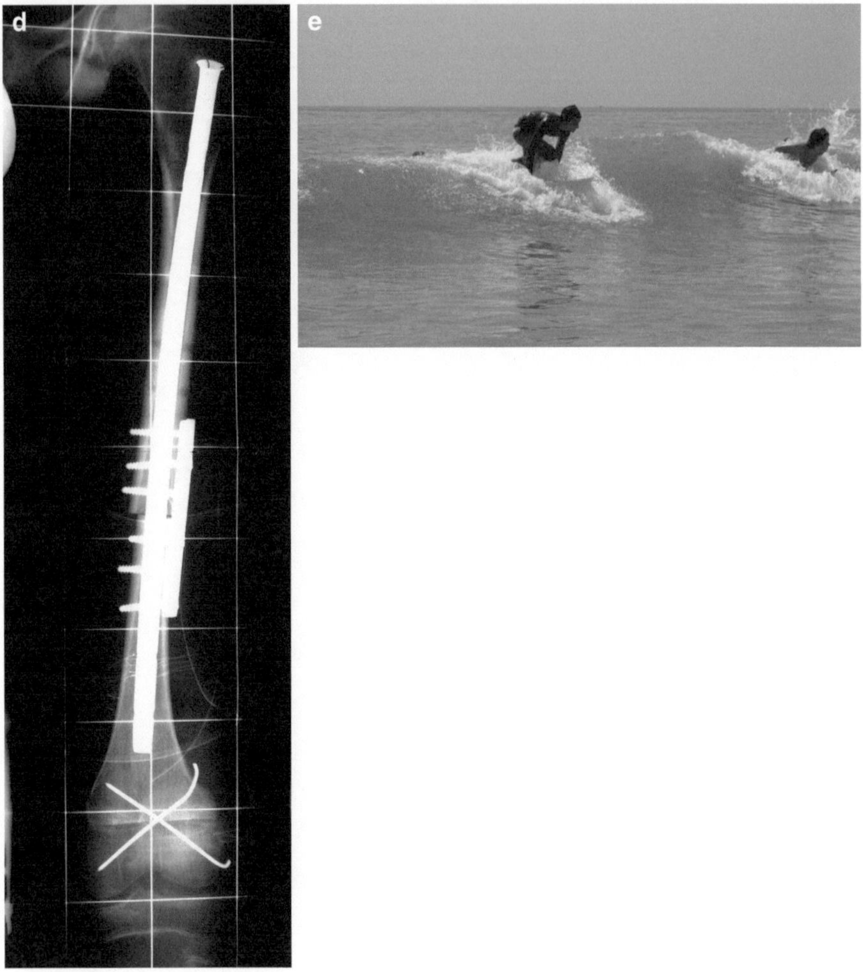

Fig. 12.9 (continued)

Bone growth retardation resulting from irradiation is clearly a dose-dependent phenomenon [2, 13, 22, 41]. We believe that if the fracture of an allograft can heal with a standard treatment for fractures, it is because the allograft is revascularized at the time of the fracture [24].

12.5.2 Isotopic Study

In 36 patients a prospective isotopic study was performed [27] with 99mTc MDP in order to evaluate the revascularization of allografts. Bone scintigraphy with 99mTc HDP was performed 3 h after injection. Anterior and posterior views over both

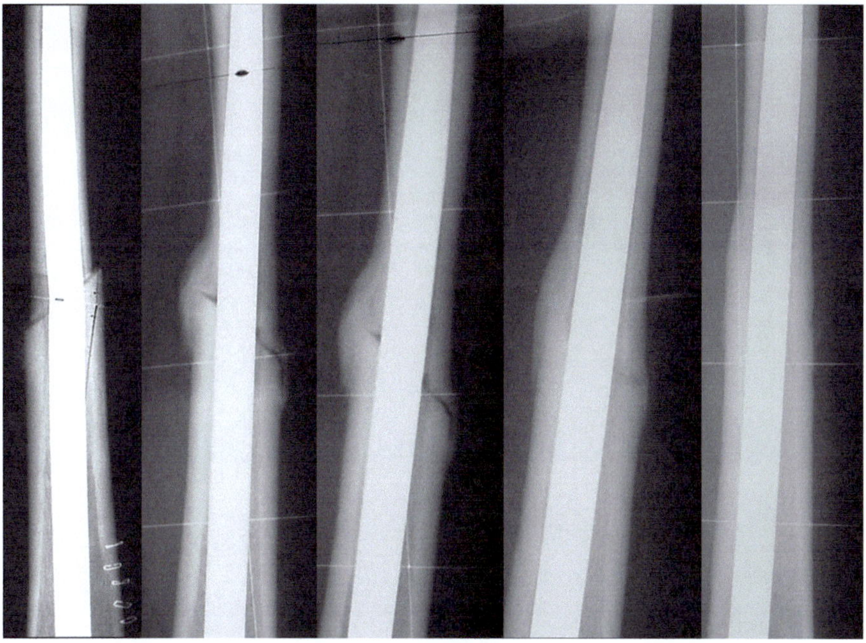

Fig. 12.10 Excellent fusion in a diaphyseal allograft-host bone junction

limbs were evaluated qualitatively by two physicians. Semi-quantitative measurements were performed with a region of interest (ROI) technique. Labeling was scored by location: over the bone allograft (A1); over the area just above the allograft (A2); as A1 but in opposite limb (A3); as (A2) but in opposite limb (A4). Background over soft tissues was considered and subtracted from all the ROIs. The allograft uptake was related with the uptake over A2 and A3, and two indices were obtained: I1 = A1/A2 and I2 = A1/A3. A further index, A2/A4, was also calculated.

All patients showed objective uptake of the 99mTc-MDP (Fig. 12.11). The values of the allograft/host bone index were conditioned by the allograft site and by the analyzed areas. As in normal bone, uptake in the metaphysis and the epiphysis was greater than in the diaphysis. Areas over an allograft with an intramedullary nail showed less uptake than the contralateral area. In areas near an allograft, uptake was greater surrounding the osteosynthesis device, due to increased metabolism. In most cases, the allograft-host bone junction showed more uptake. Five patients suffered fracture of their allograft; no relation was found between uptake indices and fracture. Uptake was greater in allografts with longer follow-ups.

The isotopic study showed objective uptake in all the allografts, and this uptake increased with time since grafting. Uptake can be related to allograft revascularization and demonstrates active metabolism in the allograft. The uptake pattern is similar to that of normal bone. The high uptake at the allograft-host bone junction in the cases subjected to study shortly after grafting can be attributed to metabolic processes associated with the healing process. This study also allowed us to evaluate activity of the retained growth plate (Fig. 12.11).

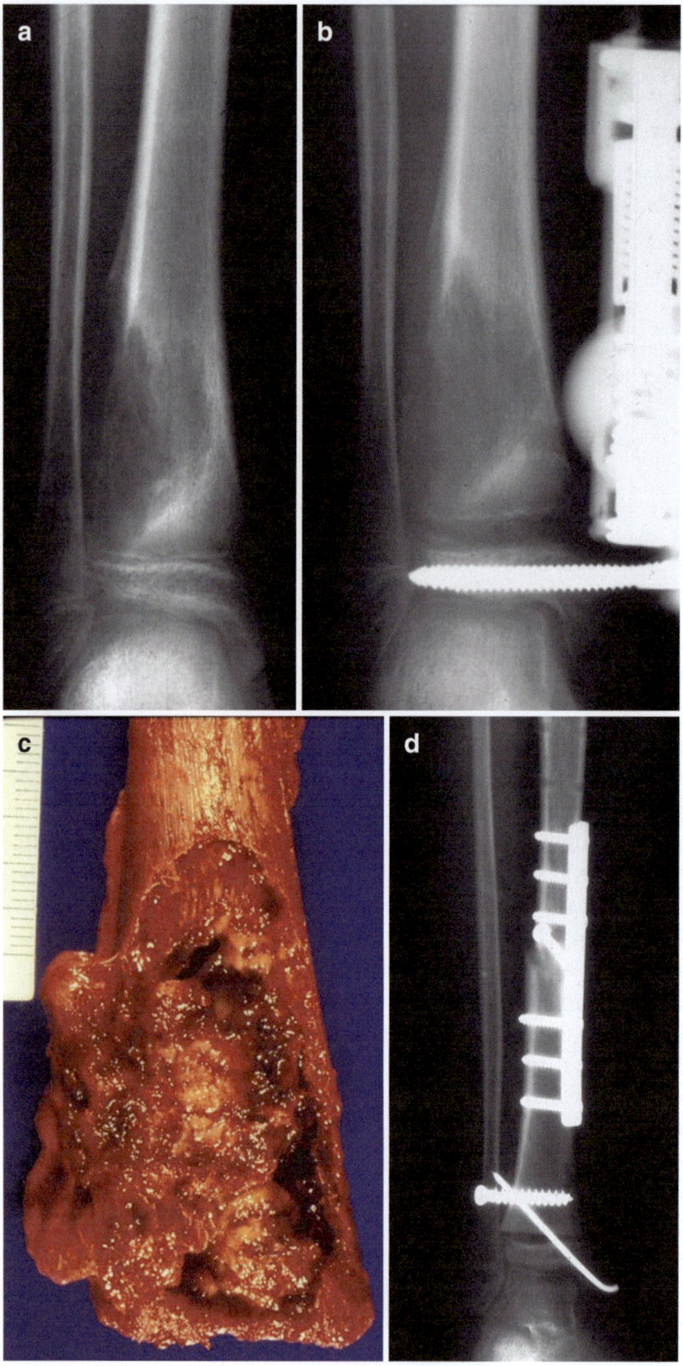

Fig. 12.11 (**a**) Telangiectatic osteosarcoma in the distal tibia of a 10-year-old girl. (**b**) Physeal distraction was performed before excision (**c**) of the tumor. (**d**) Reconstruction was carried out with an intercalary allograft. (**e**) Three years after surgery, the growth plate remains active. Isotopic uptake in the allograft is similar to that in the contralateral tibia. (**f**, **g**) This patient has no dissymmetry 12 years after treatment

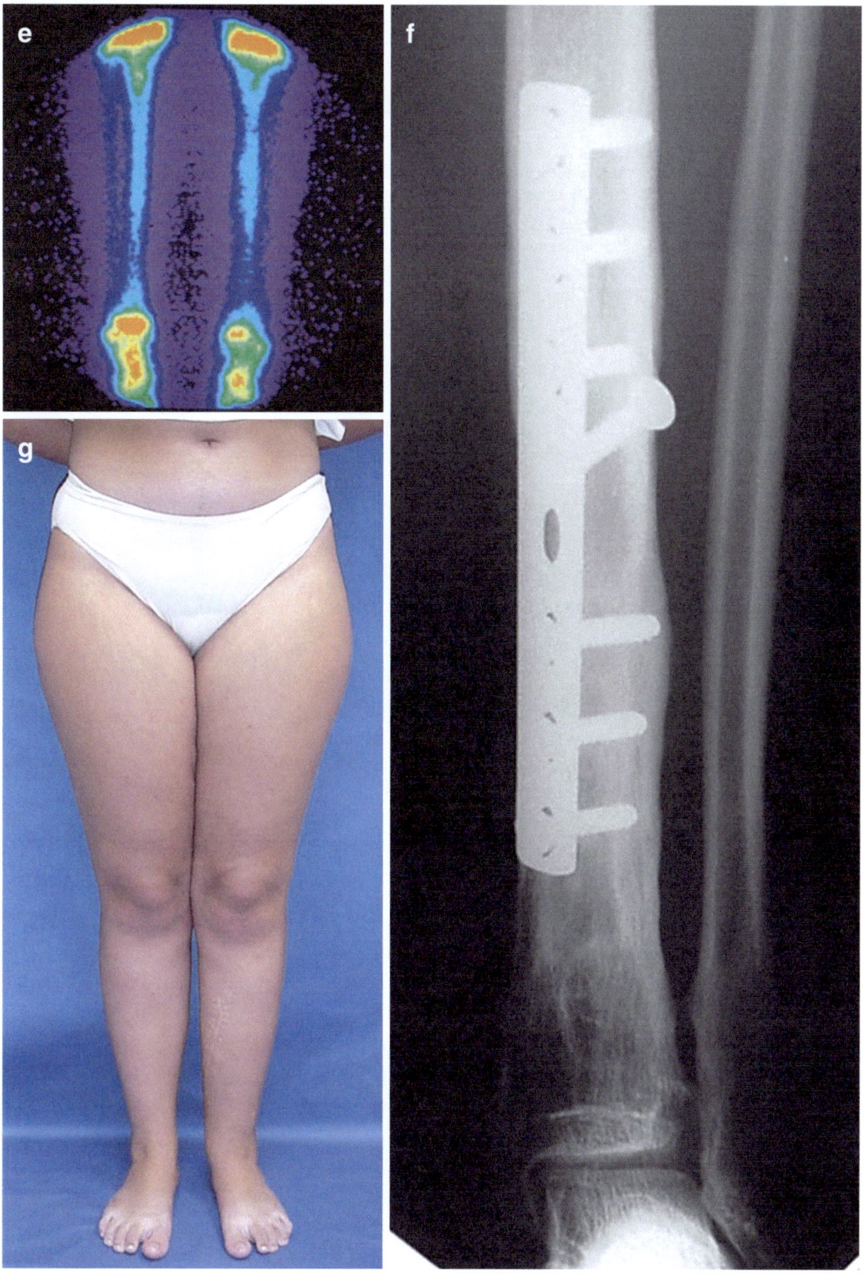

Fig. 12.11 (continued)

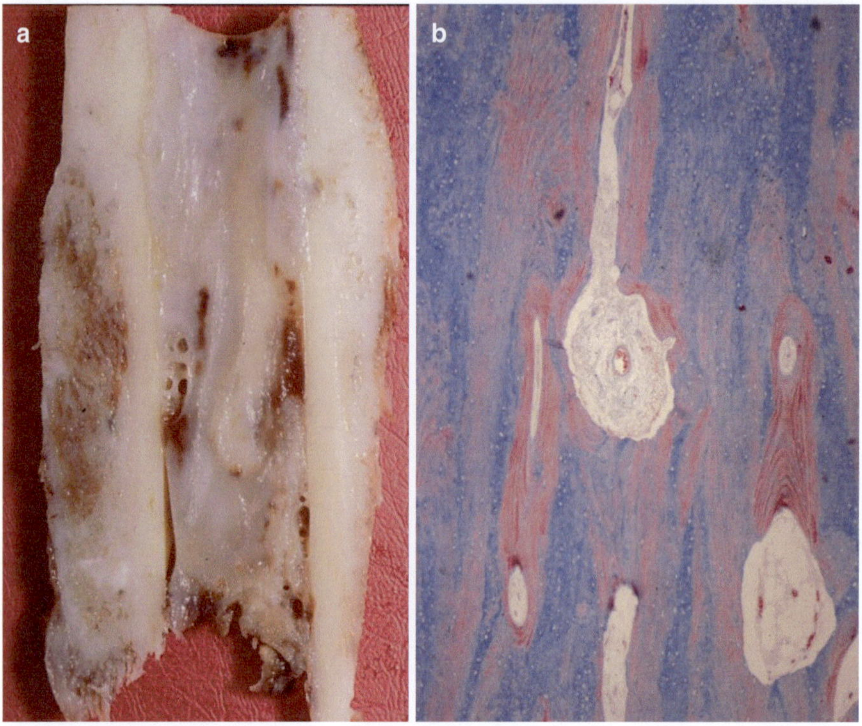

Fig. 12.12 (**a**) Macroscopic image of the periosteal callus at the allograft-host bone junction. (**b**) Masson's Trichrome staining of a retrieved allograft, showing vessels into the cortex of the graft

12.5.3 Histological Study

In order to study allograft incorporation, retrieved allografts and especially their allograft-host bone junction area were examined histologically. In some cases, patients received tetracycline (Tetra-Hubber®) for 4–6 days before removal of the allograft.

In all cases, the healing process at the allograft-host bone junction involved periosteal callus from the receptor bone (Fig. 12.12). Histological examination of allografts revealed necrotic bone, except in the areas near the host bone, and an external surface invaded by vascular buds from adjacent soft tissue.

Apart from showing healing progressing by periosteal callus, these histological studies confirmed the findings of the isotopic study regarding the revascularization of allografts from the surrounding tissue.

12.6 Subsequent Growth

When treating a bone sarcoma, an orthopedic surgeon's first concern is to preserve the life of the patient. In most cases, the surgeon can also preserve the limb, although there is little sense in preserving a limb if it will be non-functional. Better functional

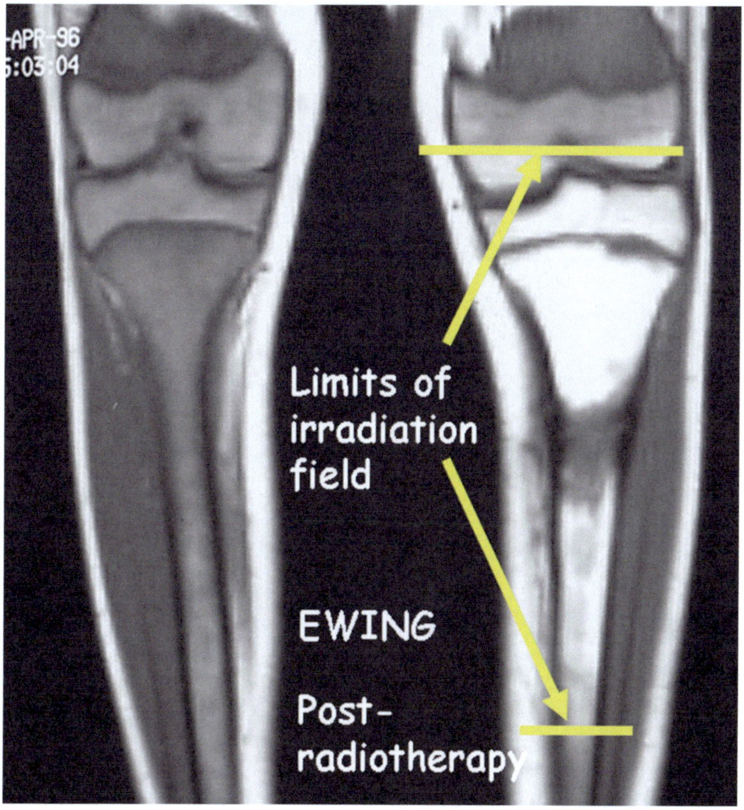

Fig. 12.13 This Ewing's sarcoma in the proximal left tibia was treated by preoperative radiotherapy. Note the limits of the irradiation field in comparison with the right tibia. The preservation of this growth plate would not prevent a limb length discrepancy

results are achieved when the joint of the patient can be preserved. When treating children and considering how to conserve functionality, it also necessary to bear in mind the future growth of the limb.

Subsequent growth of a limb is not only affected by the surgical technique employed in terms of the resection of one or more growth plates. Even in cases where the growth plate is left intact, the osteosynthesis device or radiotherapy [18–20, 35] could cause arrest of growth (Fig. 12.13). In addition, high doses of chemotherapy have been reported to cause a decrease in GH secretion.

In the last few years, various different methods to preserve the joint of a patient with a metaphyseal bone tumor have been described. Physeal distraction before excision of the tumor, as described by Cañadell in 1984, has, in our opinion, the advantage of safety: the growth plate is not a flat plane, but an irregular surface, and therefore an intra-epiphyseal osteotomy could leave parts of the tumor. Furthermore, with Cañadell's physeal distraction the whole epiphysis can be preserved, thereby increasing the joint's stability; facilitating resection and osteosynthesis of the graft; and avoiding damage to the femoropatellar joint in distal femur tumors, patellar tendon attachment in proximal tibia tumors, or the rotator cuff in

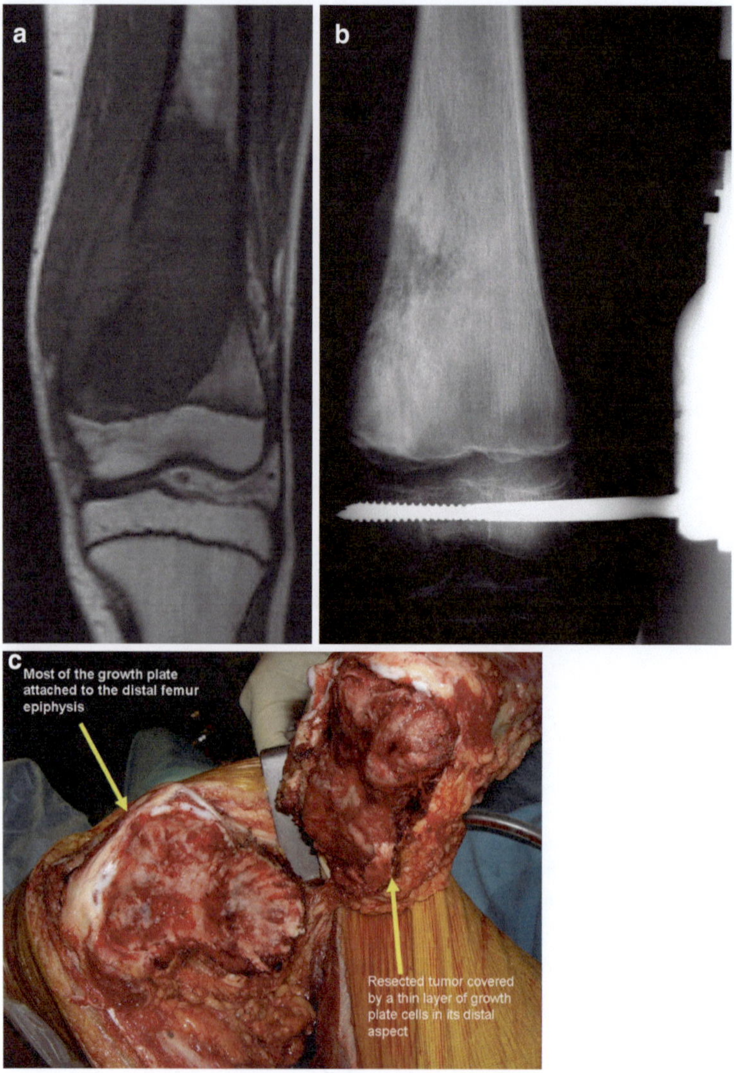

Fig. 12.14 (**a**) This osteosarcoma in the distal femur does not involve the growth plate, as shown on the MRI. (**b**) Epiphysiolysis was performed. (**c**) Intraoperative view during resection showing the epiphysis covered by a white surface, the growth plate, preservation of which can allow potential for growth. A thin layer of growth plate cells covers the resected tumor, and this constitutes a wide margin. Note the undulations in the growth plate

proximal humerus tumors. Finally, physeal distraction before excision can preserve most of the growth plate because the physis breaks in the metaphyseal border of the growth plate as a result of the degenerative lack of cells there (Figs. 12.14, 12.15, and 12.16).

Physeal distraction is indicated in cases of metaphyseal bone tumors in children when the growth plate is still open and the surgeon is sure that the tumor has not invaded the epiphysis. Other applications for external fixation in tumoral cases include distraction callotasis for limb length discrepancy, tumor resection and bone transport, combined distraction callotasis and compression for limb length discrepancy, and concurrent diaphyseal non-union.

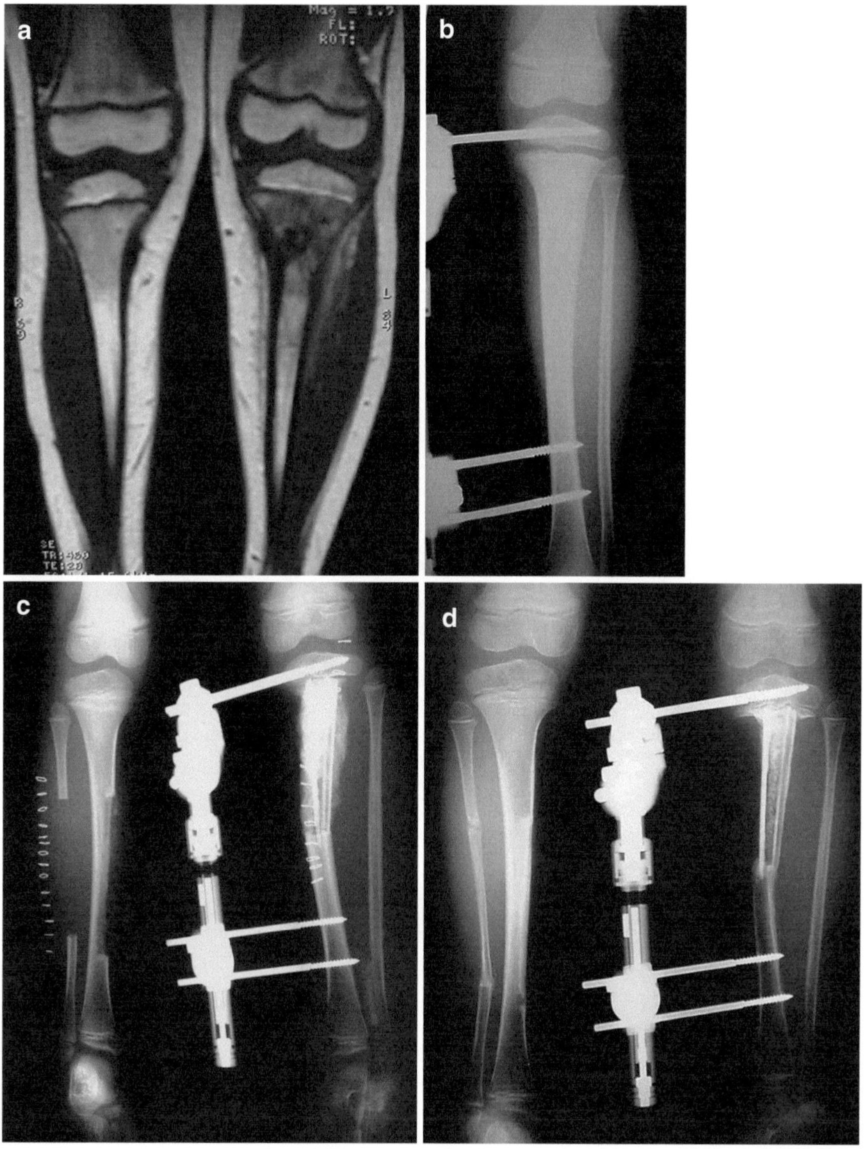

Fig. 12.15 (**a**) A Ewing's sarcoma in the proximal metaphysis of the left tibia of a 4-year-old girl. (**b**) After distraction (**c**), reconstruction was performed with an autograft from the contralateral tibia and fibula. (**d**) After healing of the graft, the external fixator was removed. Details of the preserved growth plate after resection (**e**), after healing of the graft (**f**), and 4 years later (**g**), showing normal growth. (**h**) Bone scan showing normal uptake in the distracted physis, 4 years post-op

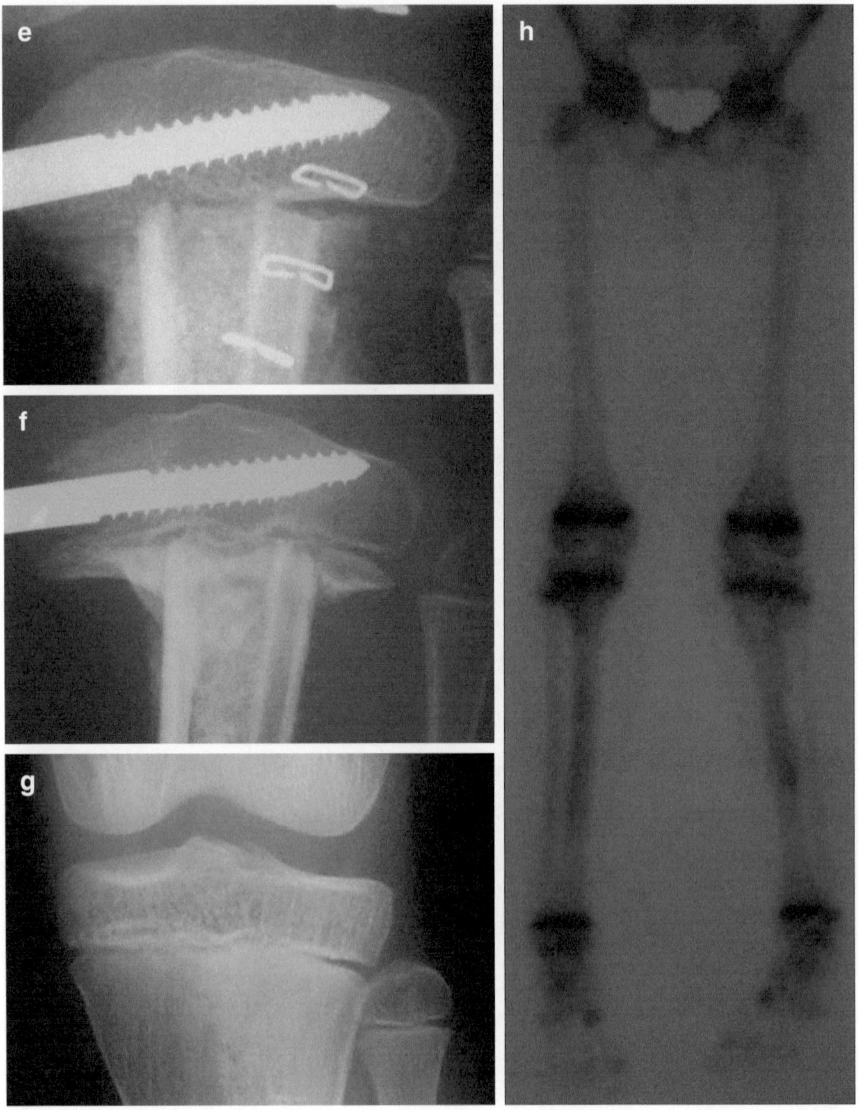

Fig. 12.15 (continued)

Distraction callotasis [23] was indicated in patients with serious dissymmetry (more than 4 cm) who had been free of disease for at least 3 years after the first limb salvage procedure [7]. The average age for this procedure was 17 years. Other patients with limb length discrepancy had equalization by other means, such as, epiphysiodesis on the contralateral limb or changing of the allograft (Fig. 12.17). The mean length gained was 9.5 cm (in the range of 7–12 cm) with an average healing index of 34 days/cm. The Mankin limb function grade was excellent or good in 63 % of the cases.

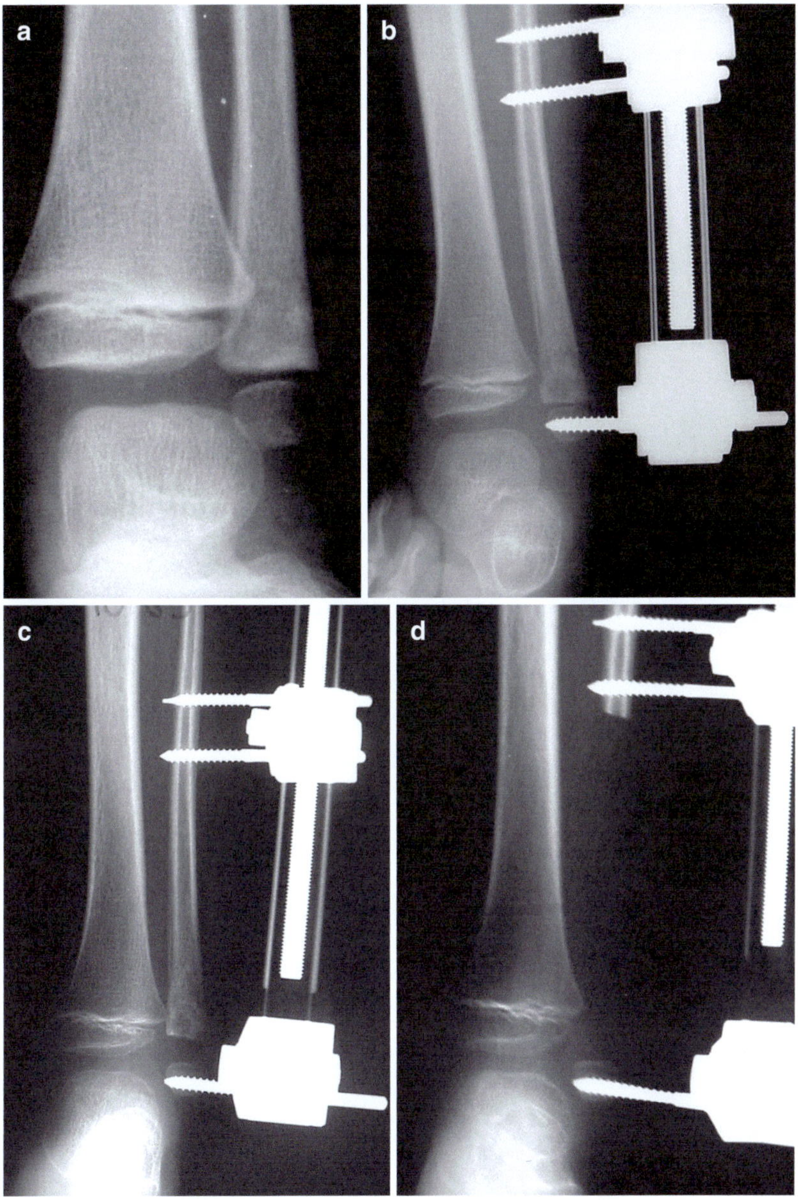

Fig. 12.16 (**a**) A Ewing's sarcoma in the distal metaphysis of the left fibula of a 4-year-old boy. In 1985, given the age of the patient, many orthopedic surgeons would have considered an amputation. (**b**, **c**) However, we performed a physeal distraction. (**d**) The tumor was resected, and the external fixator was maintained until histological assessment corroborated that the tumor did not involve the growth plate: in 1985 MRI was not available. (**e**) The limb was reconstructed with a graft. Note the Kirschner wire protruding a few centimeters below the joint. (**f**) 12 years later the ankle was still normal. The Kirschner wire has gone up, demonstrating the normal growth of this physis. (**g**) This is a comparative X-ray of the two ankles taken in 2007. (**h**–**j**) After 22 years the patient has no dis-symmetry and function is normal; the patient plays soccer for his local village team

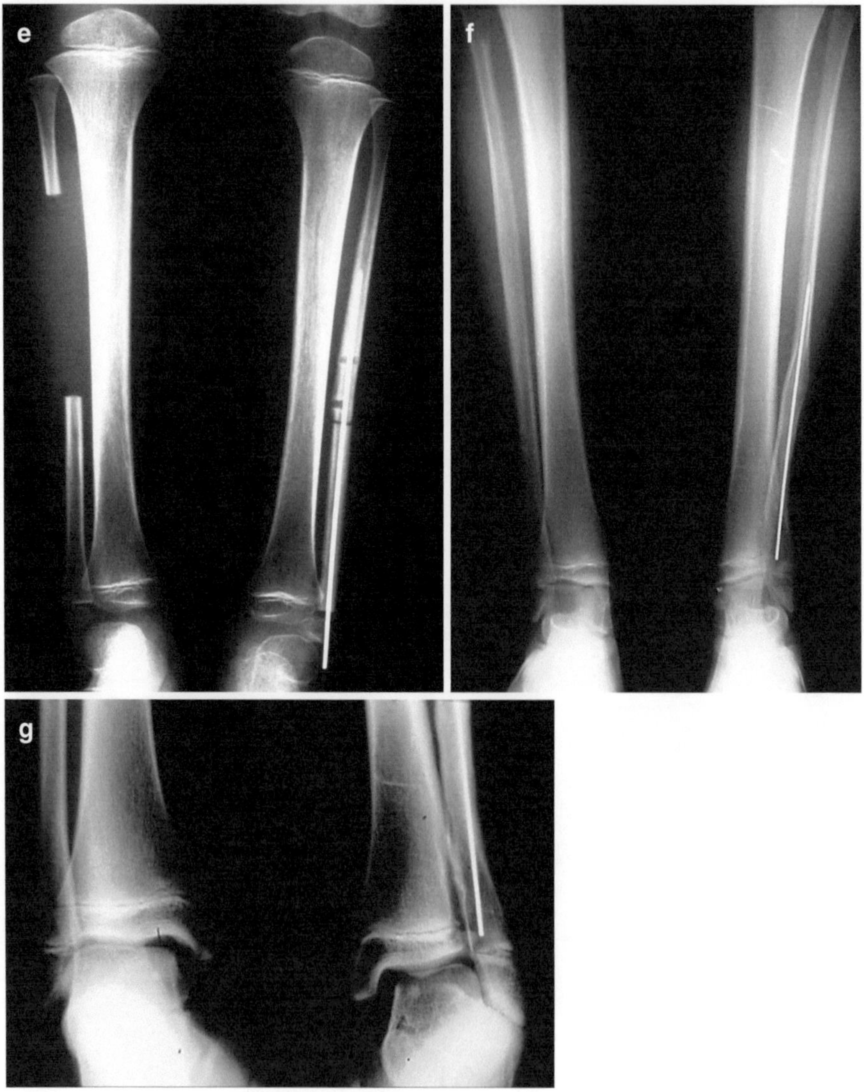

Fig. 12.16 (continued)

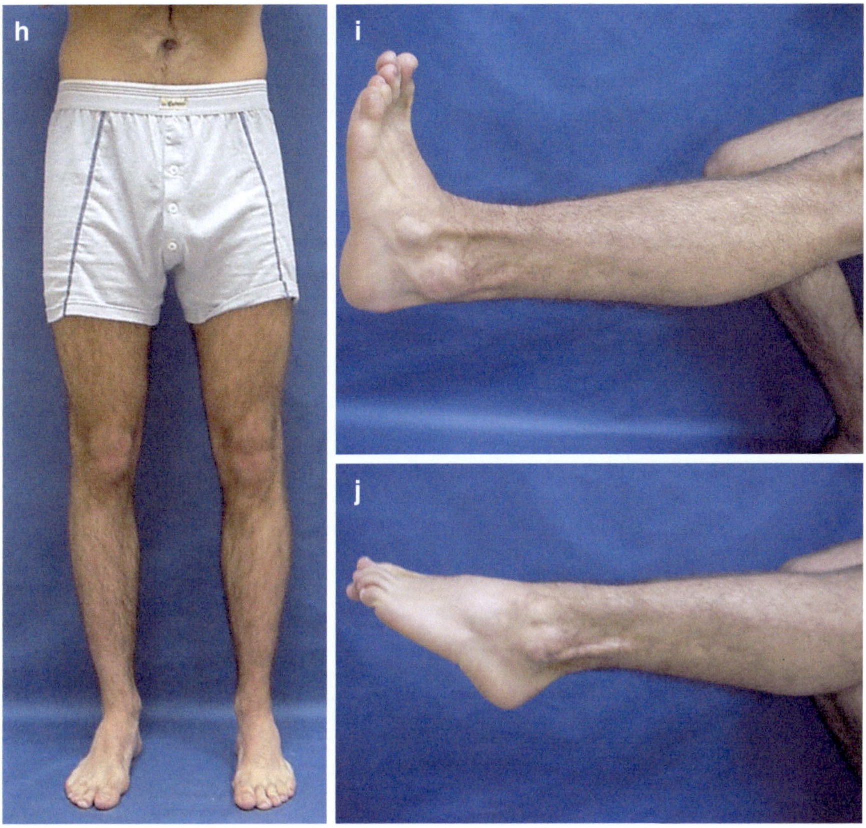

Fig. 12.16 (continued)

When the growth plate cannot be preserved, it is more difficult to avoid dissymmetry. In such cases an osteoarticular allograft can be used as a temporary solution until the end of growth (Figs. 12.18 and 12.19). Growing prostheses are another option.

12.7 Osteosynthesis of Grafts in Children

Osteosynthesis of the allograft should be borne in mind in order to prevent a final limb length discrepancy.

Previous studies in our department [26] showed that, whatever the osteosynthesis device used, consolidation in the metaphysis occurred before 6 months. At the diaphyseal end, however, consolidation often took over a year, due to chemotherapy. In addition, for the diaphyseal union when allografts are used, the "osteosynthesis *ad minimum* law" is not applicable, even in children. On the other hand, fractures of allografts are more often seen when non-intramedullary devices are used for stabilization at the allograft-host bone union [24]. Therefore, we prefer the use of locked intramedullary nails for stabilization of allografts; the nail should be locked in the epiphysis in cases of preservation of the joint. However, the locked nail will not allow growth from the preserved growth plate.

Minimal osteosynthesis devices, for example Kirschner wires, are sufficient to stabilize the metaphyseal junction and present no problems in terms of achieving union. However, such minimal devices will not allow early mobilization of the joint.

In summary, the osteosynthesis device at the diaphyseal union should be stable enough to achieve union, and, in order to avoid fracture of the allograft, intramedullary nails are preferable. Healing at the metaphyseal union can be achieved with much simpler osteosynthesis devices, which could preserve the potential for growth but will not allow for early mobilization of the joint. Therefore, when the patient is near the end of growth or radiotherapy has been or will be used, we recommend the use of locked intramedullary nails (with a locking screw in the retained epiphysis) and an allograft longer than the resected piece. In young patients, a simple osteosynthesis device could be used at the metaphyseal junction in order to preserve the growth potential of the retained growth plate.

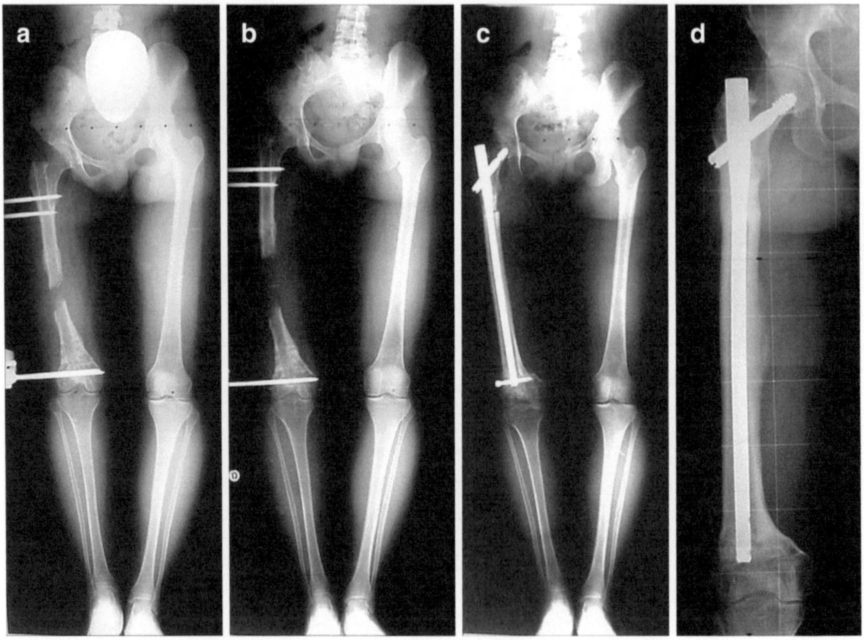

Fig. 12.17 Limb length discrepancy 6 years after intercalary reconstruction of an osteosarcoma in the distal metaphysis of the femur of an 8-year-old girl. (**a**) The osteosynthesis device was removed and distraction was performed through the shaft of the allograft. After discrepancy was corrected (**b**), a new allograft was implanted (**c**). The allograft healed (**d**) and function was excellent (**e–g**)

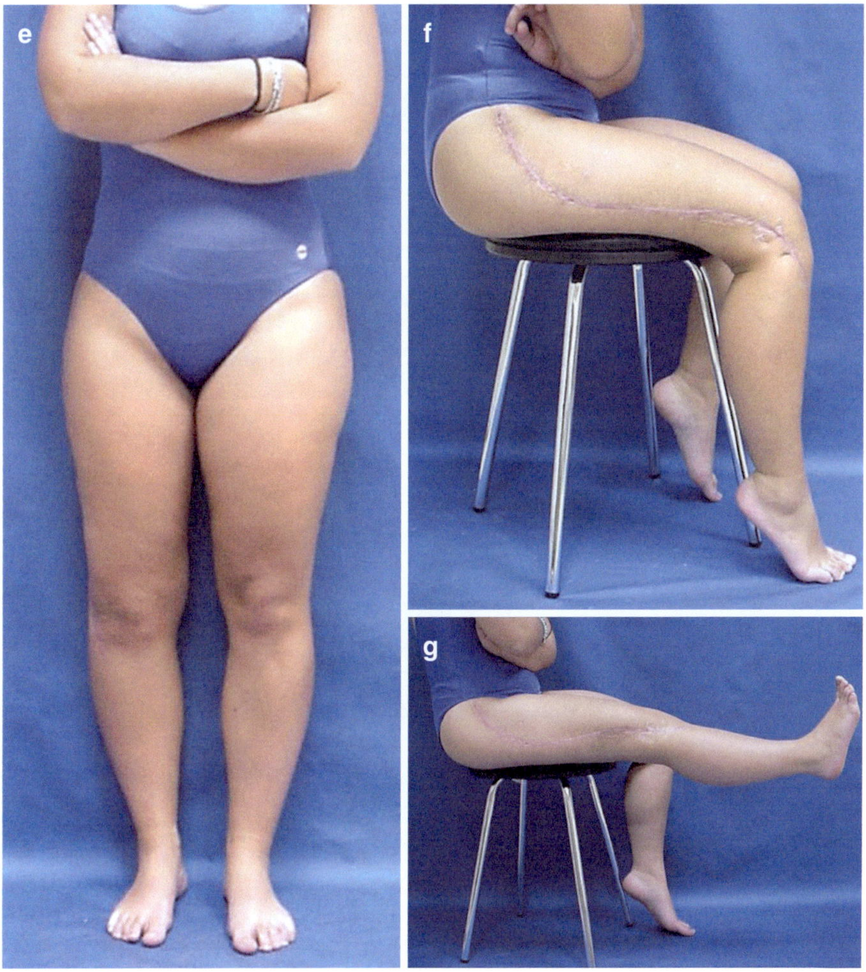

Fig. 12.17 (continued)

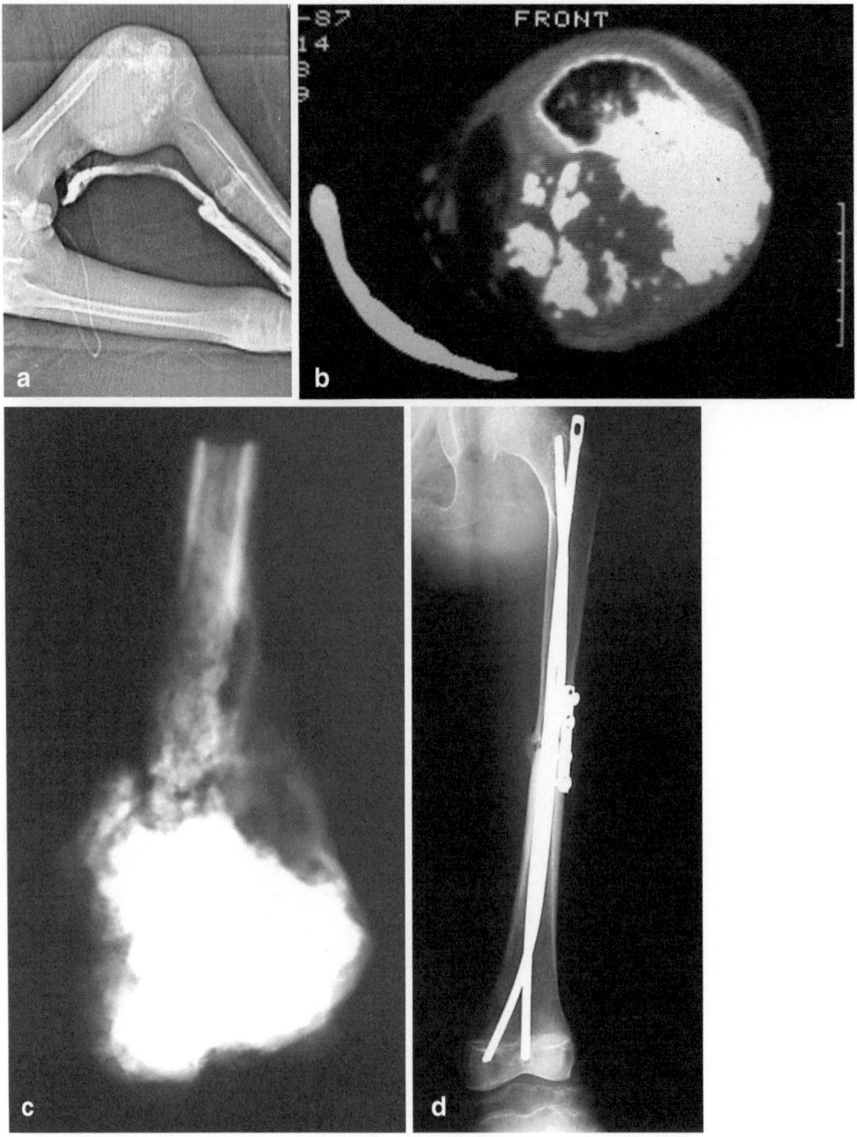

Fig. 12.18 (**a**, **b**) An 8-year-old boy with a large osteosarcoma on his left femur. (**c**) The tumor was resected (**d**), and the limb was reconstructed with an osteoarticular allograft. (**e**) Over time a leg length discrepancy developed. (**f**, **g**) After 5 years we performed bone lengthening in both the femur and the tibia. (**h**) The patient is alive and free of disease 21 years after the first limb salvage procedure

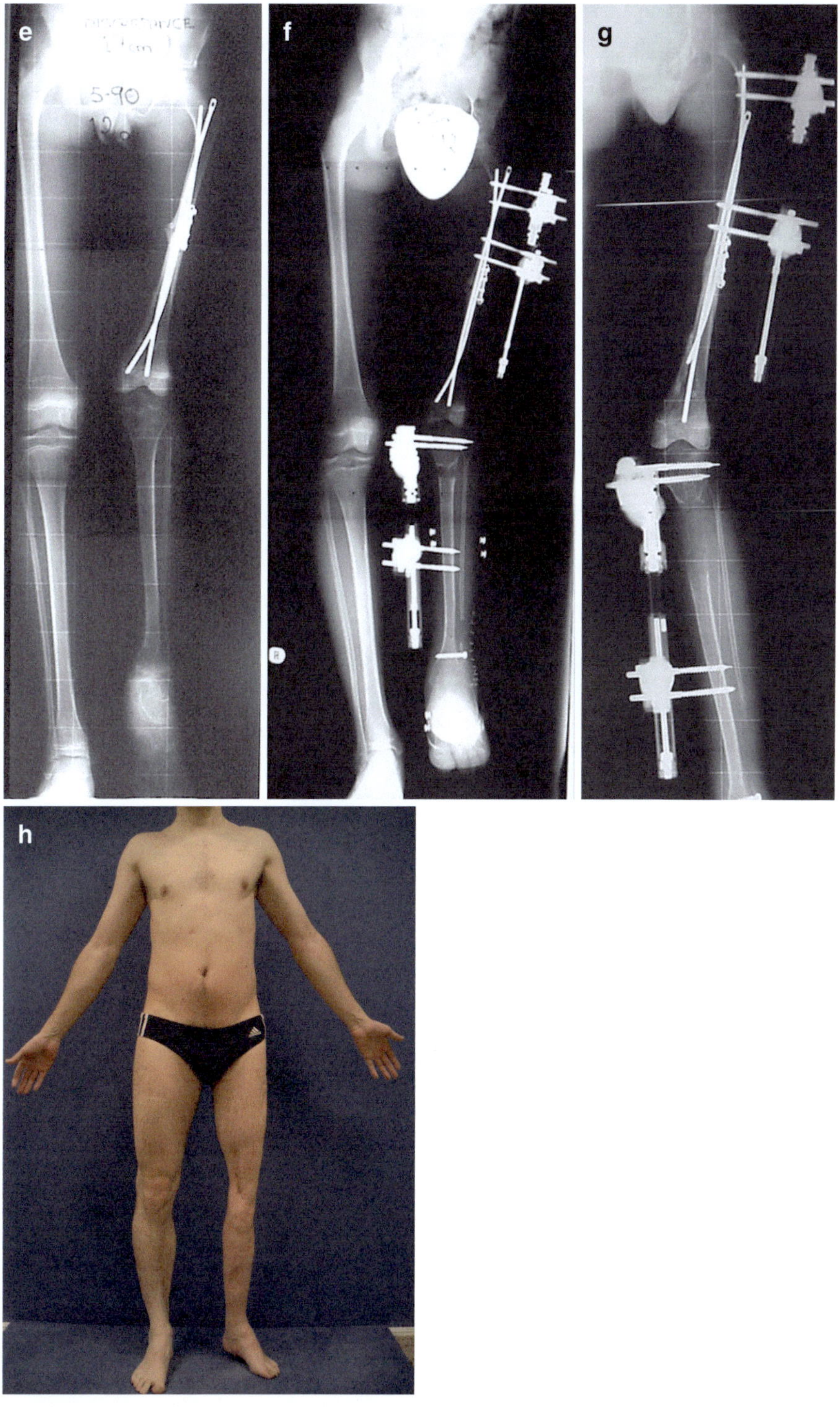

Fig. 12.18 (continued)

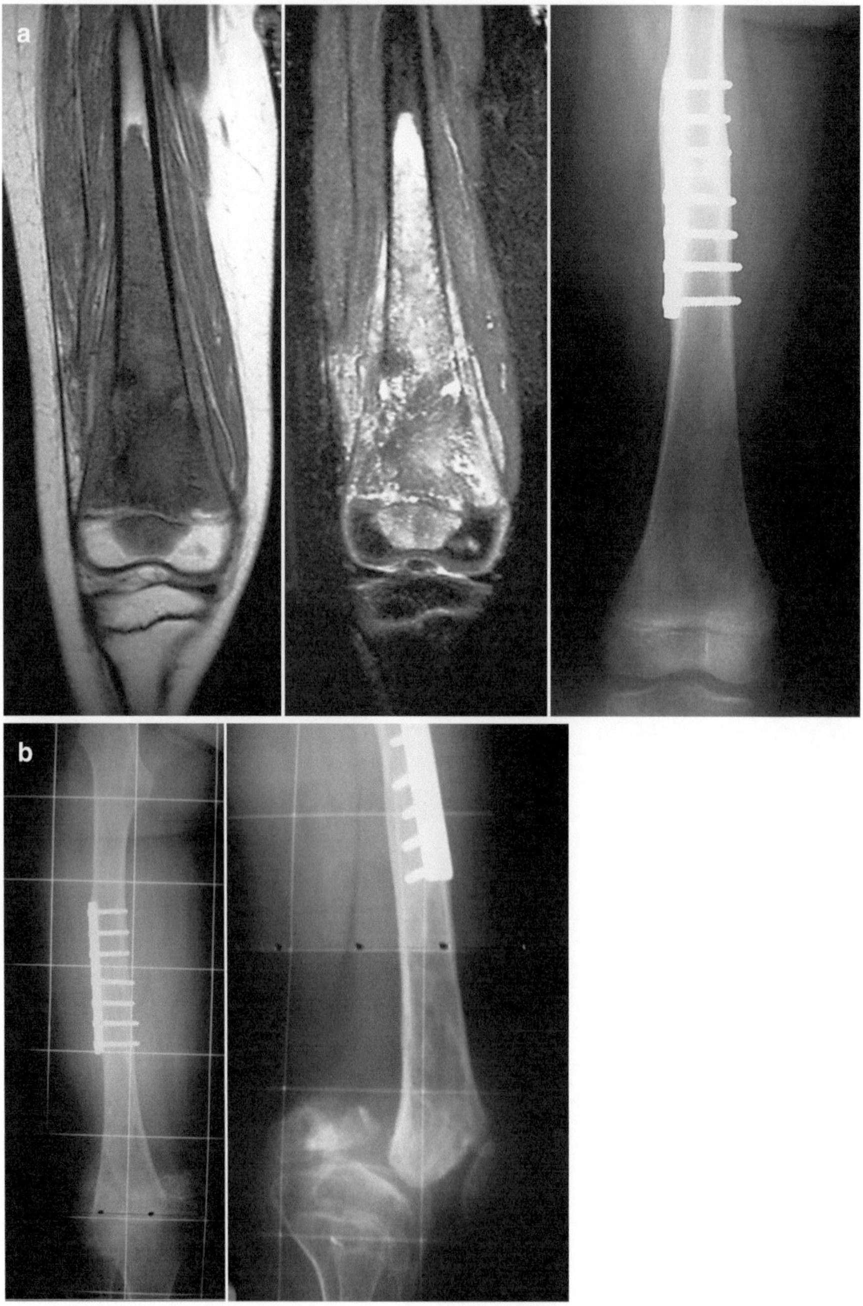

Fig. 12.19 (**a**) A 7-year-old girl with an osteosarcoma on her right distal femur; the tumor involves the epiphysis. (**b**) The tumor was resected and the limb was reconstructed with an osteoarticular allograft. (**c**) Over time, fracture of the allograft developed. (**d**) At the end of the girl's growth period, lengthening was performed, and a prosthesis was implanted (**e**) function 11 years later

Fig. 12.19 (continued)

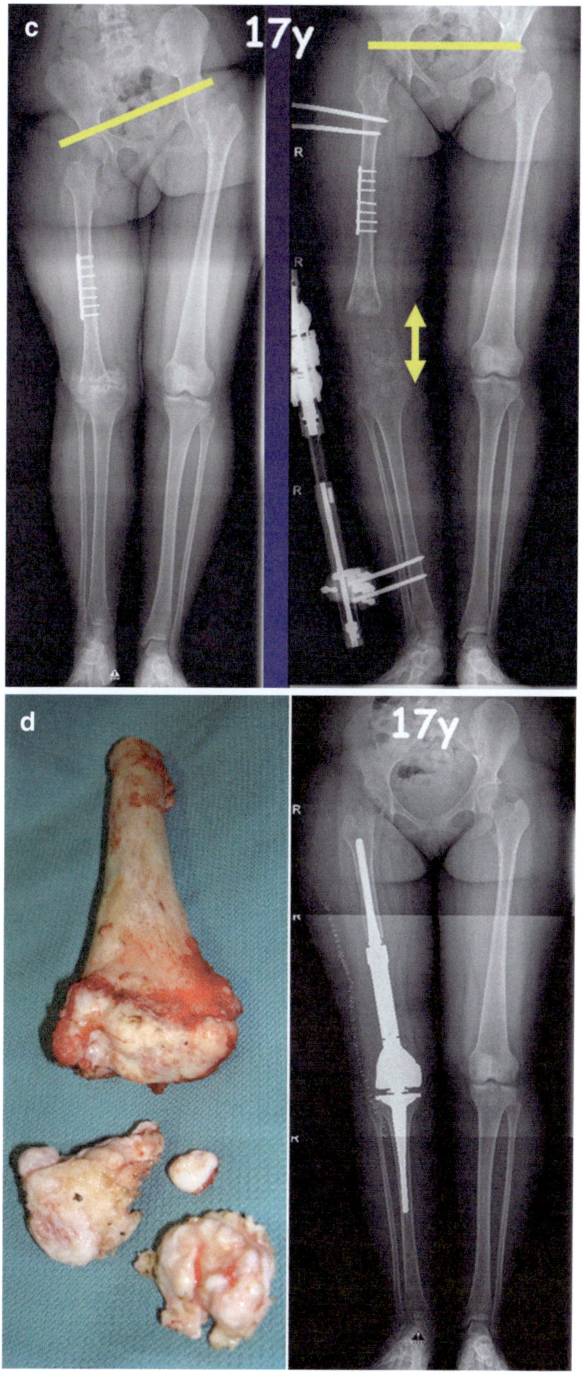

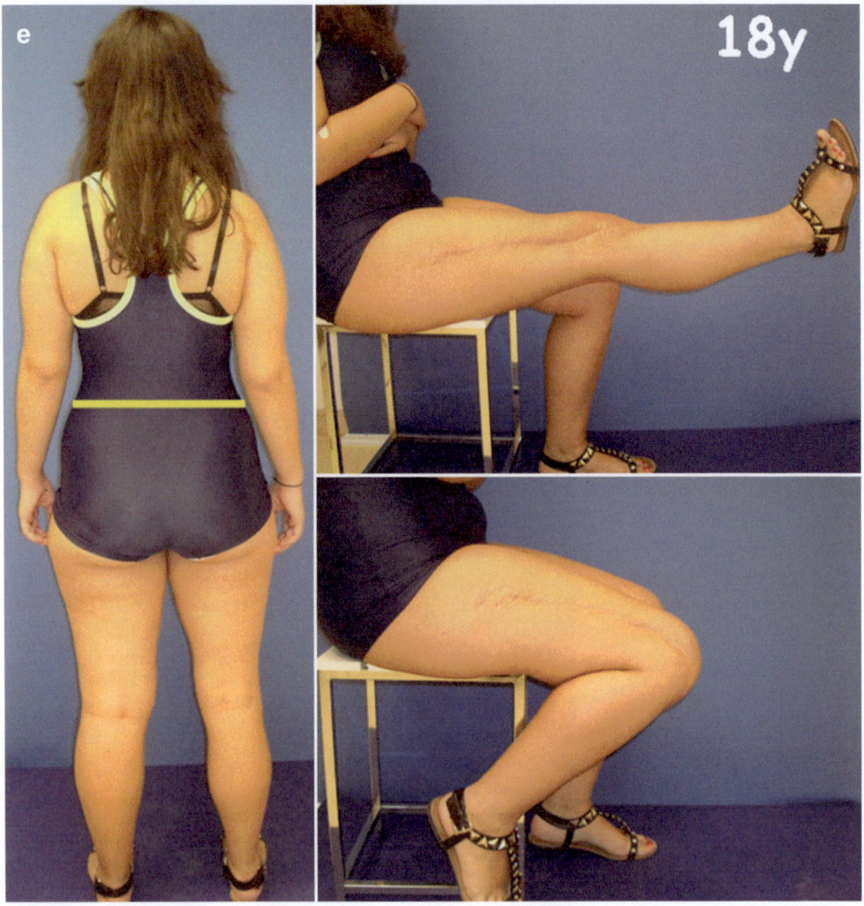

Fig. 12.19 (continued)

12.8 Conclusion

In young children, physeal distraction prior to limb salvage is a viable and safe way to preserve a normal joint. In our series of patients with a metaphyseal tumor and intact physis, limb function subsequent to limb salvage with physeal distraction was graded as excellent or good in two thirds of cases. The use of this technique does not increase the rate of local or distant tumor spread. The majority of complications encountered are due to difficulties inherent in reconstruction with structural bone grafts. Distraction callotasis can resolve leg length discrepancy following limb salvage. In our series of patients, complications and healing rates after distraction callotasis are similar to those with standard lengthening procedures. In selected cases of leg length discrepancy and non-union, external fixation may be used to compress and heal the non-union site while lengthening at another.

References

1. Aponte-Tinao L, Ayerza MA, Muscolo L, Farfalli G. Survival, recurrence, and function after epiphyseal preservation and allograft reconstruction in osteosarcoma of the knee. Clin Orthop Relat Res. 2015;473:1797–801.
2. Bisgardt JD, Hunt HB. Influence of roentgen rays and radium on epiphyseal growth of long bones. Radiology. 1936;26:56.
3. Cañadell J, San Julian M. Tumoral reconstruction in the immature knee. In: De Pablos J, editor. The immature knee. Barcelona: Ed. Masson; 1998. p. 343–9.
4. Cañadell J, San Julian M, Forriol F, Cara JA. Physeal distraction in the conservative treatment of malignant bone tumors in children. In: De Pablos J, editor. Surgery of the growth plate. Madrid: Ergon; 1998. p. 321–7.
5. Cañadell J, San Julian M. Cirugía de salvamento en el tratamiento de los tumores óseos malignos. En: Guillen P, editor. Evolución de la Traumatología y la Ortopedia en los últimos 25 años: ¡Un cuarto de siglo!. Fundación Mapfre Medicina; 1999. p. 687–92.
6. Cara JA, Amillo S, Cañadell J. Bone grafts in the treatment of malignant bone tumors: autografts vs. allografts. In: Cañadell J, San-Julian M, Cara JA, editors. Surgical treatment of malignant bone tumors, Orthopaedic monographies. Pamplona: Universidad de Navarra; 1995. p. 111–20.
7. Cara JA, Cañadell J. Forriol: bone lengthening after conservative oncologic surgery. In: Cañadell J, San-Julian M, Cara JA, editors. Surgical treatment of malignant bone tumors, Orthopaedic monographies. Pamplona: Universidad de Navarra; 1995. p. 215–25.
8. Cara JA, San-Julian M, Laclériga A, Cañadell J. Infection in grafting procedures. In: Cañadell J, San-Julian M, Cara JA, editors. Surgical treatment of malignant bone tumors, Orthopaedic monographies. Pamplona: Universidad de Navarra; 1995. p. 227–34.
9. Delépine N, Delépine G, Hernigou PH, Desbois J. Bone union of allografts and chemotherapy considerations about 55 consecutive cases. In: 5th international symposium on limb Salvage, St Malo, 5, 1989.
10. Dyck H, Malinin T, Mnaymneh W. Massive allograft implantation following radical resection of high grade tumors requiring neoadjuvant chemotherapy treatment. Clin Orthop. 1988;197:88.
11. Glasser DB, Duane K, Lane JM, Healey JH, Caparros-Sison B. The effect of chemotherapy on growth in the skeletally immature individual. Clin Orthop. 1991;262:93–107.
12. Goldwein JW. Effects of radiation therapy in skeletal growth in childhood. Clin Orthop. 1991;262:101–7.
13. Gonzales DG, Van Dijk JD. Experimental studies on the response of growing bones to X-ray and neutron irradiation. Int J Radiot Oncol Biol Phys. 1991;9:671.
14. Khoo DB. The effect of chemotherapy on soft tissue and bone healing in the rabbit model. Ann Acad Med Singapore. 1992;21:217–21.
15. Staals EL, Colangeli M, Ali N, Casanova JM, Donati DM, Manfrini M. Are complications associated to Repiphysis® expandable distal femoral prostheis acceptable for its continued use? Clin Orthop Relat Res. 2015;473(9):3014–6.
16. Mankin H, Springfield D, Gebhart M, Tomford W. Current status of allografting for bone tumors. Orthopedics. 1992;15:1147–54.
17. Mnaymneh W, Malinin T, Lackman R, Hornicek J, Ghandur-Mnaimneh L. Massive distal femoral allografts after resection of bone tumors. Clin Orthop. 1994;303:103–15.
18. Martinez-Monge R, Cambeiro M, San-Julian M, Sierrasesúmaga L. The use of braquitherapy in paediatric cancer: the search of an uncomplicated cure. Lancet Oncol. 2006;7(2):157–66.
19. Martinez-Monge R, San Julian M, Amillo S, Cambeiro M, Pardo F, Arbea L, et al. Perioperative high dose brachytherapy in high-risk resected sarcomas: initial results of a Phase I/II Trial. Radiotherapy. 2004.
20. Martinez Monge R, Garrán C, Cambeiro M, San-Julian M, Alcalde J, Sierrasesúmaga L. Feasibility report of conservative surgery, Perioperative HDR brachytherapy (PHDRB) and Low to Moderate Esternal Beam Radiation Therapy (EBRT) in pediatric sarcomas. Brachytherapy. 2004;3:196–200.

21. Neel M, Bush C, Scarborough M, Enneking W. Transepiphyseal extension of osteosarcoma. Abstract book of the 8th ISOLS. International Symposium on Limb Salvage, Florence, 10th–12th May. p. 107.
22. Rosen G, Caparros B, Niremberg A, et al. Ewing's sarcoma. Ten years experience with adyuvant chemotherapy. Cancer. 1981;47:2204–13.
23. San-Julián M, Cañadell J. Physeal distraction and bone lengthening in young children with malignant bone tumors. Acta Orthop Sand. 1997;Suppl 276:68.
24. San-Julian M, Cañadell J. Fractures in allografts for limb preserving operations. Int Orthop. 1998;22:32–6.
25. San-Julián M, Amillo S, Cañadell J. Allografts in malignant bone tumors. In: Czitrom AA, Winkler H, editors. Orthopaedic allograft surgery. Wien-New York: Springer; 1996. p. 157–63.
26. San-Julián M, Leyes M, Mora G, Cañadell J. Consolidation of massive bone allografts in limb preserving operations for bone tumors. Int Orthop. 1995;19:377–82.
27. San-Julián M, Villas A, Cañadell J, Ricther JA. Allograft revascularization scintigraphic study with 99m Tc MDP. Abstract book of the IX meeting of European Musculo Skeletal Oncology Society, Instambul, 24–25 Oct 1996. p. 14.
28. San Julian M, Diaz de Rada P, Noain E, Sierrasesúmaga L. Bone metastases from osteosarcoma. Int Orthop. 2003;27(2):117–20.
29. San Julian M. Tumores óseos malignos en la edad infantil. In: De Pablos J, Bruguera A, editors. Apuntes de Ortopedia infantil. 2nd ed. Pamplona: Ergón; 2000.
30. San Julian M, Cara JA, Cañadell J. Is amputation still really neccesary in any case of osteosarcoma? Rev Med Univ Navarra. 1999;43:13–25.
31. San Julian M, Dolz R, Garcia-Barrecheguren E, Noain E, Sierrasesumaga L, Cañadell J. Limb salvage in bone sarcomas in patients younger than age 10: A 20 years experience. Am J Pediatr Orthop. 2003;23(6):753–62.
32. San Julian M, Forriol F, Cañadell J. Investigación en banco de tejidos osteoarticulares. Monografías SECOT 4: Banco de huesos. Ed. Masson; 2002. p. 69–79.
33. San Julian M, Valentí A. Bone transplant. Transplante de órganos y tejidos. Anales del Sistema navarro de Salud. 2006;28 Suppl 2:125–36.
34. San Julian M, Moreno JL, Forriol F, Cañadell J. Integración radiológica, isotópica e histológica de los aloinjertos corticales. Estudio clínico. Rev Ortop Traum. 2000;44:436–41.
35. San Julian M, Aristu J. Sarcoma de Ewing. Luis Sierrasesúmaga. In: Antillon F, Patiño A, Bernaola E, San Julian M, editors. "Oncología Pediátrica". Luis Sierrasesúmaga. Madrid: Pearson; 2005. p. 617–36.
36. Sierrasesúmaga L, Antillón F, Cañadell J. Treatment of Ewing's sarcoma. Protocol, description, applications and results. In: Cañadell J, Sierrasesúmaga L, Calvo F, Ganoza C, editors. Treatment of malignant bone tumors in children and adolescents. Pamplona: Servicio de Publicaciones de la Universidad de Navarra S.A; 1991.
37. Silverman EN. The skeletal lesions in leukemia: clinical and roentgenographic observations in 103 infants and children, with a review of the literature. AJR. 1948;59:818.
38. Sinohara N, Sumida S, Masuda S. Bone allografts after segmental resection of tumors. Int Orthop. 1990;14:273–6.
39. Vander Griend R. The effect of internal fixation on the healing of large allografts. J Bone Joint Surg. 1994;76 A:657–64.
40. Villas C, San Julian M, Alfonso M. Autoinjertos en cirugía de los tumores óseos. Injertos, Sustitutivos óseos y materiales en la cirugía reconstructiva del aparato locomotor. Ed Masson; 2005.
41. Whitehouse WM, Lampe I. Osseous damage in irradiation of renal tumors in infancy and childhood. AJR. 1953;70:721.
42. Zart DJ, Miya L, Wolff DA, Mackley JT, Stevenson S. The effects of cisplatin on the incorporation of fresh singenic and frozen allogenic cortical bone grafts. J Orthop Res. 1993;11:240–9.

Chapter 13
Other Techniques for Epiphyseal Preservation

Mikel San-Julian

Abstract Most pediatric bone sarcomas are located at the metaphysis of long bones. In selected cases, the epiphysis can be preserved by metaphyseal or intra-epiphyseal osteotomy. Compared to intra-epiphyseal osteotomies, physeal distraction before excision of the tumor has some advantages, but in some cases osteotomy is indicated.

Keywords Limb salvage • Metaphyseal osteotomy • Intraepiphyseal osteotomy • Joint preservation

13.1 Metaphyseal Osteotomy

With diaphyseal tumors, preservation of the epiphysis is not a problem. With metaphyseal tumors, however, preservation of the epiphysis is not always possible although there are still some metaphyseal locations from which a tumor can be safely excised by metaphyseal osteotomy, thus avoiding damage or resection of the growth plate.

In young children, the biological impetus towards growth and bone formation is so strong that even chemotherapy does not stop it; a tumor that is originally near or in contact with the growth plate can be displaced by new bone formation to the diaphysis during the neoadjuvant chemotherapy period, and thus intra-epiphyseal osteotomy can preserve not only the joint, but also the entire growth plate (Figs. 13.1 and 13.2).

13.2 Intra-epiphyseal Osteotomy

Prior to the first publications of our work, the possibility of preservation of the epiphysis in metaphyseal bone tumors was apparently largely overlooked, and alternative techniques, such as intra-epiphyseal osteotomy [9], have only been

M. San-Julian, MD, PhD
Department of Orthopaedic Surgery, University of Navarra, Pamplona, Navarra, Spain
e-mail: msjulian@unav.es

M. San-Julian (ed.), *Cañadell's Pediatric Bone Sarcomas: Epiphysiolysis before Excision*, DOI 10.1007/978-3-319-24220-0_13

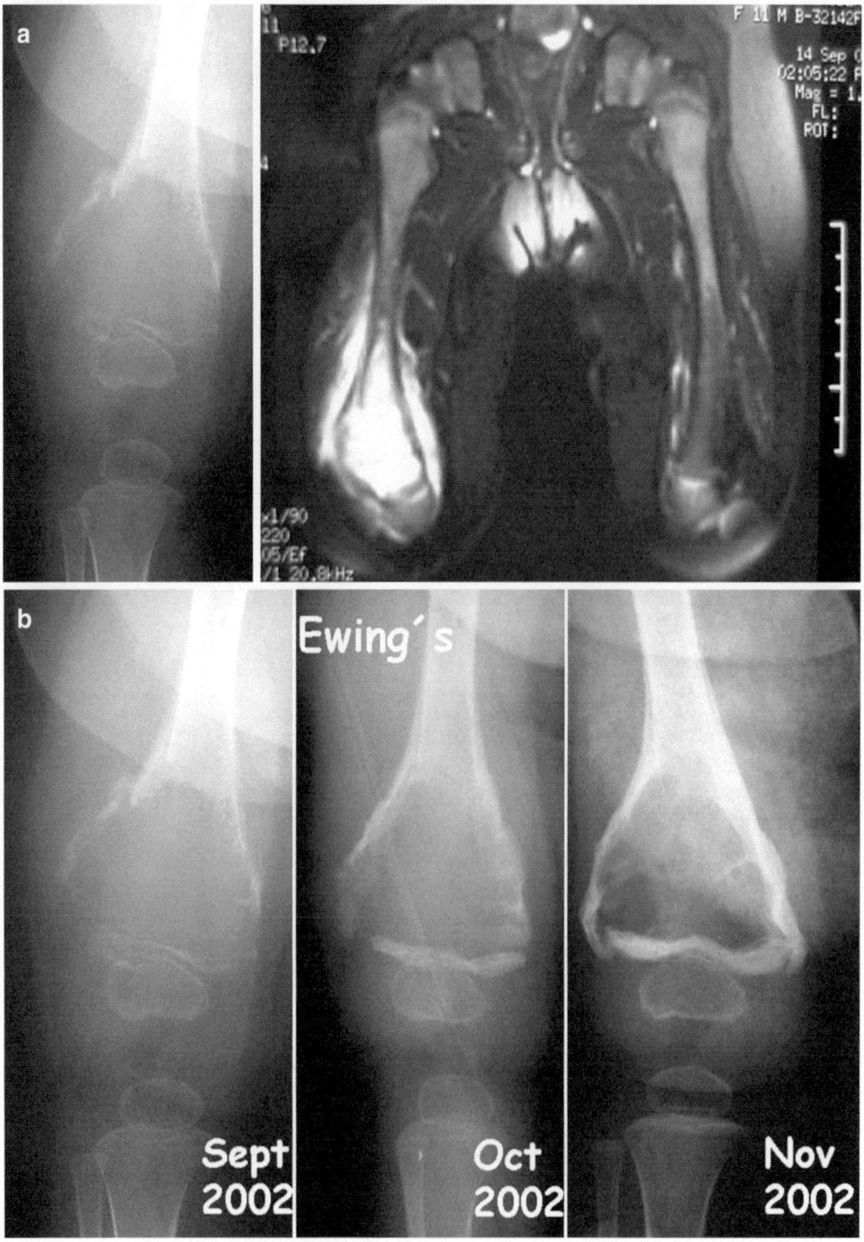

Fig. 13.1 (**a**) Ewing's sarcoma in the distal metaphysis of the femur of a 9-month-old baby. MRI shows is in contact with the physis. Most of our colleagues dealing with bone tumors would advise an amputation. (**b**, **c**) Neoadjuvant treatment was very succesful. Note the new bone formation from the distal femur growth plate. (**d**, **e**) Resection was performed through metaphyseal and diaphyseal osteotomies in order to preserve the joint. Autografts from ipsilateral fibula and tibia were used for reconstruction. (**f**) Follow-up: 13 years later, limb function is excellent (Reproduction from San-Julian et al. [14])

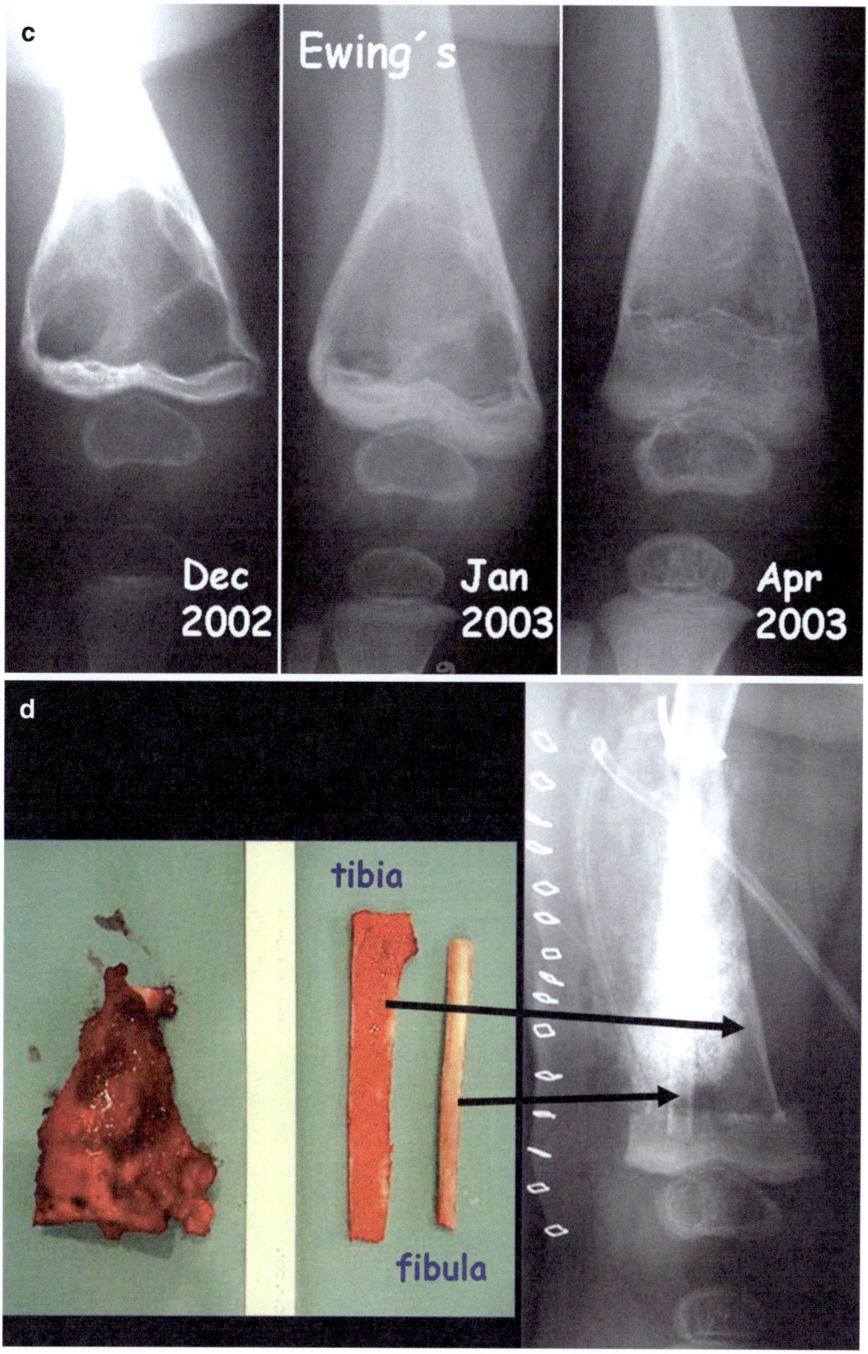

Fig. 13.1 (continued)

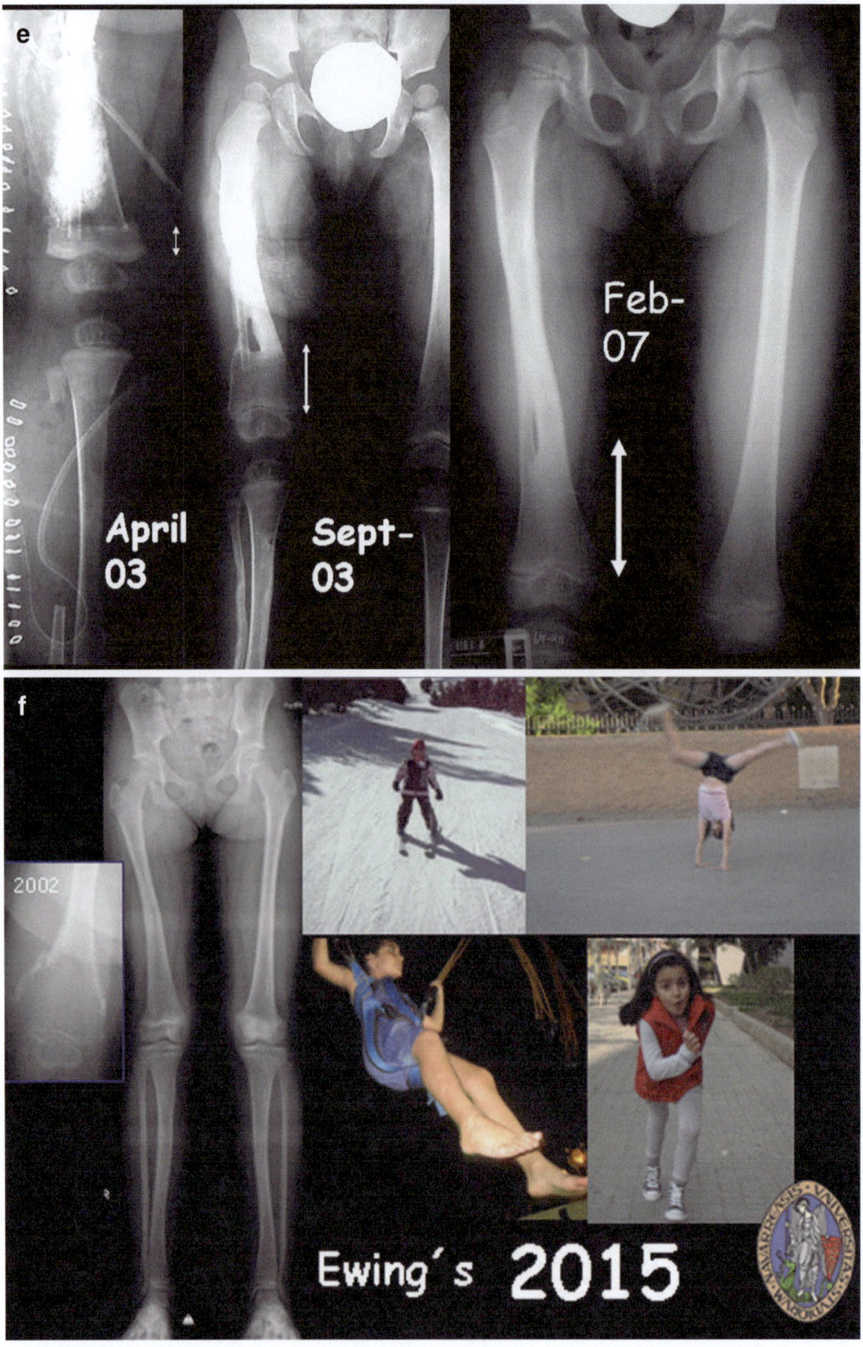

Fig. 13.1 (continued)

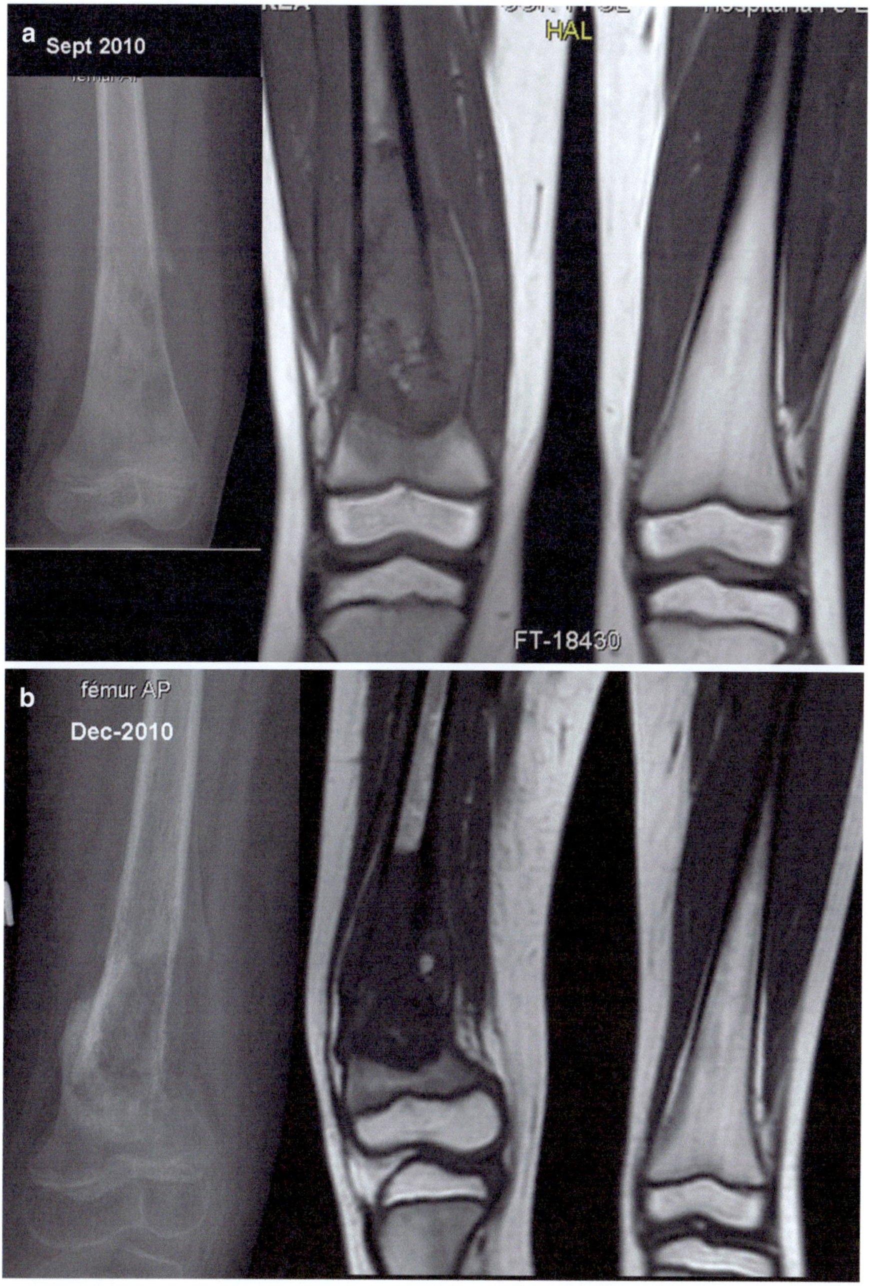

Fig. 13.2 (**a**) Osteosarcoma in the distal metaphysis of the femur of 8-year-old girl. (**b**) She started chemotherapy elsewhere and suffered a pathological fracture. (**c**) After neoadjuvant chemotherapy in our center. Note the growth in the distal femur growth plate that has displaced the tumor to the diaphysis. (**d**) Resection and reconstruction with an allograft. Good healing was obtained

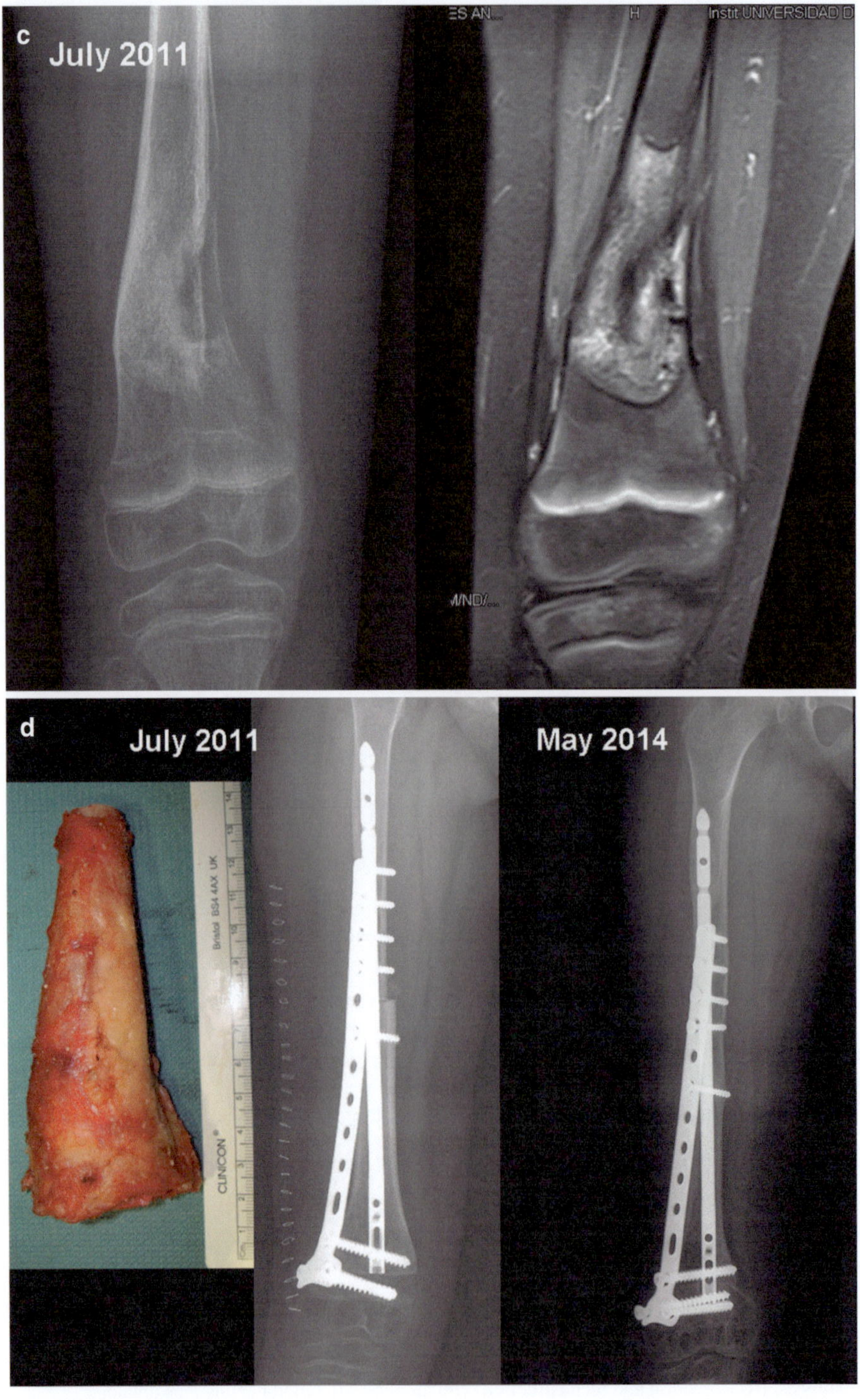

Fig. 13.2 (continued)

suggested subsequently. We have used intra-epiphyseal osteotomy in some cases, in which epiphysis could be preserved but physeal distraction was contraindicated (Figs. 13.3 and 13.4).

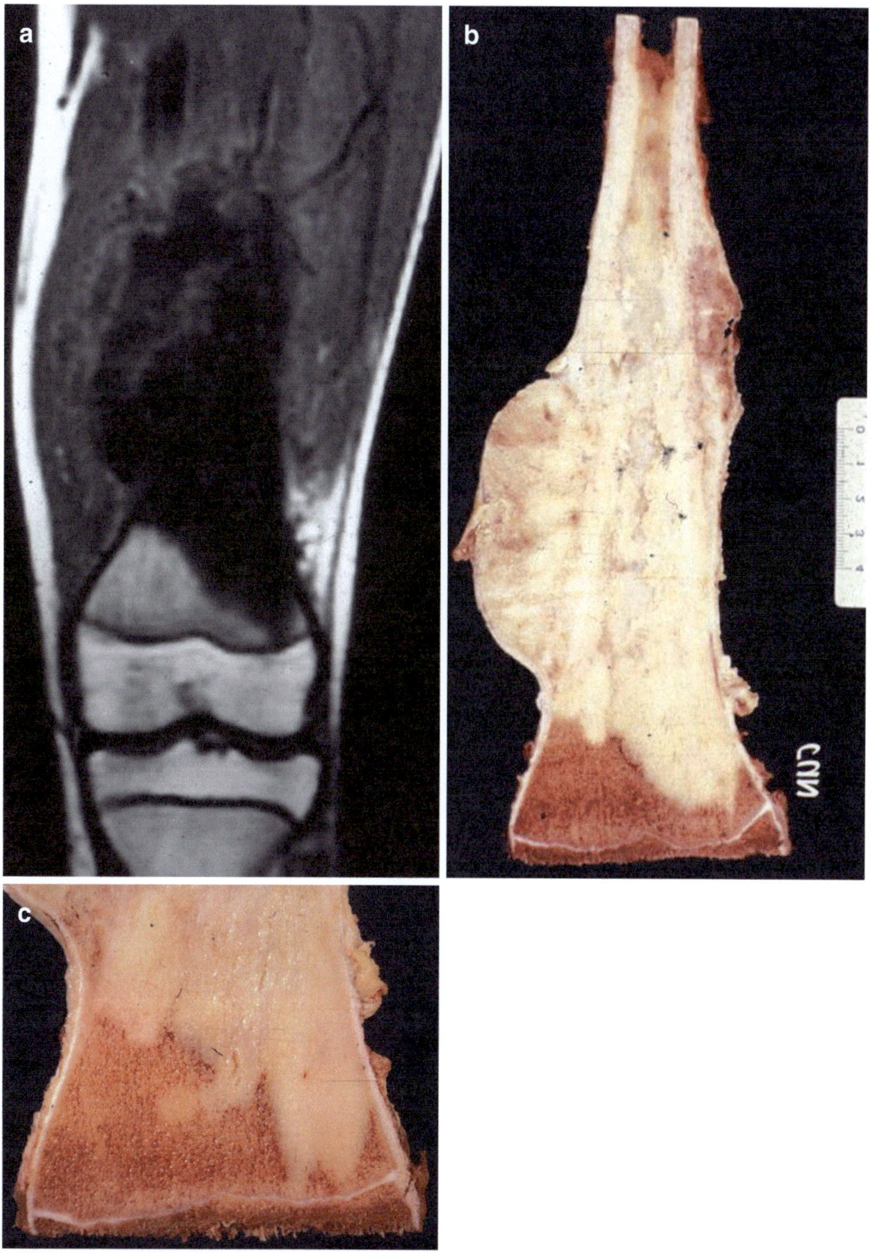

Fig. 13.3 (**a**) Osteosarcoma in the distal metaphysis of the femur of a 16-year-old boy. MRI shows the tumor in contact with the physis. This patient was treated in 1987. (**b**, **c**) Intra-epiphyseal osteotomy was performed in order to preserve the joint. Note that the growth plate is very thin

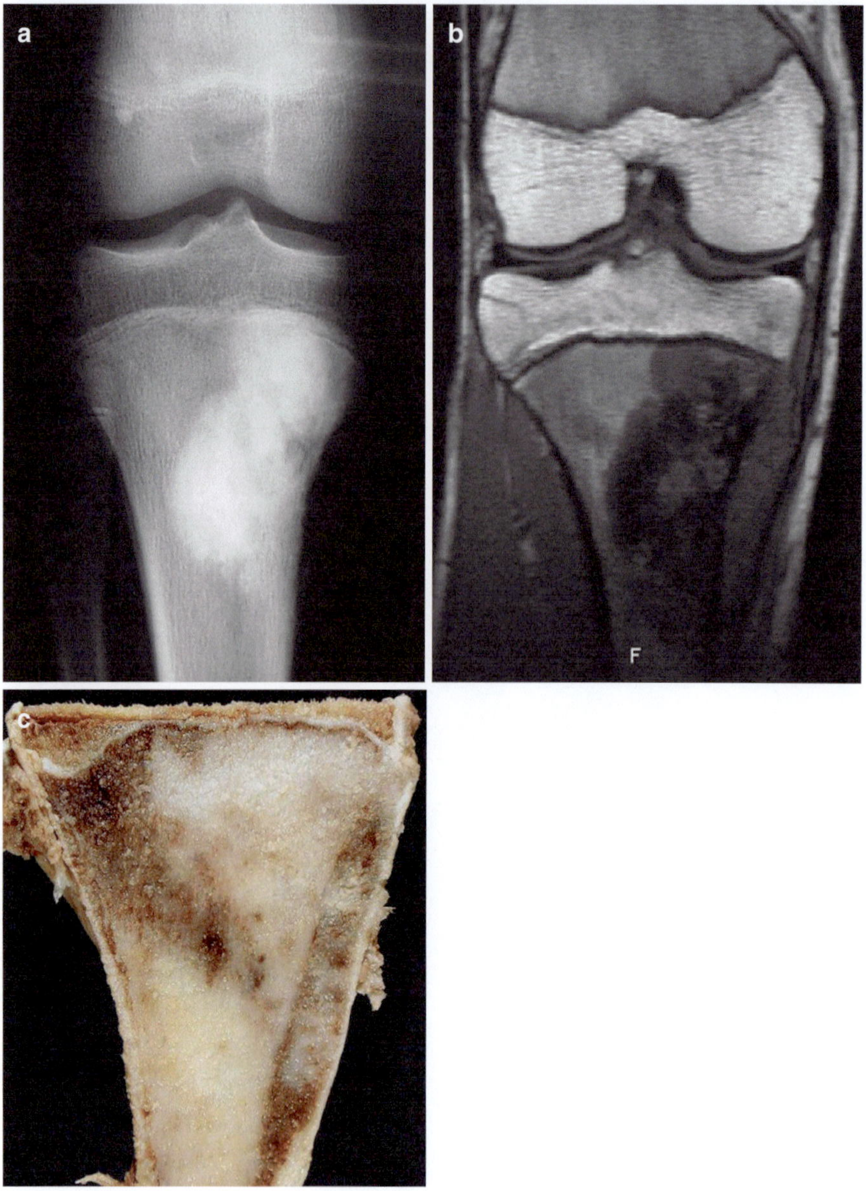

Fig. 13.4 (**a**, **b**) Osteosarcoma in the proximal metaphysis of the tibia of a 17-year-old boy. The tumor is in contact with the growth plate. (**c**) After careful consideration of epiphysiolysis before resection, we chose intra-epiphyseal osteotomy in view of the age of the patient. (**d**, **e**) Reconstruction with an intercalary allograft stabilized with both a plate and a nail

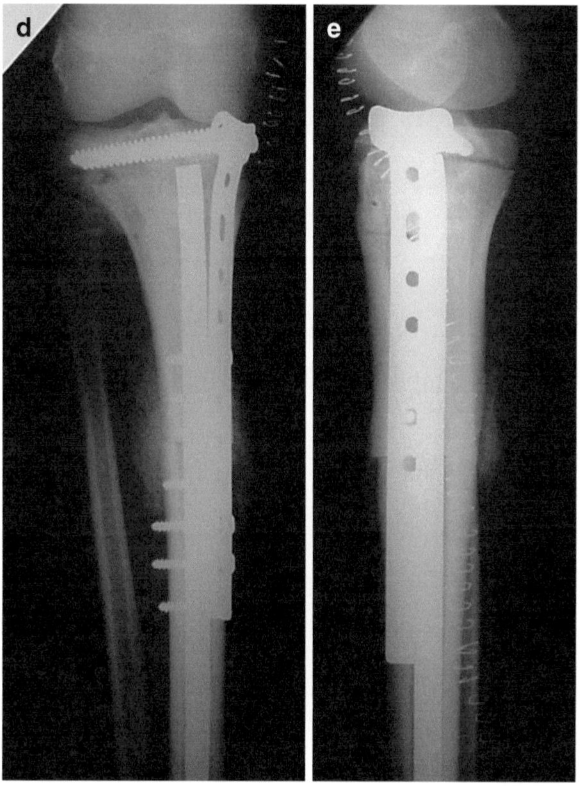

Fig. 13.4 (continued)

In the more recent reports of intra-epiphyseal osteotomy [2, 6–8, 10–12], the technique has been used mainly in proximal tibia locations. Tumor involvement of the physis is assessed by preoperative MRI. If intra-epiphyseal osteotomy is indicated, it is done under X-ray control in order to include the growth plate in the resected specimen. The residual epiphyseal bone segment is less than 2 cm thick and reconstruction is by a combination of vascularized fibula and allograft [3]. Authors report that local recurrence has not been observed to occur in the retained epiphysis [2, 13]. Other authors [1, 5] have employed metallic implants for reconstruction of the intercalary region, but follow-up is not yet long enough to know the long-term results with such implants. An epiphyseal osteotomy is fixed with small fragment screws.

In our opinion, the advantages of physeal distraction over intra-epiphyseal osteotomy are:

1. ***Safety***. The growth plate is not a flat surface – it has indentations and protuberances (Figs. 13.5 and 13.6) – and consequently intra-epiphyseal osteotomy could leave bits of tumor.
2. ***Easier resection***. Physeal distraction before excision of a metaphyseal bone tumor removes the need for metaphyseal osteotomy. Therefore, resection requires only one osteotomy – the diaphyseal one.

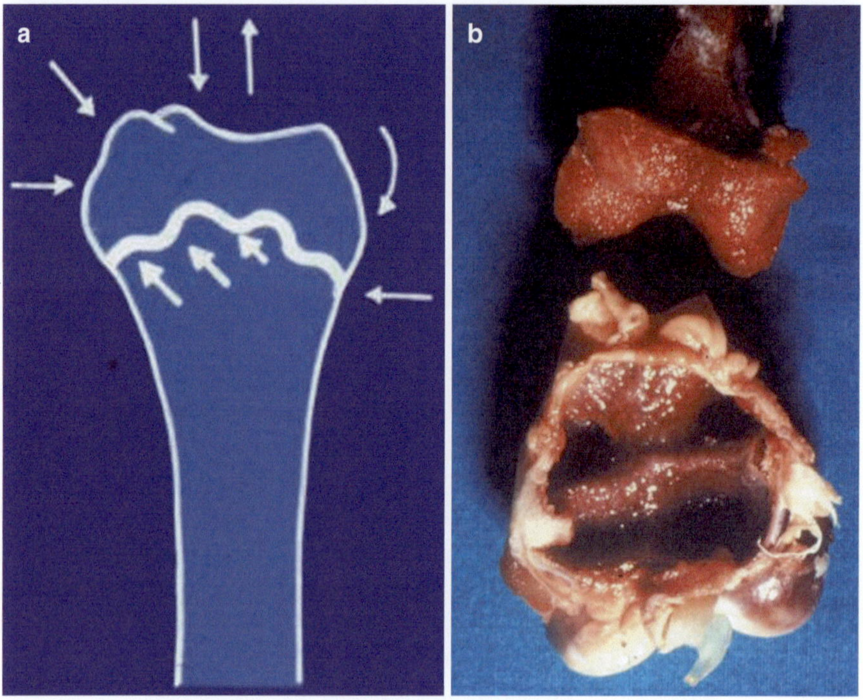

Fig. 13.5 (**a**) Because of the morphology of the growth plate, intra-epiphyseal osteotomy could leave tumor cells in the hollows of the surface. (**b**) Experimental epiphysiolysis in a lamb. Note the undulate appearance of the growth plate

Fig. 13.6 The morphology of the growth plate in the proximal humerus contraindicates, in our opinion, intra-epiphyseal osteotomy

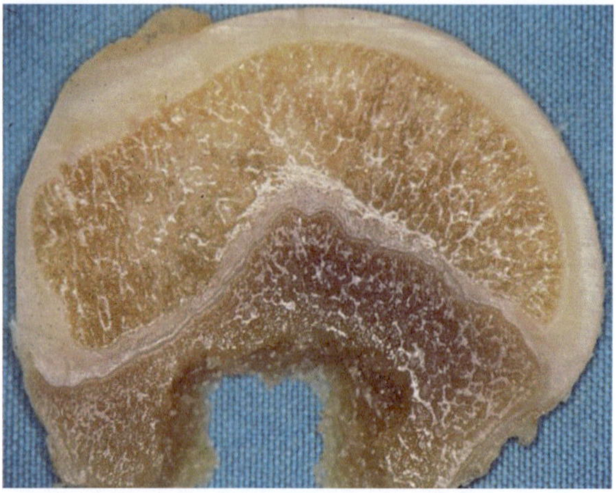

3. ***Preservation of the whole epiphysis***. This has several advantages:

   - Joint stability is better maintained because most ligaments, tendinous attachments, capsules, etc. are preserved (Fig. 13.7).

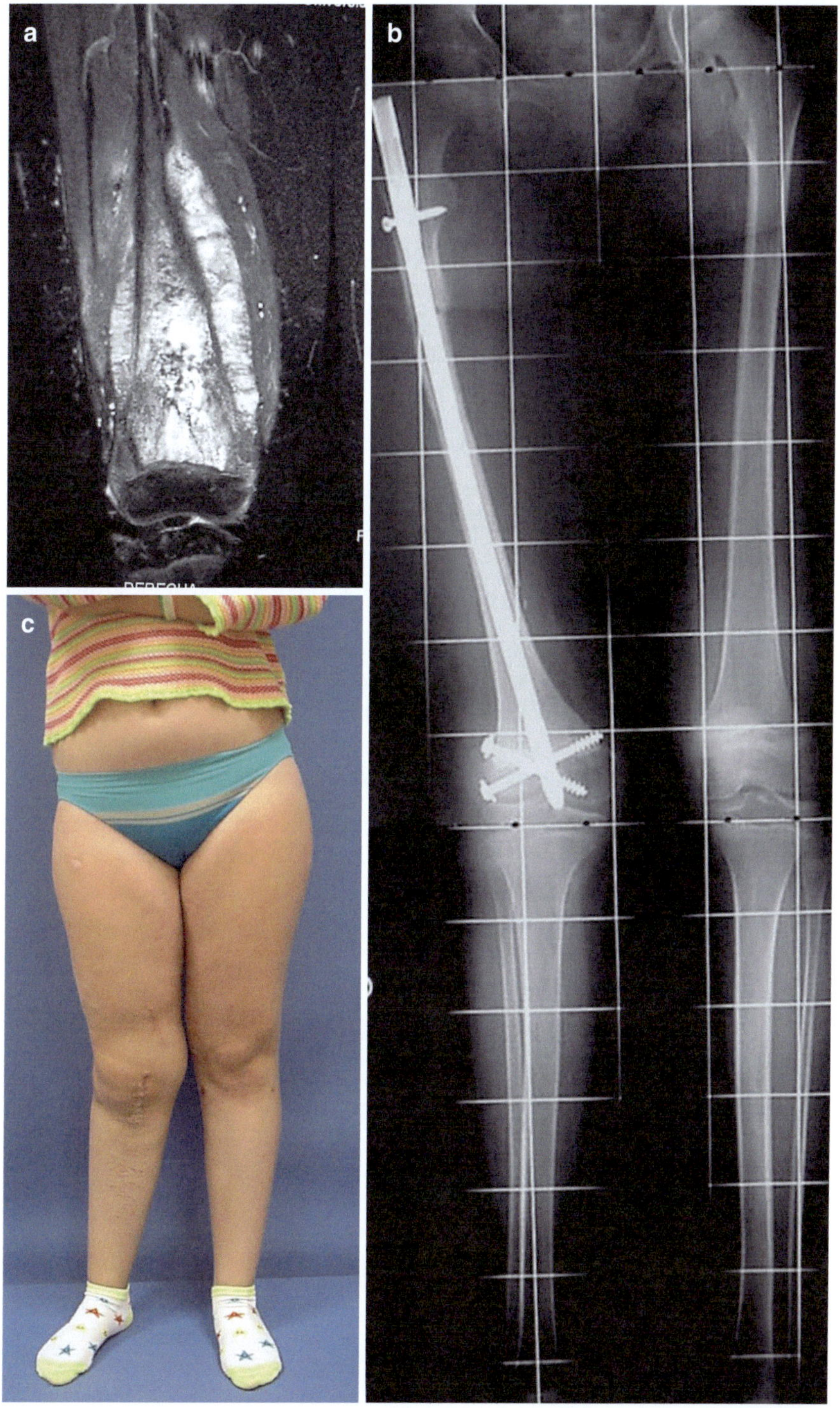

Fig. 13.7 (**a**) Osteosarcoma in contact with the whole physis. (**b**) Intra-epiphyseal osteotomy and reconstruction with an allograft. (**c**) Note the limb length discrepancy and the valgus instability

- Graft osteosynthesis is facilitated because the epiphyseal segment of bone is bigger.
- In distal femur locations, the *trochlea femoralis* is preserved. Intra-epiphyseal osteotomy implies the loss of part of the *trochlea femoralis* (Fig. 13.8), which can lead to a loss in knee function. Similarly, the patellar tendon attachment in the proximal tibia (Fig. 13.9) and the rotator cuff in the shoulder can be preserved.

4. ***Preservation of most of the growth plate***. Epiphysiolysis occurs through the layer of degenerative cells on the metaphyseal side of the growth plate. Therefore, most of the growth plate is retained, together with the epiphysis (Fig. 13.10). When the distraction procedure is performed at a rate of 1–1.5 mm/day, the retained physis remains active [4].

We believe that intra-epiphyseal osteotomy is indicated in the following situations:

- For resection of metaphyseal tumors with no involvement of the physis in which a pathological fracture has occurred. In such cases, unless the fracture heals during neoadjuvant treatment, physeal distraction is contraindicated because of the risk of distraction through the tumor instead of the growth plate (Fig. 9.9).
- For resection of metaphyseal tumors in contact with part of the growth plate. In this scenario, intra-epiphyseal osteotomy could be an alternative to the standard Cañadell technique (see Chap. 10).
- For resection of metaphyseal tumors without involvement of the physis, but in patients who are close to the end of growth: in such patients it is more difficult to achieve physeal distraction.

Some example cases relating to the second and the third of these criteria are shown in Figs. 13.3 and 13.4.

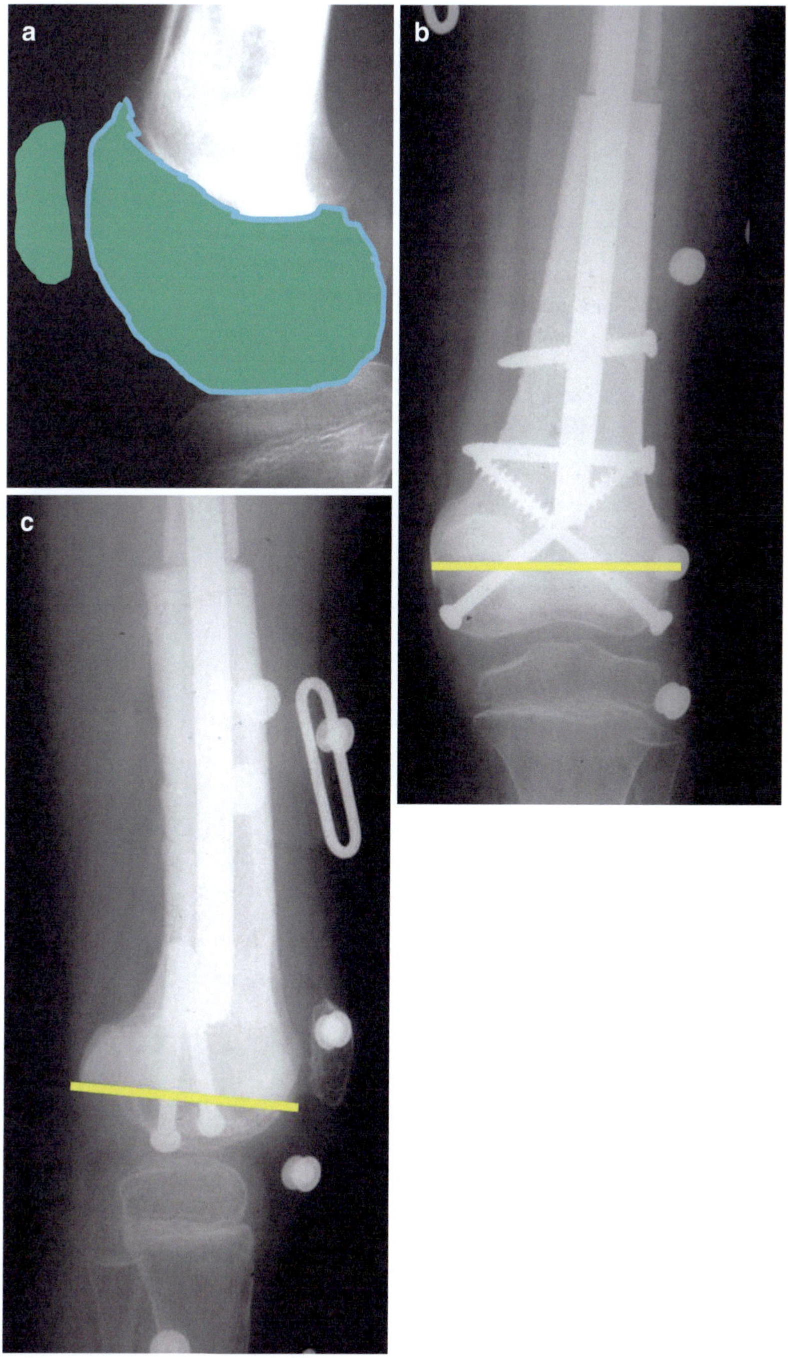

Fig. 13.8 (**a**) The growth plate extends to the cartilage of the condyles and trochlea femoralis. (**b**, **c**) The patient came to our hospital after pulmonary metastases had been detected by another institution. The previous X-rays were not available to us. Apparently, intra-epiphyseal osteotomy had been performed to preserve the joint. The functional result was poor because the osteotomy line cut the trochlea

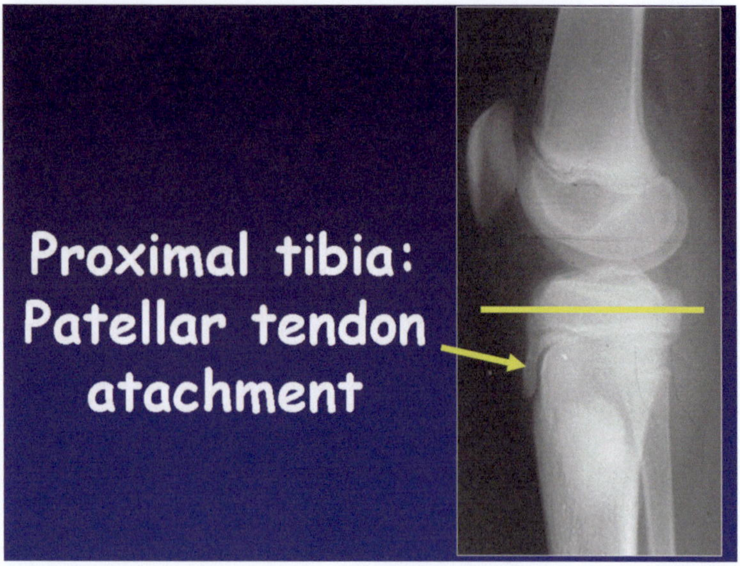

Fig. 13.9 Intra-epiphyseal osteotomy does not allow for preservation of the patellar tendon attachment

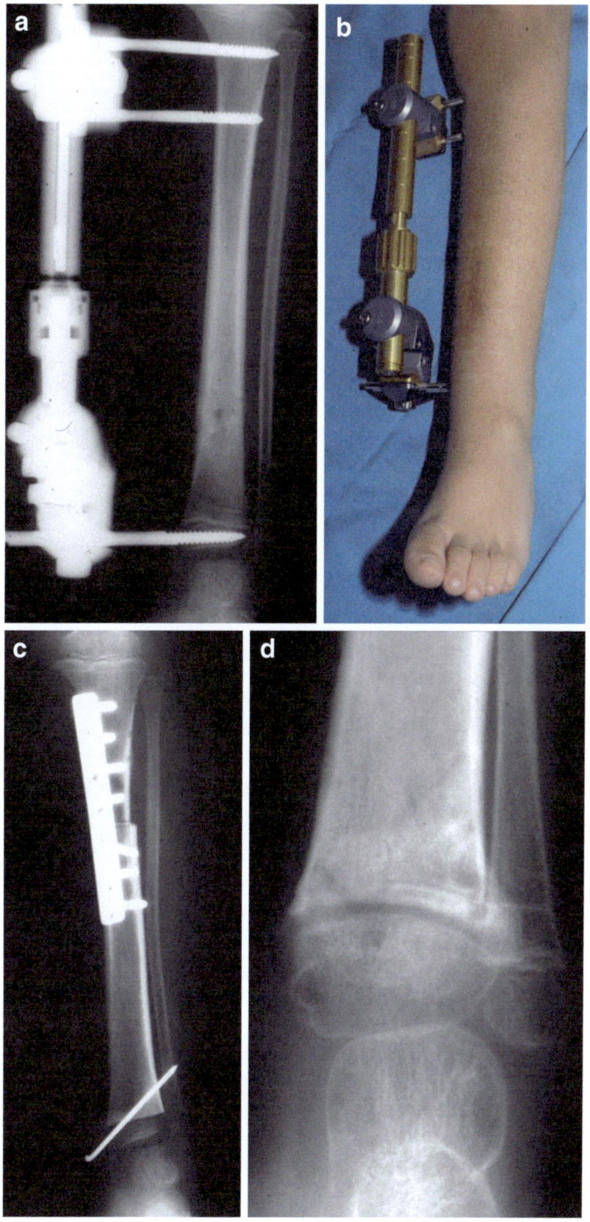

Fig. 13.10 (**a**, **b**) Physeal distraction before excision of a Ewing's sarcoma in the distal tibia of a 3-year-old boy. (**c**, **d**) The growth plate remains active after removal of the distal Kirschner wire

References

1. Andreou D, Henrichs MP, Gosheger G, Nottrott M, Streitbürger A, Hardes J. Neue Operationsverfahren bei Knochentumoren. Pathologe. 2014;35 Suppl 2:232–6 (German).
2. Aponte-Tinao L, Ayerza MA, Muscolo L, Farfalli G. Survival, recurrence, and function after epiphyseal preservation and allograft reconstruction in osteosarcoma of the knee. Clin Orthop Relat Res. 2015;473(5):1797–801.
3. Capanna R, Manfrini M, Ceruso M, et al. A new reconstruction for metaphyseal resections: a combined graft (allograft shell plus vascularized fibula). Preliminary results. In: Brown KL, editor. Complications in limb salvage. Prevention, management and outcome. Montreal: Publisher ISOLS; 1991. p. 319.
4. De Pablos J, Cañadell J. Experimental physeal distraction in immature sheep. Clin Orthop. 1990;250:73–80.
5. Yang D, Hongliang Y, Zhichang Z, Weiping J, Qingcheng Y, Shu Q. Reconstruction with preservation of the epiphysis by using custom-made prosthesis in children with distal femoral osteosarcomas. Chin J Orthop. 2015;35(2):121–6 (Chinese).
6. Fang B, YI C, Zhang H, Zhang Q, LI Y, Wei Q, He W, Zeng Z. Combined epiphyseal preservation and autograft bone transfer in treatment of children osteosarcoma. Chin J Reparat Reconstr Surg. 2013;27(1):45–9 (Chinese).
7. Hayashi K, Tsuchiya H, Yamamoto N, Takeuchi A, Tomita K. Functional outcome in patients with osteosarcoma around the knee joint treated by minimised surgery. Int Orthop (SICOT). 2008;32:63–8.
8. Jing L, Lei S, Guo-jing C. Image navigation assisted joint-saving surgery for treatment of bone sarcoma around knee in skeletally immature patients. Surg Oncol. 2014;23:132–9.
9. Manfrini M. Intraepiphyseal resection. In: Albiñana J, editor. Bone tumors in children and adolescents. Rev Mapfre Medicina. 1997;8(Suppl I):282–3.
10. Xu S, Yu X, Xu M, Fu Z, Chen Y, Sun Y, Su Q. Limb function and quality of life after various reconstruction methods according to tumor location following resection of osteosarcoma in distal femur. BMC Musculoskelet Disord. 2014;15(453):1–9.
11. Tsuchiya H, Abdel-Wanis ME, Sakurakichi K, Yamashiro T, Tomita K. Osteosarcoma around the knee Intraepiphyseal excision and biological reconstruction with distraction osteogenesis. J Bone Joint Surg [Br]. 2002;84-B:1162–6.
12. Yoshida Y, Osaka S, Tokuhashi Y. Analysis of limb function after various reconstruction methods according to tumor location following resection of pediatric malignant bone tumors. World J Surg Oncol. 2010;8:39.
13. Zhang P, Feng F, Cai Q, Yao W, Gao S, Wang J, Wang X. Effects of metaphyseal bone tumor removal with preservation of the epiphysis and knee arthroplasty. Exp Ther Med. 2014;8:567–72.
14. San-Julian M, Vázquez-García BL, Sierrasesúmaga L. Limb salvage in children. In: European surgical orthopaedics and traumatology. Berlin/Heidelberg: Springer; 2014. p. 4251–80.

Chapter 14
Worldwide Experience with the Cañadell Technique

SongFeng Xu, WeiTao Yao, ZhaoQiang Chen, XiuChun Yu, QiQing Cai, YongCheng Hu, Zhen Wang, G. Ulrich Exner, Charles E. Dumont, Antonio Marcelo G. de Souza, Màrius Aguirre-Canyadell, and Roberto Vélez

Abstract Cañadell's technique for limb preserving surgery in pediatric bone sarcoma treatment was developed at the *Clínica Universidad de Navarra* in Pamplona, Spain and first presented in 1984. Recently, teams at many hospitals all over the world (for example, in China, Switzerland, Brazil, the Netherlands, Germany, Hungary, and Turkey) have successfully used the technique and published their results. Only now is it becoming clear that the positive results reported by Cañadell

S. Xu, MD, PhD • X. Yu, MD, PhD
Department of Orthopedics, General Hospital of Ji'Nan Military Region, Ji'Nan, ShanDong Province, People's Republic of China
e-mail: xusongfeng@gmail.com

W. Yao, MD, PhD • Q. Cai, MD, PhD
Department of Bone and Soft Tissue Cancer, HeNan Cancer Hospital, ZhengZhou, HeNan Province, People's Republic of China

Z. Chen, MD, PhD • Y. Hu, MD, PhD
Department of Orthopedic Oncology, TianJin Hospital, TianJin Medical University, TianJin, People's Republic of China

Z. Wang, MD, PhD
Department of Orthopedic Oncology, XiJing Hospital, the Fourth Military Medical University, Xi'an, ShanXi Province, People's Republic of China

G.U. Exner • C.E. Dumont
Department of Orthopaedics, Orthopaedie Zentrum Zuerich, Zuerich, Switzerland

A.M.G. de Souza, MD, PhD
Orthopaedic Oncology Service, Cancer Hospital of Pernambuco, Recife, Brazil

M. Aguirre-Canyadell, MD, PhD (✉) • R. Vélez, MD, PhD
Department of Orthopaedic Surgery and Traumatology, Orthopaedic Oncology Unit, Hospital Universitari Vall d'Hebron, Universitat Autònoma de Barcelona, Barcelona, Spain
e-mail: maguirre@vhebron.net

M. San-Julian (ed.), *Cañadell's Pediatric Bone Sarcomas: Epiphysiolysis before Excision*, DOI 10.1007/978-3-319-24220-0_14

at the beginning of the 1990s can be easily achieved by other experts in the field. To illustrate this point, we present here some of the results obtained with this technique by teams based in hospitals other than that of Cañadell in Pamplona

Keywords Bone sarcoma • Limb salvage • Epiphyseal preservation • Cañadell's technique • Cryosurgery • Recycled bone

14.1 Application of Cañadell's Technique in Four Chinese Hospitals

Cañadell's technique involving epiphysiolysis before tumor excision [1] in order to preserve the epiphysis in limb salvage surgery associated with treatment for malignant bone tumors in adolescents has been widely accepted and used in clinical practice all over the world. Since April 2010 and especially since the publication of the Chinese edition of "Pediatric Bone Sarcoma" [2] in December 2011, the technique has gradually been used more and more in China. We report on 15 patients who have undergone epiphysiolysis in four Chinese hospitals up to January 2015.

14.1.1 Methods

The four Chinese hospitals whose experiences are reported here are the General Hospital of Ji'Nan Military commanding Region (Ji'Nan, China)(JN), HeNan Cancer Hospital (ZhengZhou, China)(ZZ), TianJin Hospital (TianJin, China)(TJ), and XiJing Hospital (XJ) (Table 14.1).

In JN from July 2012 to October 2014, five patients were treated with epiphysiolysis before tumor excision; there were three boys and two girls, with median age of 8 years (6–11 years) at surgery. Three neoplasms were located in distal femur and two in proximal tibia. On the basis of the Enneking staging system [3], in all five patients the disease was in stage IIB. All tumors were pathologically diagnosed as osteosarcoma, with four being of the osteoblastic type and one of the chondroblastic type. Preoperative chemotherapy was given in two courses on a neoadjuvant basis with cisplatin, Adriamycin and ifosfamide [4]. The reconstruction methods after tumor resection were distraction osteogenesis in one patient, alcohol inactivated autograft replantation in one patient, and microwave inactivation with external fixation in three patients.

In ZZ, between April 2010 and November 2012 [5], five patients were treated with epiphysiolysis before tumor excision; there were two boys and three girls, with median age of 13 years (9–15 years) at surgery. All five neoplasms were located in left distal femur. On the basis of the Enneking staging system, disease was at stage IIB. All tumors were pathologically diagnosed as osteosarcoma. Preoperative chemotherapy, which was given twice on a neoadjuvant basis, was with methotrexate,

Table 14.1 General information of 15 patients in four Chinese hospitals

No.	Hospital	Birth	Age	Gender	MRI type	Epiphysiolysis surgery	Site	Resection surgery	Reconstruction method	Chemo	Follow-up (months)	MSTS	Limb length (L/R cm)	Compli-cation	Pathology
1.	JN	2001/4/21	11	Male	2	2012/7/11	Left proximal tibia	2012/8/2	Distraction osteogenesis	Cisplatin, adriamycin and ifosfamide	30	29	82/81	None	Osteo-sarcoma
2.	JN	2004/9/6	7	Female	2	2012/7/30	Left distal femur	2012/8/29	Alcohol inactivated autograft replantation	Cisplatin, adriamycin and ifosfamide	17	28	82/84	Autograft fracture	Osteo-sarcoma
3.	JN	2008/7/12	6	Female	2	2014/8/18	Right distal femur	2014/8/27	Microwave inactivation with external fixation	Cisplatin, adriamycin and ifosfamide	5	28	74/74	None	Osteo-sarcoma
4.	JN	2005/8/20	9	Male	2	2014/9/1	Right proximal tibia	2014/9/24	Microwave inactivation with external fixation	Cisplatin, adriamycin and ifosfamide	6	30	77/77	None	Osteo-sarcoma (chon-droblast)
5.	JN	2006/1/10	8	Male	1	2014/10/17	Left distal femur	2014/11/7	Microwave inactivation with external fixation	Cisplatin, adriamycin and ifosfamide	3	30	72/72	None	Osteo-sarcoma
6.	ZZ	1996/11/27	15	Female	3	2011/7/9	Left distal femur	2011/8/4	Allograft replantation	Methotrexate, pirarubicin, carboplatin and ifosfamide	41	23	69/69	Joint stiffness	Osteo-sarcoma
7.	ZZ	1994/9/1	15	Female	2	2010/4/30	Left distal femur	2010/5/13	Allograft replantation	Methotrexate, pirarubicin, carboplatin and ifosfamide	21	29	76/76	Pulmonary metastasis	Osteo-sarcoma

(continued)

Table 14.1 (continued)

No.	Hospital	Birth	Age	Gender	MRI type	Epiphysiolysis surgery	Site	Resection surgery	Reconstruction method	Chemo	Follow-up (months)	MSTS	Limb length (L/R cm)	Compli-cation	Pathology
8.	ZZ	2003/4/10	9	Female	1	2012/11/22	Left distal femur	2012/11/22	Inactivated autograft replantation	Methotrexate, pirarubicin, carboplatin and ifosfamide	21	25	58/58	Autograft nonunion	Osteo-sarcoma
9.	ZZ	1995/4/14	15	Male	1	2010/7/21	Left distal femur	2010/7/29	Allograft replantation	Methotrexate, pirarubicin, carboplatin and ifosfamide	54	24	70/74	Infection and allograft rejection	Osteo-sarcoma
10.	ZZ	1995/9/15	11	Male	2	2010/1/19	Left distal femur	2010/2/6	Allograft replantation	Methotrexate, pirarubicin, carboplatin and ifosfamide	59	29	81/84	Pulmonary metastasis	Osteo-sarcoma
11.	TJ	2004/9/1	9	Male	3	2013/9/23	Left distal tibia plus lung mets	2013/10/21	Distraction osteogenesis	Doxorubicin and cisplatin	17	18	Unknown	Recurrence and amputation	Osteo-sarcoma
12.	TJ	2008/1/30	6	Female	1	2014/5/16	Left distal tibia	2014/6/17	Distraction osteogenesis	Doxorubicin and cisplatin	7	22	Unknown	Delayed union	Ewing's sarcoma
13.	TJ	2006/1/5	8	Male	2	2014/8/14	Left distal femur	2014/9/10	Distraction osteogenesis	Doxorubicin and cisplatin	4	21	Unknown	Infection	Osteo-sarcoma
14.	TJ	2004/11/18	6	Male	1	2012/6/28	Right distal tibia	2012/8/20	Distraction osteogenesis	Doxorubicin and cisplatin	22	30	Equal	None	Osteo-sarcoma
15.	XJ	2003/8/12	8	Male	1	2012/5/25	Left proximal tibia	2012/6/21	Allograft replantation with pedicled fibula	Methotrexate, cisplatin, adriamycin and ifosfamide	26	30	Equal	Skin ulcer and local infection	Osteo-sarcoma

pirarubicin, carboplatin and ifosfamide. The reconstruction methods after tumor resection were inactivated autograft replantation in one patient, and allograft replantation with internal fixation in four patients.

In TJ from June 2012 to August 2014, four patients were treated with epiphysiolysis before tumor excision. The patients were three boys and one girl; median age at surgery was 7 years (6–9 years). One neoplasm was in the left distal femur, and three were in the proximal tibia. Three patients were in Enneking stage IIB; one boy was in stage III with pulmonary metastasis. The tumors of the three boys were pathologically diagnosed as osteosarcoma; the girl had a Ewing's sarcoma. Preoperative chemotherapy was doxorubicin and cisplatin, which were given in three courses on a neoadjuvant basis. The method chosen for reconstruction after tumor resection was distraction osteogenesis in all four patients.

In XJ, one 8-year-old boy with a neoplasm in his left proximal tibia received epiphysiolysis before tumor excision, in May 2012. Disease was at stage IIB and pathologically diagnosed as osteosarcoma. Preoperative chemotherapy was in three courses, on a neoadjuvant basis, and with methotrexate, cisplatin, Adriamycin and ifosfamide. The method chosen for reconstruction was allograft replantation with vascularized fibula.

All patients received postoperative courses of neo-adjuvant chemotherapy. The follow-up schedule involves revisions every 3 months in the first and second year, and then every 6 months for the next 3 years. Postoperative results were evaluated according to the MSTS limb function score system. Statistical analysis involved calculation of the correlation between related factors, survival, and postoperative function.

14.1.2 Results

In JN, after a mean follow-up of 12 months (3–30 months), all children were alive and four patients were disease-free. One girl experienced fracture of an inactivated autograft and required a second operation with internal fixation. This girl, who was 7 years old at the initial surgery, was the only of the patients to suffer any limb discrepancy. The other four children showed equal lower limb length of 82, 74, 77 and 72 cm [6] (Fig. 14.1). At the most recent follow-up, no cases of recurrence or metastasis were found, and the mean MSTS score was 29 (ranging between 28 and 30).

Of the ZZ patients, one died of pulmonary metastasis 6 months after start of treatment (epiphysiolysis). After a mean follow-up of 39 months (21–59 months), the other four children treated at ZZ were alive [5] but with certain complications: one girl had knee joint stiffness (30 months after epiphysiolysis); one boy was found to have pulmonary metastasis (31 months after epiphysiolysis (Fig. 14.2); one girl suffered non-union of an inactivated autograft, which required a second round of surgery with bone grafting (4 months after epiphysiolysis); and one boy suffered allograft infection (7 months after epiphysiolysis). The four surviving patients all have a degree of limb discrepancy: from 3 to 5 cm. At the most recent follow-up, no cases of recurrence were found, and the mean MSTS score was 26 (from 23 to 29).

In TJ, after a mean follow-up of 12 months (4–22 months), all four children were alive. One, a 6-year-old boy, had no recurrence, no complications, limb equivalence,

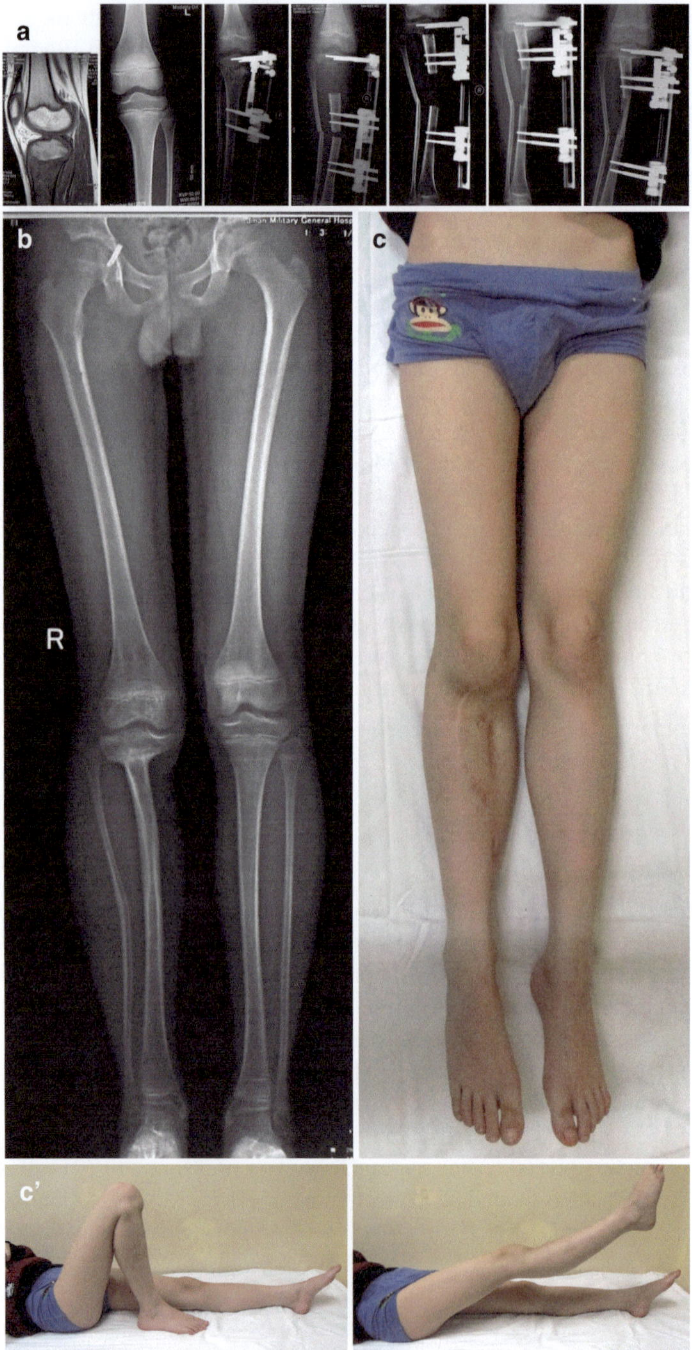

Fig. 14.1 (**a**) The preoperative MRI showed the tumor to be in contact with the physis. Physeal distraction was achieved, and reconstruction was made through bone transport. After 30 months, X-ray showed full bone union. (**b**, **c**) The boy showed limb equivalence with MSTS score of 30 (Endorsed by Pro.XiuChun Yu)

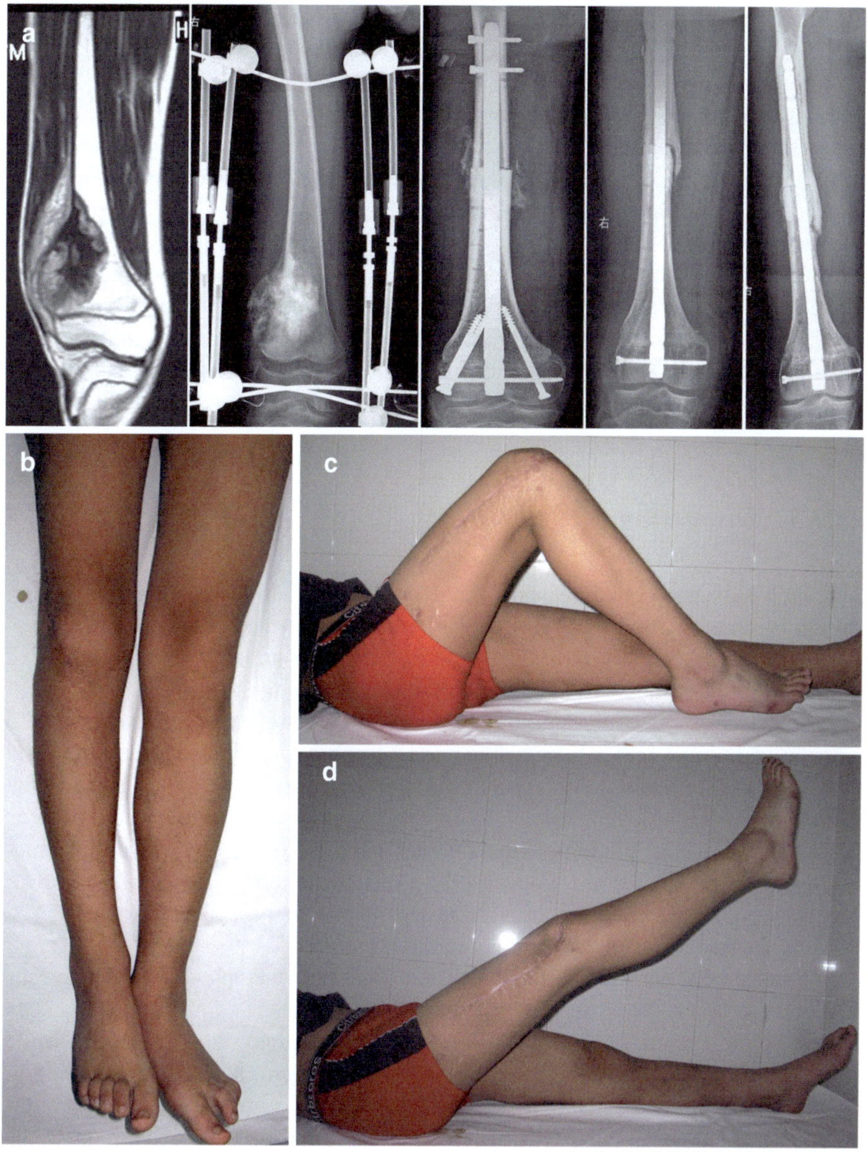

Fig. 14.2 (**a**) Eleven year boy. The preoperative MRI showed the tumor to be nearly in contact with epiphysis, classified as Type 2. After epiphysiolysis, the patient underwent tumor resection and allograft reconstruction. Twelve months later, X-ray study showed full bone union; After 29 months, pulmonary metastasis was detected; treatment was thoracoscopic resection of pulmonary nodule. After 54 months, (**b–d**) the patient was alive with no metastasis; lower limb discrepancy was 4 cm. MSTS score was 29 (Endorsed by Pro.QiQing Cai)

and an MSTS score of 30. One boy suffered tumor recurrence above the epiphysis and underwent a second operation, with above-knee amputation. One boy had wound infection (3 months after epiphysiolysis); limb length discrepancy has not been recorded. One, the girl, had delayed union of the distal tibia and limb length discrepancy has not yet been recorded. At the most recent follow-up, the mean MSTS score was 23 (from 18 to 30).

After a follow-up of 26 months, the 8-year-old boy with OS treated at XJ was without recurrence, disease-free, and had limb equivalence. However, he experienced skin ulceration and local infection 1 year after the first operation and underwent further surgery to remove the internal fixation and perform transposition of the muscle flap. At the latest follow-up, the MSTS score was 30.

In summary, of the 15 patients, after a mean follow-up of 22 months (4–59 months), 12 (80 %) showed no evidence of disease, and eight (53 %) showed limb equivalence. Just one patient experienced local recurrence above the epiphysis. Seven patients (47 %) suffered complications, such as, skin ulceration, infection, delayed union, autograft fracture, and joint stiffness. Pooling evaluations of the most recent follow-ups, the mean MSTS score was 26.4, ranging between 18 and 30.

14.1.3 Discussion

The limb salvage procedure should not delay adjuvant therapy; reconstruction should be enduring and not be associated with a large number of local complications requiring secondary procedures and frequent hospitalization; and function of the limb should be at least as good as that obtained by amputation [7].

In most cases of osteosarcoma, especially in young patients, resection of a metaphyseal tumor with a 3–5 cm safe margin implies loss of the adjacent joint and such loss usually leads to limb length discrepancy. However, a safe margin in the context of a metaphyseal tumor can be obtained without sacrificing the epiphysis: as described by Cañadell, in tumors that do not cross the growth plate, physeal distraction provides a safe margin while averting loss of the epiphysis [2]. The growth cartilage itself is believed to provide a dependable margin of safety and so the 3–5 cm margin suggested by most authors is unnecessary.

The absence of anastomoses between epiphyseal and metaphyseal vessels means that in those cases where imaging methods indicate that the epiphysis has not been affected by the tumor, it is possible to conserve the epiphysis and the joint while resecting the tumor [2]. This is made possible by physeal distraction according to Cañadell's technique [1]. Note that physeal distraction is not used for bone lengthening, but rather as the first part of tumor resection: it effects a separation of the epiphysis from the tumor-bearing metaphysis.

The indications for physeal distraction in pediatric bone sarcoma treatment are that the tumor must be located in the metaphysis, that the physis must be open, and that the tumor must not have transgressed the physis. If the tumor is in contact with part of the physis, physeal distraction can be tried. MRI is the imaging method of choice in evaluating physeal tumor involvement, and enables categorization of tumors near the epiphysis into three types [8]. As described by San-Julian, if all of the physis is affected, there is a great possibility that tumor cells have passed across it and consequently physeal distraction is contraindicated [8]. Crucial factors in the success of physeal distraction are a positive response to chemotherapy, accurate preoperative assessment of tumor extension to the epiphysis by MRI, and appropriate reconstruction techniques.

In the group of 15 patients reported here who underwent Cañadell's technique, 12 (80 %) experienced no recurrence or metastasis, and eight (53 %) showed limb equivalence. However, four patients (47 %) had recorded limb discrepancy of between 1 and 4 cm and for a further three patients (33 %) limb lengths were not recorded or not relevant. Differences may exist in the details of how epiphysiolysis was carried out in the four hospitals considered. Seven of the 15 patients (47 %) had complications, some of which may be associated with different reconstruction methods in the four hospitals. In general, for all patients, limb function was acceptable in the most recent follow-up; the mean MSTS score was 26.4 (18–30).

14.1.4 Conclusion

In China, Cañadell's limb salvage procedure involving epiphysiolysis before tumor excision for skeletally immature patients has gradually been adopted in clinical practice. All of the patients reported here, who were treated at four Chinese hospitals, can be seen to have benefitted from undergoing the technique. Naturally, variations in management of the technique and different reconstruction methods after tumor resection are expected to affect clinical results.

14.2 Preservation of Joints in Pediatric Diaphyseal and Metaphyseal Bone Sarcomas by Gradual Separation through the Physis. Management of Reconstruction Problems

14.2.1 Introduction

The artificial joint reconstructions currently available are prone to failure with time and are imperfect substitutes for natural biological joints. While diaphyseal bone structures can be anatomically reconstructed by relatively simple techniques and measures, the reconstruction of joints poses a much more complex problem. The goal in children and young people with normal life expectancy must be biologic reconstructions that can have lifelong durability.

In treating sarcomas it is crucial to remove the tumor completely, leaving no living tumoral cells within the body. How to achieve uncontaminated margins is one of the great challenges in tumor surgery, and how much distance is necessary between the surgical cut and the tumor being removed is a matter of debate. Without pathologic examination, delineation of tumor boundaries depends on the macroscopic imaging techniques currently available. The decision of how much apparently healthy tissue to excise around a tumor ("wide" and "marginal" margins according to Enneking) is, unfortunately, in most cases still "experience based" if the dissection planes are not determined by anatomic structures (in which case "radical" margins are indicated according to Enneking).

Joint preservation depends primarily on preservation of the cartilaginous components of a joint. Ligaments can be partially reconstructed. To preserve a joint there are principally three possible resection planes:

- Metaphyseal resection with preservation of the physis. This is comparable to osteotomy.
- Trans-physeal resection by slow distraction. This is the so-called Cañadell technique or Pamplona technique (Canadell/San Julian 8, 9).
- Trans-epiphyseal resection.

Excellent results have been obtained with and reported for the Cañadell/Pamplona technique [8, 9] when appropriately indicated. Surprisingly, then, the approach is still regarded by some in the Americas and Europe as controversial; it has, however, received acceptance in China [10, 11].

We have used the Pamplona technique in six patients since 1988 and have not encountered any case of local recurrence. Our results were published in 2012 [12]. The technique has been applied when the growth plate was judged not to have been crossed by the tumor, even if the tumor was in contact with up to three quarters of the length of the growth plate. One patient in our series died from metastases, while all others continue to do well at the time of writing (April 2015). None had local recurrence. At 8-years follow-up, four patients have Musculoskeletal Tumor Rating Scale (MSTS) scores of 30 points, the other patient has a score of 25 points. In all cases the MSTS score excludes the point "emotional acceptance"; all patients, however, express complete satisfaction with their reconstructions in long term follow-up.

While we found the technique of physeal distraction reliable and useful, we have still had to struggle with the reconstruction and wish to discuss here several aspects of difficulty encountered in three patients.

14.2.2 Patients, Methods and Results

Patient 1. (N.S.; born in 1994; Fig. 14.3). A girl diagnosed with high-grade osteosarcoma at age 11 years (Fig. 14.3a). Despite her young age, the patient insisted on a wholly biologic reconstruction of her leg. To the treating staff physician, physeal distraction appeared to have progressed uneventfully. However, on reviewing all the images on the eve of surgery, the surgeons (the authors of this paper) recognized that laterally part of the physis had remained intact and a fracture through the tumor bearing metaphysis had occurred (Fig. 14.3b). Trans-epiphyseal resection was performed (Fig. 14.3c). The defect was reconstructed with free microvascular fibula transfer (Fig. 14.3d). The patient expressed satisfaction with her leg reconstruction, but died from systemic metastases (that had already been evident at the time of tumor surgery) 8 months later.

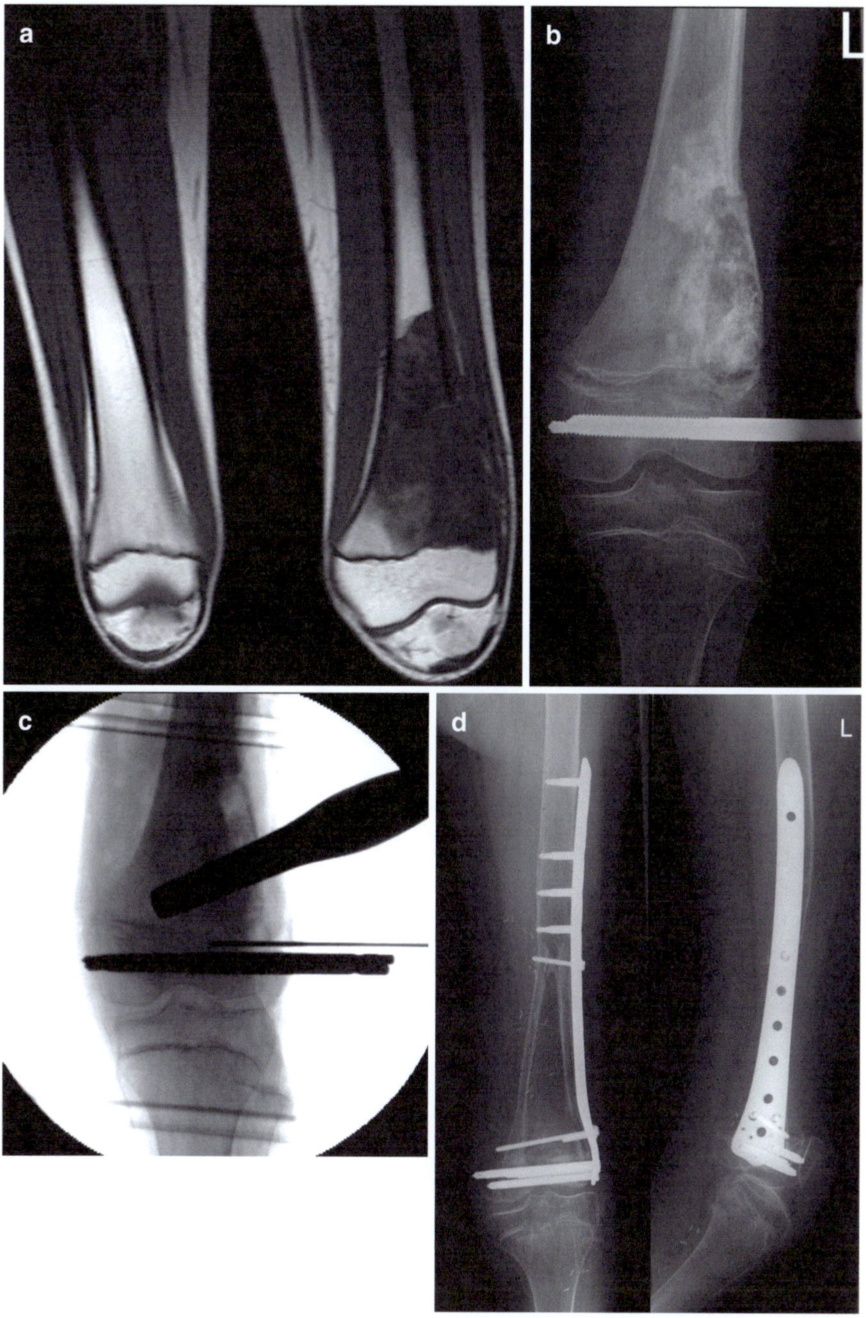

Fig. 14.3 (**a**) Patient 1. Osteosarcoma. The MRI shows the extent of the tumor, which is in contact with two thirds of the distal femoral physis. (**b**) This X-ray taken after 12 days of distraction for physeal separation shows the fracture through the metaphyseal part of the femur; part of the osteosarcoma remains attached to the epiphysis. (**c**) This intra-operative X-ray shows the K-wire placed for guidance of the saw between the K-wire and the Schanz screws used for fixation of the external distractor. (**d**) Postoperative documentation of the reconstruction with free microvascular fibula

Patient 2. (F.H.; born in 1995; Fig. 14.4). A 10-year-old boy diagnosed with high-grade osteosarcoma in the right femur (Fig. 14.4a) and treated in 2005. Chemotherapy was according to COSS 96. Physeal distraction was carried out (Fig. 14.4b). Initial reconstruction was with free microvascular double barrel fibula (Fig. 14.4c). Because of partial failure and lack of signs of bone formation, an allograft was added 8 months after the initial reconstruction, leaving part of the fibula (Fig. 14.4d). At age 14 years, the patient underwent epiphysiodesis for the contralateral knee. At the time of writing, the patient is 19 years old, disease free, has 130°-0°-0° flexion/extension of the knee, and a MSTS score of 30.

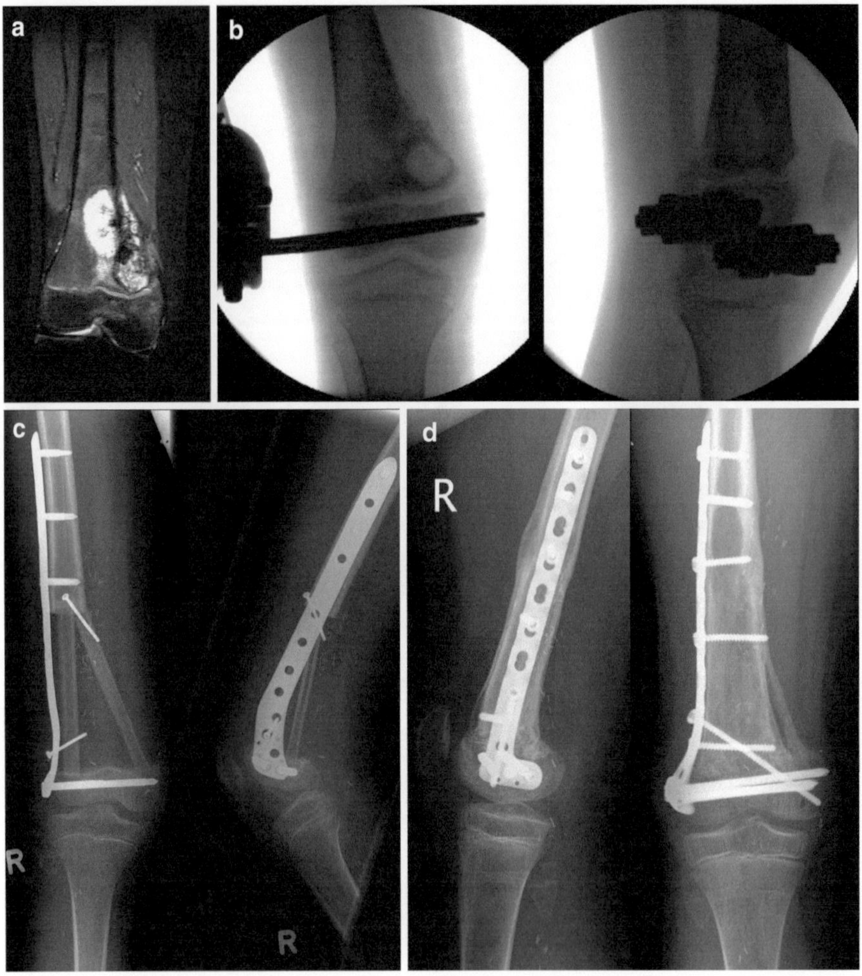

Fig. 14.4 (**a**) Patient 2. Osteosarcoma in the distal femur. MRI after preoperative chemotherapy. (**b**) Physeal separation before definitive surgery. (**c**) Post-operative X-ray after reconstruction with a free microvascular allograft. (**d**) Definitive healing after additional allograft

Patient 3. (R.K.; born in 1993; Fig. 14.5). A 15-year-old girl diagnosed with high grade osteosarcoma in the right femur (Fig. 14.5a). Chemotherapy was according to EURAMOS. Physeal distraction was carried out (Fig. 14.5b). The tumor was resected

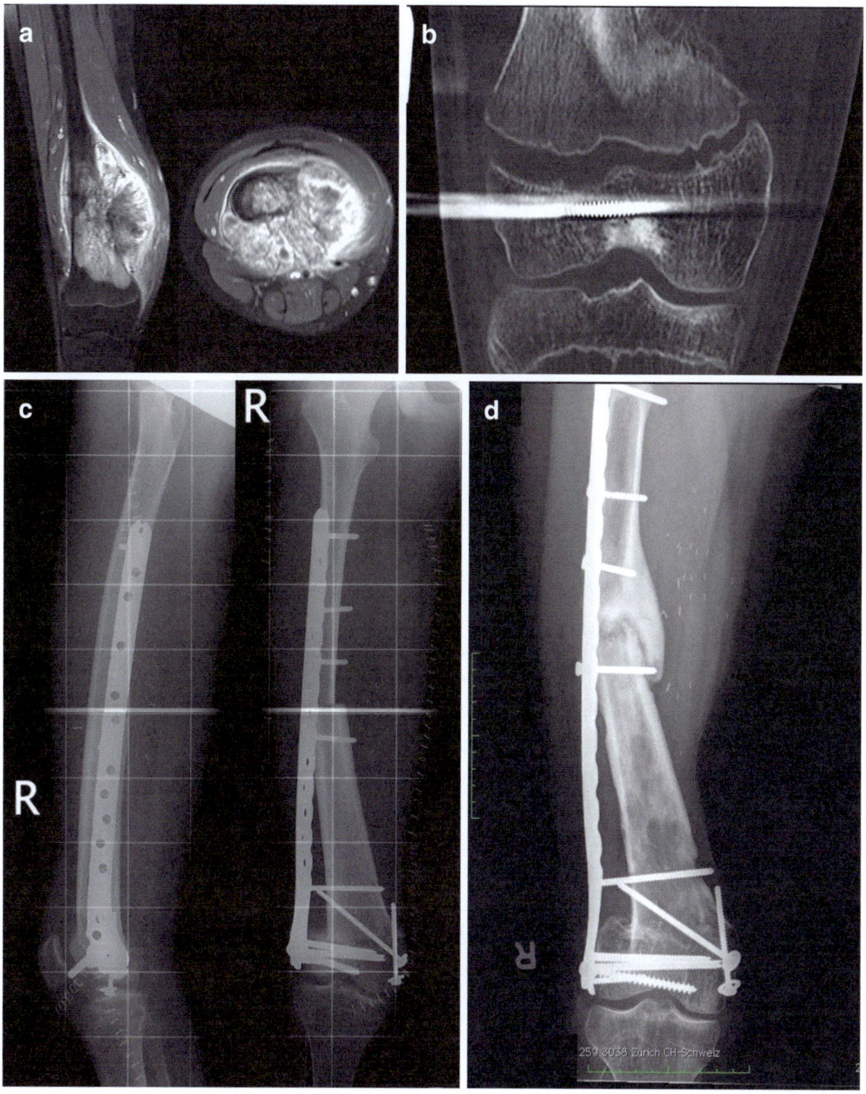

Fig. 14.5 (**a**) Patient 3. MRI showing the extensive involvement of the region of the Hunter canal. (**b**) CT reconstruction after physeal distraction showing correct rupture of the physis. (**c**) Initial reconstruction with allograft and reconstruction of the femoral vessels with autograft from the contralateral *Vena saphena magna*. (**d**) Failed allograft due to low grade infection with *Staphylococcus epidermidis*. (**e**) Temporary cement spacer. (**f**) Vessel loop formed with ipsilateral vein for arterial and venous anastomosis of the free microvascular fibula. (**g**) Final stable biologic reconstruction with allograft and "onlay" vascular fibula

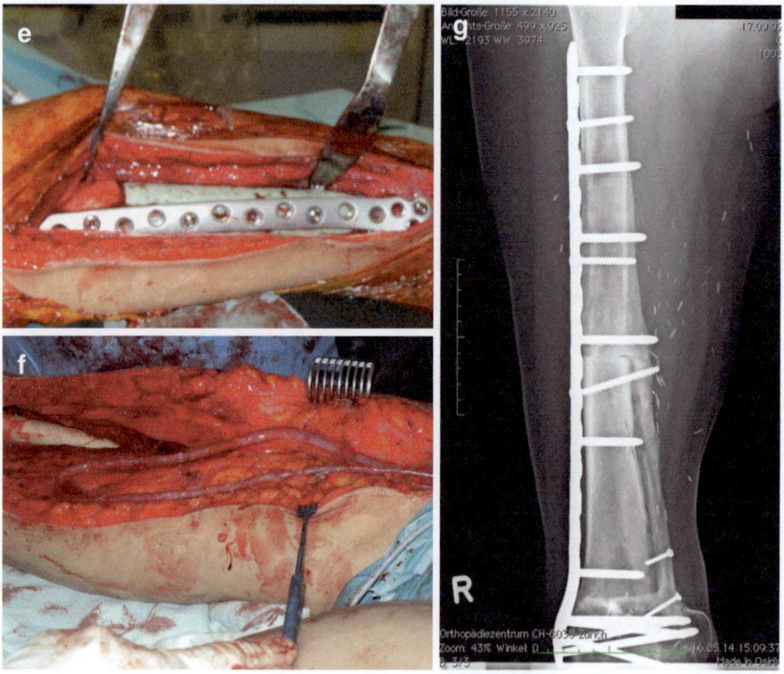

Fig. 14.5 (continued)

with the adjacent femoral vessels. Reconstructing of both the artery and vein was by contralateral saphenous vein graft. Reconstruction of the bone was with fresh frozen allograft (Fig. 14.5c). As a result of low grade infection with *Staphylococcus epidermidis*, the allograft did not fuse and fractured 3 years later (in 2010) (Fig. 14.5d). The allograft was removed and an antibiotic loaded cement spacer was implanted (Fig. 14.5e). Three weeks later the cement spacer was replaced by an allograft with simultaneous free microvascular fibula transfer using the initially preserved ipsilateral saphenous vein for arterial anastomosis to the femoral artery below the inguinal ligament (Fig. 14.5f). This allograft also failed and was replaced 3 years later (in 2013) leaving the transplanted fibula. This led to final definitive healing (Fig. 14.5g). Currently (2015), the patient is disease free and feels unlimited in spite of restricted flexion in the knee joint (flexion/extension is 110°-0°-0°). MSTS score is 25.

14.2.3 Discussion

The case of patient one, in which physeal separation was incomplete and fracture occurred in the tumor bearing metaphysis, illustrates the importance of careful analysis of the progress of physeal separation. If radiography is not unequivocally clear, it is necessary to consider using magnetic resonance (MRI) or computed tomography (CT) to assess whether separation has occurred within healthy bone. Note, however, that MRI is limited by the possibility of artifacts arising from the implants and device used for distraction.

In the case of patient two, because of the relatively short segment of excised bone and the young age of the patient, we opted for double barrel fibular reconstruction, which has greater potential for remodeling and thickening of the vascularized fibula. Subsequent secondary augmentation with an allograft resulted in full biologic healing, in spite of at the fact that there had been at least a partial failure of the initially transplanted fibula.

The situation in patient three was especially difficult because of the necessity at the time of tumor surgery to reconstruct not only the bone but also the arterial and venous vessels. In view of the complexity of the procedure, we considered it inappropriate to put at further risk the circulation in the extremity by augmenting the bone reconstruction with free fibula transfer. The failure of the allograft was most likely related to a low grade infection. The patient, who had chosen her biologic reconstruction, has persevered through many demanding reoperations and revisions but is finally satisfied with a fully biologically-reconstructed functional and stable leg.

14.2.4 Conclusion

Replacement of bone after tumor resection can be achieved through demanding procedures to establish biologic reconstructions or through relatively simple techniques with artificial implants. Apart from the much simpler and quicker procedures, another advantage of artificial implants is that rehabilitation is much shorter than that with biologic reconstructions. However, only biologic reconstructions have the potential to last for a lifetime; artificial reconstructions are prone to failure.

In our view, each patient is unique and the mode and material chosen for reconstruction must consider how to maximize potential future quality of life, that is, the quality added life years (QUALY) for the individual patient.

In carefully selected cases, the Cañadell or Pamplona technique of physeal distraction has contributed greatly to improve the long-term functional results in growing children subjected to resection of bone tumors. Whenever the technique is feasible, it should be considered.

14.3 The Experience in Brazil: Epiphyseal Distraction Combined with Autograft of Cryogenically Recycled Tumoral Bone. A New Method for Epiphyseal Sparing Surgery in Malignant Bone Tumors

14.3.1 Introduction

Patients with an open metaphysis and bone sarcomas that have not invaded the metaphysis can present a challenge to the orthopedic surgeon. In some cases, trans-epiphyseal resection osteotomy would not enable adequate future osteosynthesis because the remaining epiphyseal bone tissue would be too scarce, soft and thin.

The possibility of maintaining the epiphysis intact whilst maintaining (or even increasing) the resection margins through a previous separation of the diaphysis from the epiphysis was first described by Cañadell in 1984 and published in an international journal in 1994 [13]. Originally Cañadell and his co-workers reconstructed the bone defect with an autograft or an allograft. In Kanazawa, H. Tsuchiya and colleagues developed a simple method of recycling malignant bone tumor by freezing the specimen in liquid nitrogen; the method was described in 2005 [14]. We visited Kanazawa in 2004, and since then we have been using this method at our hospital. We have also had the opportunity to see San Julian presenting his technique at the ISOLS in Hamburg in 2007 and later also visited his department in Pamplona. Since then we have used, whenever indicated, these two techniques in combination. We have found no mention in the literature of this combined approach and, therefore, describe the method here.

14.3.2 Materials and Methods

From May 2008 to April 2010, three patients fulfilled the criteria for treatment by epiphyseal distraction and bone freezing. Epiphyseal distraction was undertaken following the descriptions of Cañadell and San Julian [8, 13, 15]. In all three cases we used a linear type LRS Orthofix external fixator inserting two pins proximally and two distally to the tumor limits. According to the tumor site, the two pins inserted at the epiphysis were always inserted parallel to the metaphyseal line. Fluoroscopy was used in all cases. Distraction started the day after placement, and separation of the epiphysis from the diaphysis took place around the 12th–14th day; the separation was felt by the patients, who referred pain and/or a click at the fixator. Definitive resection of the bone tumor was then scheduled.

The freezing technique consisted of en bloc excision of the tumor as a section of bone, removal of soft tissue, curettage of the medullary canal and any lytic part of the tumor and then incubation of the bone graft for 20 min in liquid nitrogen (the first 5 min intermittently and the other 15 continuously), thawing at room temperature for 10 min and finally thawing in distilled water for more 10 min. The graft was then ready to be re-implanted and fixed according to conventional osteosynthesis methods.

14.3.3 Case Reports

Case 1 (GSS)

This was a 12-year-old girl with a type IIB proximal right tibia osteosarcoma. The patient was sent to our hospital with pain in her right leg that had been ongoing for almost 5 months. She had difficulty in walking and a growing mass. She had been radiographed at her town of origin, and referred directly to our unit when the X-ray revealed a huge bone tumor. Image based staging was performed, and 4 days later a biopsy was obtained to confirm the diagnosis. The X-ray and the MRI showed a huge bone mass, mostly extra-compartmental, growing to the medial side of the tibia but not crossing the metaphysis.

Neo-adjuvant chemotherapy was administered in accordance with the Brazilian protocol. Four months later, an external fixator was installed and distraction initiated; epiphyseal separation occurred on the 14th day. Two days later, the tumor was resected by means of a distal tibia osteotomy. The resected specimen was then treated in liquid nitrogen according to the Kanazawa protocol and re-implanted and fixed to the distal tibia diaphysis with two stainless steel plates and a spongiosa screw.

The extra compartmental tumor tissue was sent for pathological analysis; the report described it as extra-compartmental tumor tissue with possible viable tumor in regression. Almost 3 weeks later, adjuvant chemotherapy was started. Four months later, still on chemotherapy, the patient developed an infection at the distal site of osteotomy. The infection was treated with drainage and antibiotics and resolved easily, within 1 month. Nine months after tumor resection surgery, non-union was diagnosed at the distal osteotomy, and an iliac crest bone graft was performed.

During this period, the patient used an external articulated brace, which enabled her to put her full weight on her operated leg and enabled her to make active knee flexion and extension during gait and physiotherapy exercises.

Two years after tumor resection a solitary lung osteosarcoma metastasis was detected, and the patient underwent lung segmentectomy followed again by chemotherapy. Seven months after the lung operation, she developed another infection at the same site as the previous one. Five months later, local recurrence of the tumor was detected in the metaphyseal-diaphyseal area and the limb was amputated above the knee. Before amputation, despite all the complications, the patient had normal knee and ankle function. At the time of writing, 6 years after the initial tumor surgery, the patient is free of disease and walking with her lower limb prosthesis.

Case 2 (MFBS)

This is the case of an 8-year-old boy with a type IIB osteosarcoma in the distal right femur. The patient initially reported injury for 2 months and then pain. Finally, he could no longer walk. After biopsy and confirmation of diagnosis, neo-adjuvant chemotherapy was begun.

Three months later and after another biopsy, the case was evaluated for surgical planning. Although the radiologic evidence was not clear on one of the formal indications prescribed by Cañadell and San Julian [13, 15], epiphyseal distraction of the distal femoral epiphysis was considered opportune and a linear external fixator was installed. Separation occurred after 12 days of distraction. Five days later, the tumor was resected, the resected segment of bone was treated according to the Kanazawa protocol, and the frozen autograft was re-implanted. Because the graft was too big and because, at that time, there was no adequate fixation system covered by the national health system, we were obliged to fix the graft with a straight stainless steel plate and two crossed screws distally.

Pathology analysis of the extra-compartmental tumor tissue found no viable tumor cells.

Consolidation at the distal site of reconstruction failed; this can be attributed to the inadequate fixation method and also, possibly, to the freezing of the bone. The original plate and screws were removed, and the non-union stabilized with an external brace that facilitated knee flexion and extension. A fibrous callus has since developed, and the patient is able to walk and do sports such as bicycle riding without the orthosis. He uses a shoe lift for discrepancy compensation. Knee function has been conserved. Currently, we are planning the placement of an external fixator to correct distal pseudo-arthrosis and to lengthen the femur.

Case 3 (IBB)

This was an 11-year-old boy with a stage IIB osteosarcoma in the distal left femur (Fig. 14.6). The patient reported pain for almost a year before he was X-rayed and the bone tumor was diagnosed. An incisional biopsy confirmed the diagnosis.

After finishing the conventional neo-chemotherapy protocol, and after establishing that the tumor had not invaded the epiphysis, epiphyseal distraction was undertaken. Separation occurred after 13 days.

Bone tumor resection was performed 7 days later. The resected segment of bone was then treated and frozen. The extra-compartmental tumor tissue sent to pathology revealed no viable tumor. The remaining bone was re-implanted and fixed with an angled stainless steel 90° plate.

Three weeks after being discharged from hospital, the patient was provided with an orthosis with knee and ankle flexion/extension; rehabilitation involved physiotherapy and walking with partial weight bearing.

Proximal and distal consolidation was observed in X-rays taken about 4 months after surgery, but the orthosis was maintained for 2 years as an external support to the plate and to avoid metal fatigue. At the time of writing, 6 years after the resection and reconstruction surgery, this patient has absolutely normal knee function and appearance of the knee is normal; there is only a slight growth reduction, of about 1.5 cm, in the operated leg. We plan to wait for the boy's skeletal maturation before removing the plate.

14.3.4 Results

All three patients were successfully submitted to epiphysiolysis before excision and separation occurred at an average time of 13 days. Graft consolidation to the host bone (as evaluated by X-ray) took an average of about 6 months to reach the status of being "good" (according to the ISOLS criteria regarding fusion of allografts (Table 14.2)).

In all cases, the long-term disadvantages of endoprosthesis substitution were avoided.

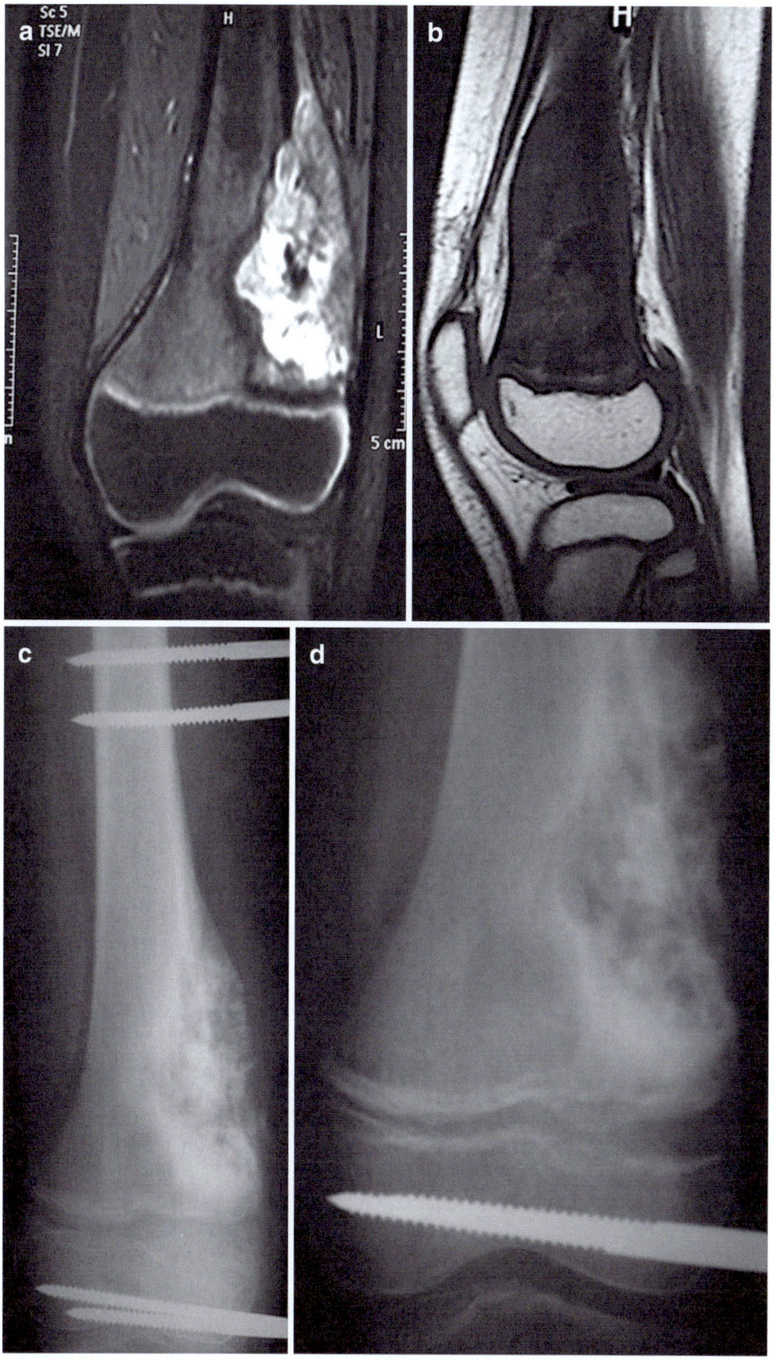

Fig. 14.6 (**a**, **b**) Stage IIB osteosarcoma. The epiphysis is preserved. (**c**, **d**) Epiphyseal separation. (**e**) Tumor specimen with extra compartmental tissue. (**f**) Remaining bone after dissection of extra compartmental tumoral tissue. (**g**) Frozen graft. (**h**) Post-operative X-ray showing fixation with 90° angled plate. (**i**) Four years post-op. (**j**, **k**) Six years post-op. Six years post-op., functional result with full weight bearing (**l**) and (**m**, **n**) normal knee flexion-extension

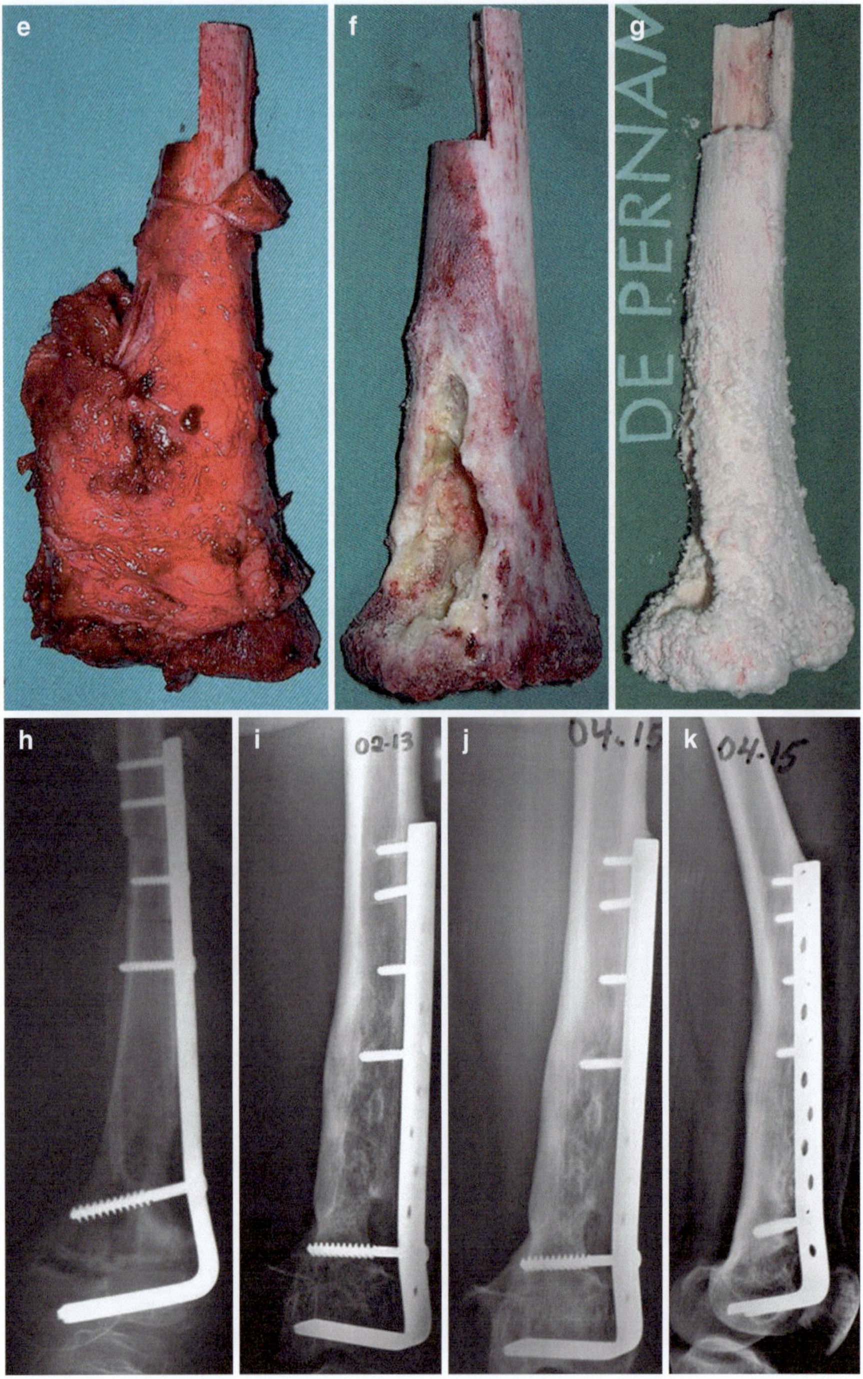

Fig. 14.6 (continued)

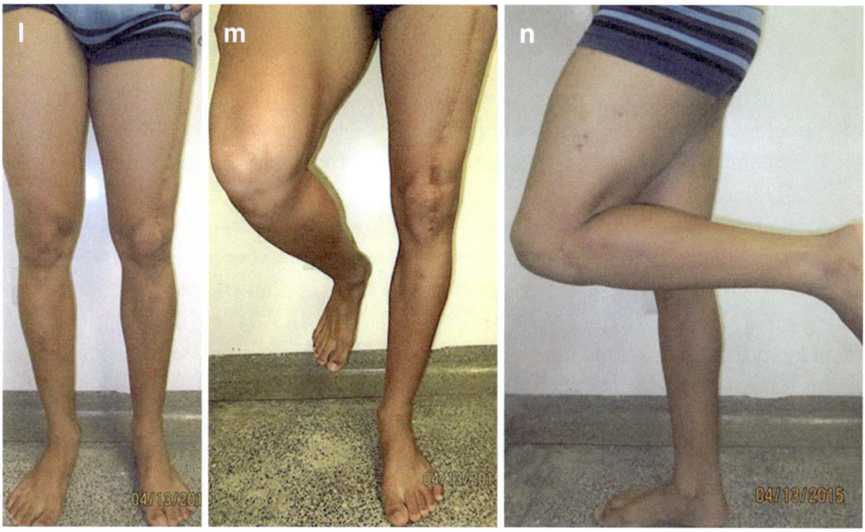

Fig. 14.6 (continued)

Table 14.2 ISOLS criteria regarding fusion of allografts

Excellent	Fusion complete. Osteotomy line not visible
Good	Fusion >75 %. Osteotomy line still visible
Fair	Fusion 25–75 %
Poor	Fusion <25 %. No evidence of callus

14.3.5 Discussion

Each of the three patients whose cases are described were operated on using exactly the same techniques and respecting the oncologic parameters for bone tumor surgery regarding margins. We followed the technique for epiphyseal distraction as described by Cañadell, and we followed the technique of biologic bone tumor reconstruction using recycled frozen bone as originally described by Tsuchiya.

We believe that local recurrence is neither related to epiphyseal distraction nor to the freezing method; local recurrence is absolutely related to the margins achieved during tumor resection. The higher incidence of recurrence in the leg can be attributed to the lack of soft tissue cover in the leg and extra-compartmental spread of tumors.

Unfortunately, we were unable to adhere completely to the principles of stable osteosynthesis because our public health system lacks provision for certain implants, and this limitation could explain the non-union in two of the cases reported here.

The combination of epiphysiolysis before tumor excision and reconstruction with recycled frozen bone as an autogenous graft constitutes a safe approach to the treatment of certain patients with bone sarcomas. The combination can preserve the growth potential of the limb in skeletally immature patients and provides the possibility of excellent long-term functionality.

14.4 Experience of the Hospital Vall d'Hebron of Barcelona

The aim of this commentary is to report the experience of the Hospital Vall d'Hebron of Barcelona with the surgical technique of physeal distraction before excision for the treatment of pediatric bone sarcomas as an alternative limb salvage procedure in skeletally immature patients.

At the Hospital Vall d'Hebron of Barcelona, from July 2006 to October 2013, five patients were treated by physeal distraction before tumor excision (Table 14.3); there were three girls (cases 1, 4 and 5) and two boys (cases 2 and 3). Age at the time of surgery was between 4 and 13 years (Figs. 14.7 and 14.8). All the tumors were located in metaphysis; three were in the proximal tibia (cases 1, 2 and 3), one was in the distal radius (case 4), and one in the proximal humerus (case 5). A histological diagnosis of Ewing's sarcoma was established in four patients (cases 1, 2, 4 and 5) and of osteosarcoma in one (case 3). Neoadjuvant chemotherapy was given to all patients.

The first surgical procedure, attaching the external fixator, involved the insertion of two pins into the epiphysis and another two into the diaphysis at least 4 cm from the diaphyseal tumor margin. The external fixator was then attached. In three cases we used a Blue Monotube (cases 1, 2 and 3) and in two cases a Yellow Monotube (cases 4 and 5). Distraction began in the operating room and was continued at a rate of 0.75–1 mm daily until rupture of the growth plate, which manifested with local pain and was confirmed by radiographic control.

The reconstruction methods after tumor resection were vascularized fibular free flap in one patient (case 1), intercalary bone allograft in three (cases 2, 3 and 5) and contralateral fibular autograft in one (case 4). After reconstruction, we maintained the external fixator in its place in four patients (cases 1, 2, 4 and 5). In one case (case 3), a medial gastrocnemius flap was transferred anteriorly, to cover the intercalary bone allograft.

Histological examination of the resection specimen confirmed in all cases that the margins were negative and also that the tumor had not involved the growth plate margins.

There were no cases of local recurrence in the retained epiphysis, but one patient (case 5) is currently undergoing chemotherapy treatment in another institution after local soft tissue recurrence and lung metastasis that was detected 14 months after the operation. At present, the rest of the patients (cases 1, 2, 3 and 4) are being followed up at our center, show no evidence of disease, and have excellent radiological and functional outcomes.

The patients presented the following orthopedic complications. Two patients with proximal tibial tumor (cases 1 and 2) suffered non-union of the graft that required a further operation to achieve union between the allograft and the host bone. One patient (case 1) had a 6 cm limb length discrepancy 85 months after surgery, and this disparity was resolved by contralateral epiphysiodesis with "8" plates. The patient with a tumor in the distal radius (case 4) suffered a fracture of the united allograft, which has been successfully treated by exchange osteosynthesis and autologous graft.

We believe that what has enabled us to apply the technique of physeal distraction before excision for the treatment of pediatric bone sarcomas with satisfactory results

Table 14.3 General information of the five patients of the Hospital Vall d'Hebron of Barcelona

No.	Birth	Age	Gender	Epiphysiolysis surgery	Site	Resection surgery	Reconstruction method	Chemo	Follow-up (months)	Limb length (R/L cm)	Complication	Pathology
1.	2003/7/16	4	Female	2007/10/18	Right proximal tibia	2007/11/12	Vascularized fibular free flap	VIDE VAC	89	73/79	None	Ewing
2.	1999/12/2	9	Male	2009/7/23	Right proximal tibia	2009/8/10	Intercalary allograft	VIDE VAC	60	84/85	Delayed union	Ewing
3.	1999/3/14	13	Male	2013/1/7	Right proximal tibia	2013/1/28	Intercalary allograft	Cisplatin, adriamycin and methotrexate	25	91/93	Soft tissue recurrence	Osteosarcoma
4.	2006/7/15	6	Female	2013/5/31	Left distal radius	2013/6/13	Contralateral fibular autograft	VIDE VAC	24	–	Autograft osteolysis	Ewing
5.	2008/10/22	5	Female	2013/10/10	Left proximal humerus	2013/11/14	Intercalary allograft	VIDE VAC	20	–	Autograft fracture	Ewing

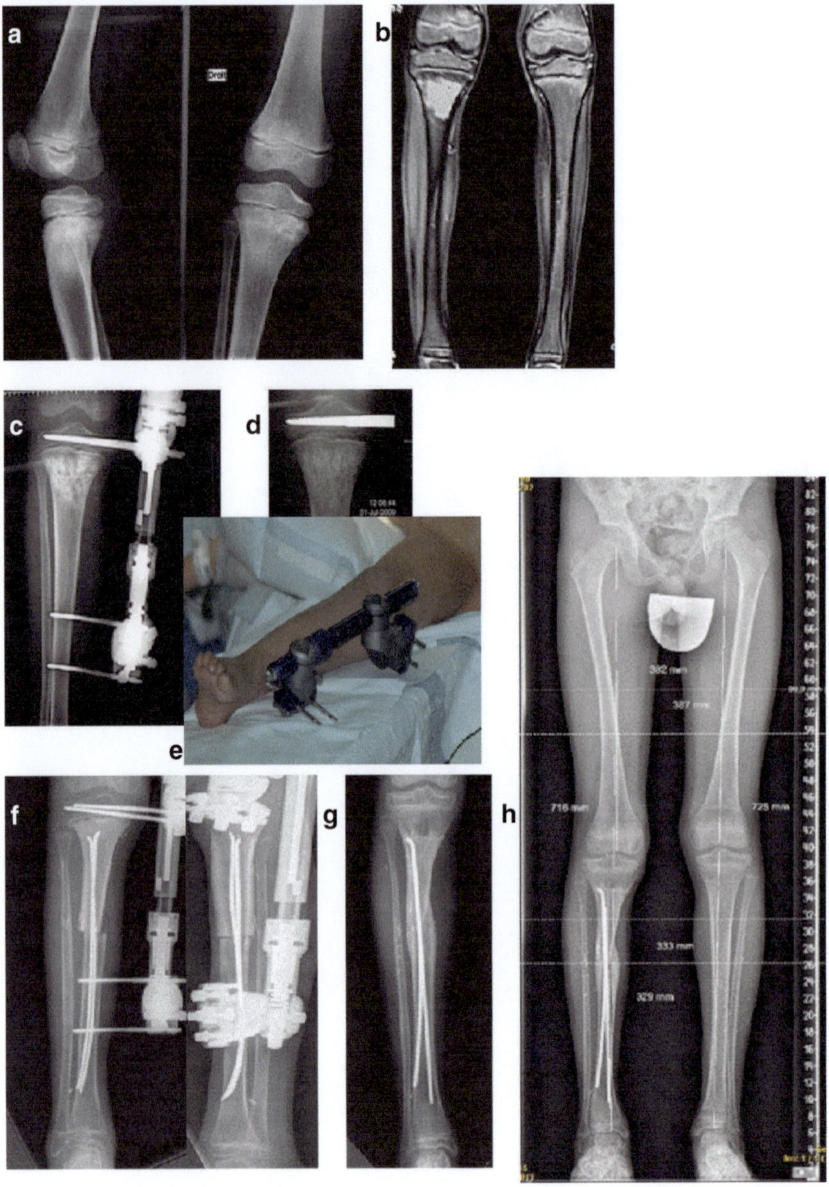

Fig. 14.7 (**a**, **b**) X-ray and MRI of a Ewing's sarcoma in the proximal tibia of a 9-year-old boy. (**c–e**) Physeal distraction before excision. (**f**, **g**) After reconstruction with an intercalary bone allograft. The growth plate in this patient currently remains active (**h**), 60 months after surgery

in our center is the combining of the expertise of specialists in pediatric orthopedics and in orthopedic oncology. We usually kept external fixation in place until consolidation of the bone graft with the epiphysis; this did not result in complications. Although the main goal of physeal distraction before excision is to preserve the

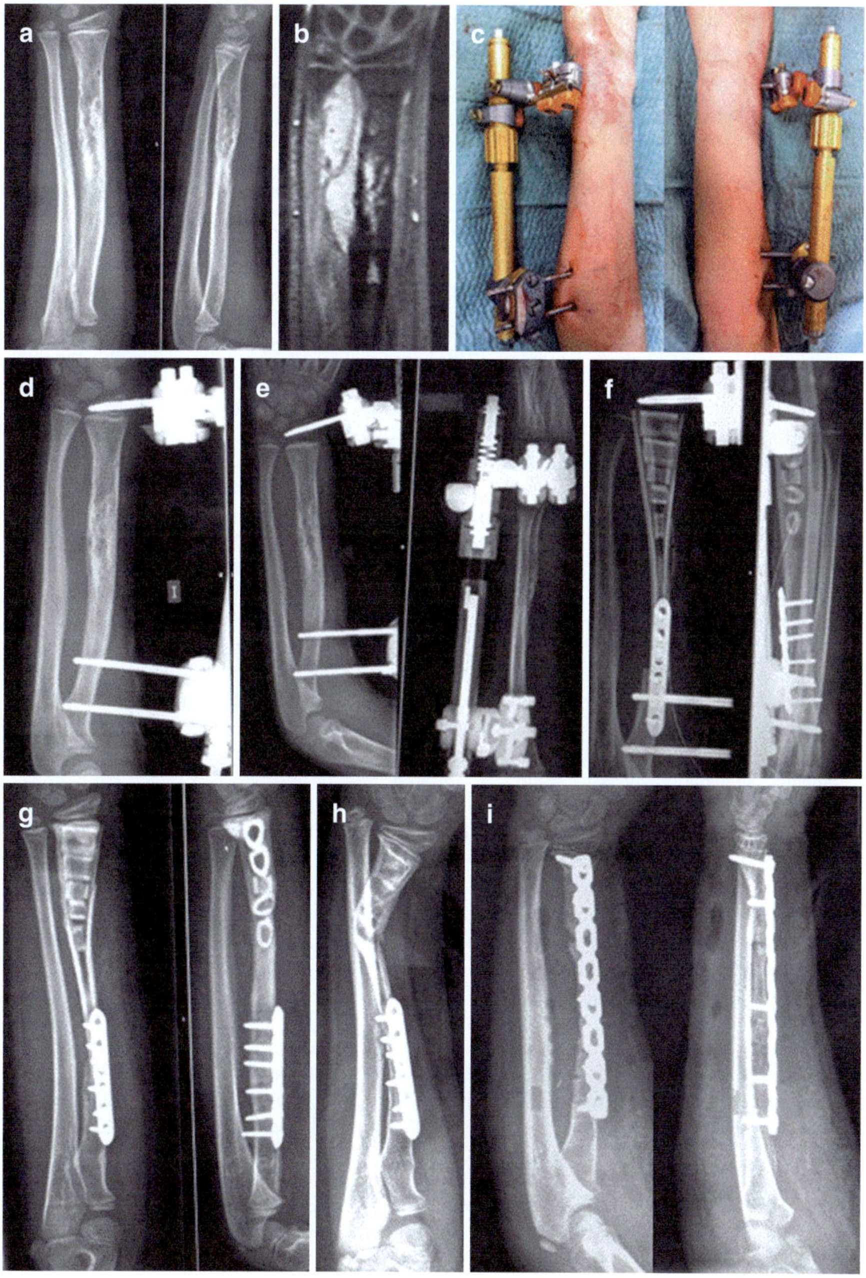

Fig. 14.8 (**a**, **b**) X-ray and MRI of a Ewing's sarcoma in the distal left radius of a 6-year-old girl. (**c–e**) Physeal distraction before excision. (**f**) After reconstruction with a contralateral fibular autograft. (**g**) Union of the autograft with active growth plate 6 months after surgery. (**h**, **i**) Fracture of the graft and treatment of this fracture

epiphysis and thus the joint, we have found that a low rate of distraction allowed us to maintain growth capacity in some of our patients. Consequently, the technique has enabled us to obtain good functional outcome for the joint and also a reduced degree of limb discrepancy.

References

1. Canadell J, Forriol F, Cara JA. Removal of metaphyseal bone tumours with preservation of the epiphysis. Physeal distraction before excision. J Bone Joint Surg. 1994;76(1):127–32.
2. Cañadell J, San-Julian M, Cara JA, et al. Conservation of the epiphysis while removing metaphyseal bone tumours: epiphysiolysis before excision. In: Cañadell J, San-Julian M, editors. Pediatric bone sarcomas: epiphysiolysis before excision. New York: Springer; 2009. p. 101–8.
3. Enneking WF, Dunham W, Gebhardt MC, Malawer M, Pritchard DJ. A system for the functional evaluation of reconstructive procedures after surgical treatment of tumors of the musculoskeletal system. Clin Orthop Relat Res. 1993;286:241–6.
4. Xu M, Xu SF, Yu XC. Clinical analysis of osteosarcoma patients treated with high-dose methotrexate-free neoadjuvant chemotherapy. Curr Oncol. 2014;21(5):e678–84.
5. Yao W, Cai Q, Gao S, et al. Epiphysis preserving operations for the treatment of lower limb malignant bone tumors. Eur J Surg Oncol. 2012;38(12):1165–70.
6. Xu SF, Yu XC, Xu M, et al. Successful management of a childhood osteosarcoma with epiphysiolysis and distraction osteogenesis. Curr Oncol. 2014;21(4):658–62.
7. Simon MA. Limb salvage for osteosarcoma in the 1980s. Clin Orthop Relat Res. 1991;270:264–70.
8. San-Julian M, Aquerreta JD, Benito A, et al. Indications for epiphyseal preservation in metaphyseal malignant bone tumors of children: relationship between image methods and histological findings. J Pediatr Orthop. 1999;19(4):543–8.
9. Cañadell J, de Pablos J. Breaking bony bridges by physeal distraction. A new approach. Int Orthop. 1985;9:223–9.
10. Weitao Y, Qiqing C, Songtao G, Jiaqiang W. Epiphysis preserving operations for the treatment of lower limb malignant bone tumors. Eur J Surg Oncol. 2013;38:1165–70.
11. Zhang P, Feifei F, Qiqing C, Weitao Y, Songtao G, Wang J, Wang X. Effects of metaphyseal bone tumor removal with preservation of the epiphysis. Exp Ther Med. 2014;8(3):567–73.
12. Betz M, Dumont CE, Fuchs B, Exner GU. Physeal distraction for joint preservation in malignant metaphyseal bone tumors in children. Clin Orthop Relat Res. 2012;470(6):1749–54.
13. Cañadell J, Forriol F, Cara JA. Removal of metaphyseal bone tumours with preservation of the epiphysis. Physeal distraction before excision. J Bone Joint Surg Br. 1994;76:127–32.
14. Tsuchiya H, Wan SL, Sakayama K, Yamamoto N, Nishida H, Tomita K. Reconstruction using an autograft containing tumour treated by liqid nitrogen. J Bone Joint Surg (Br). 2005;87-B:218–25.
15. Cañadell J, Forriol F, Cara JA, San-Julian M. Removal of metaphyseal bone tumors with preservation of the epiphysis. Physeal distraction before excision. In: Cañadel J, San-Julian M, Cara JA, editors. Surgical treatment of malignant bone tumors. Pamplona: Ediciones Universidad de Navarra; 1995. p. 153–60.

Chapter 15
Questions and Answers

Mikel San-Julian

Abstract The technique of physeal distraction before tumor excision has been described at several national and international meetings, where it has invariably aroused considerable interest. This chapter deals with some of the questions put forward at these meetings.

- **Does this technique mean any delay in the protocol for treatment of the tumor**?
  Answer: No.
  You can place the external fixator during the course of pre-operative chemotherapy. You need only 15 min. to place the external fixator, 15 days before the established date for surgery. The external fixator allows the patient to continue with his or her normal life, and it does not impede adherence to chemotherapy protocols, even intra-arterial procedures.

- **Do you employ the technique in all cases of metaphyseal bone tumors**?
  From: Antonie Tamineau, University of Leyden, The Netherlands In: SICOT, 1996 Meeting, Amsterdam
  Answer: No.
  It is a technique for selected cases: those cases of metaphyseal bone tumors in which the tumor has not crossed the growth plate. If the tumor has crossed the growth plate, the joint will require reconstruction surgery (arthrodesis, prosthesis, or osteoarticular allograft).

- **What is the reason for the distraction technique**?
  From: Zdenek Matejowsky Sr., Praga
  In: EMSOS, 1994 Meeting, Amsterdam
  Answer: The anatomy of the growth plate.
  The growth plate, which is what seems to represent a temporary barrier to tumor spread, is not a flat surface but is rather convoluted, and so, when performing

M. San-Julian, MD, PhD
Department of Orthopaedic Surgery, University of Navarra, Pamplona, Navarra, Spain
e-mail: msjulian@unav.es

M. San-Julian (ed.), *Cañadell's Pediatric Bone Sarcomas: Epiphysiolysis before Excision*, DOI 10.1007/978-3-319-24220-0_15

intra-epiphyseal osteotomy, it is difficult to be sure that the section has not passed through the tumor and left tumoral tissue behind.

- **What about the risk of infection**?
  From: Mario Campanacci, Bologna
  In: ISOLS, 1995 Meeting, Firenze
  Answer: The risk is the same as with other reconstructive surgery.
  The risk of infection is no higher in tumor pathology than it is in other scenarios of reconstructive surgery. Obviously, patients are immuno-suppressed as a result of the chemotherapy, but the external fixator is only used for 10–15 days. Not even in cases where we used an external fixator as a support for autografting or bone transport (see Chap. 9), have we had any problems related with infection. Seven percent of our series suffered an infection of the reconstruction during the follow-up; this rate is no higher than that in our own overall series of allografts or prostheses, or that reported by other authors.
- **Do you employ antibiotics during the distraction procedure**?
  From: Cristina Alves, Portugal
  In: Pediatric OrthopaedicMeeting, Aveiro, Portugal, 2015
  Answer: No
- **Could you exploit the procedure to achieve some lengthening before resection**?
  From: Marco Manfrini, Bologna
  In: EMSOS, 1997 Meeting, Münster
  Answer: No.
  The technique is just an epiphysiolysis in order to achieve a good margin for resection of the tumor. It is not a lengthening procedure. The tumor should be resected as soon as possible. Other techniques exist for avoiding or correcting limb-length discrepancies after tumor resection.
- **Could this technique stimulate tumor growth**?
  From: Wilfred Winkelman, Münster
  In: EMSOS, 1997 Meeting, Münster
  Answer: No.
  The disruption of the growth plate occurs suddenly after several days of distraction. We do not believe that this stimulates tumor growth.
- **Does chemotherapy influence callus formation**?
  From: Wilfred Winkelman, University of Münster
  In: EMSOS, 1997 Meeting, Münster
  Answer: What callus?
  Chemotherapy has an important effect on the consolidation of allografts and callus formation in bone transport procedures (see Chap. 9), but epiphysiolysis before resection of the tumor is not a procedure concerned with callus formation: it is simply a way to get a good resection margin, and so there is no need to wait for callus formation.

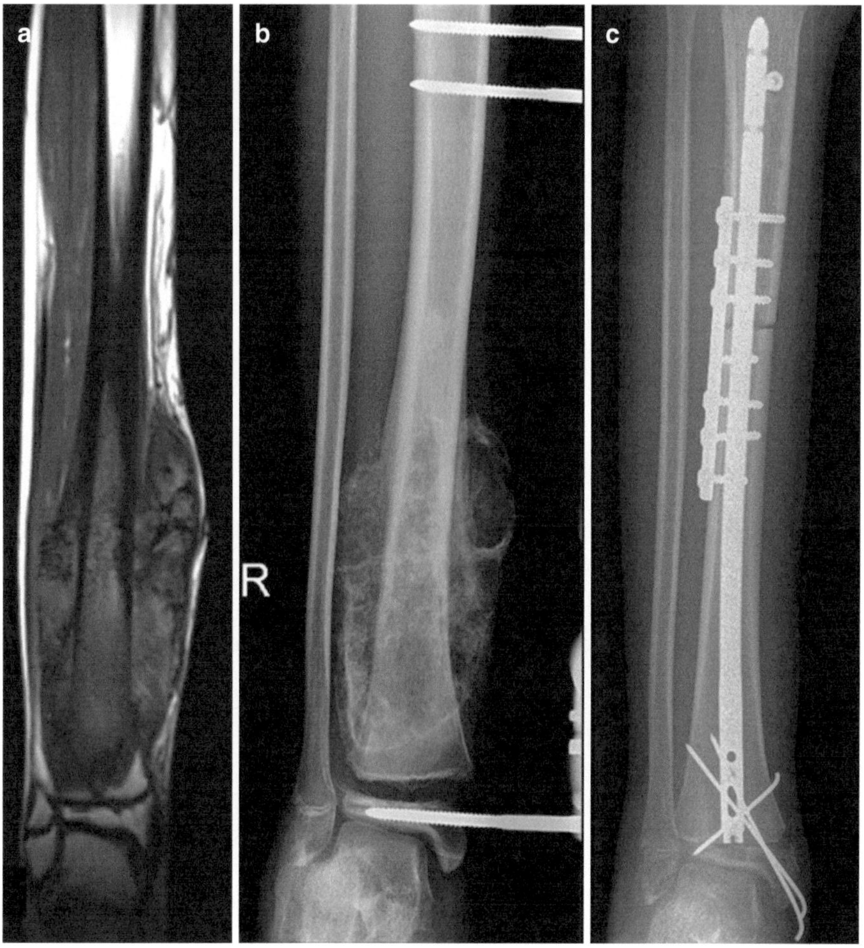

Fig. 15.1 (**a–c**) The oldest patient in our series was 15 y-o

- **Are there any age limits for the procedure**?
  From: Name unknown
  In: EMSOS, 1997 Meeting, Münster
  Answer: Appropriacy has to be determined on a patient by patient basis.
  The youngest patient in which the technique has been used was 3 years old (see Fig. 12.8), but malignant bone tumors are not frequently seen in children so young. The oldest patient in the series was 15 years old (Fig. 15.1). Before applying the technique, one has to ascertain that the growth plate is still active and that the patient has not finished growing.
- **Has the technique been employed in lytic lesions**?
  From: Becker, Münster
  In: EMSOS, 1997 Meeting, Münster

Answer: Yes.
Osteogenic sarcoma and Ewing's sarcoma, the two bone tumors most frequently seen in childhood, are not usually lytic lesions. However, we have successfully used the technique with lytic lesions such as telangiectatic osteosarcoma (see Fig. 11.11). In such cases, it is important to be sure that there is no pathological fracture.

- **Has the technique been employed in metaphyseal tumors which were seen to be in contact with the growth plate in the MRI scans**?
From: Name unknown
In: SICOT, 1996 Meeting, Amsterdam
Answer: Yes.
The most important thing is to be sure that the tumor has not crossed the growth plate.

- **Has the technique been employed in benign lesions**?
From Gabriel Mato, Portugal
In: Pediatric OrthopaedicMeeting, Aveiro, Portugal, 2015
Answer: We have not used the technique in such cases, but other colleagues (for instance, Julio de Pablos and colleagues at the Rizzoli Institute) have done so.

- **Does the retained growth plate remain active after the distraction procedure**?
From: Marco Manfrini, Bologna
In: EMSOS, 1997 Meeting, Münster
Answer: In some cases.
As reported by De Pablos et al. from our department, if physeal distraction is used as a lengthening procedure, the growth plate may continue growing when lengthening is performed at a rate of 1–1.5 mm/day. In cases of epiphysiolysis for preserving the epiphysis, it is also possible that the growth plate will continue growing; Chap. 9 presents some cases that demonstrate subsequent growth. However, arrest of growth could be caused by other factors, such as, radiotherapy, delayed weight bearing, and the osteosynthesis device used for stabilization of the retained epiphysis (see Chap. 9).

- **Osteosynthesis of the allograft with a locked nail will not allow subsequent growth**!
From: Rodolfo Capanna, Firenze
In: ISOLS, 1996 Meeting, Firenze
Answer: True.
We used this kind of osteosynthesis device in patients who were nearing the end of growth. Allografts which were 1.5–2 cm longer than the resected piece were employed in an attempt to minimize the final limb-length discrepancy. We preferred this approach to osteosynthesis for the older patients in our series because it eliminates the risk of allograft fracture. However, in young children, we prefer minimal osteosynthesis devices of the epiphysis, such as Kirschner wires or the distal end of two Enders, to permit later growth (see Chap. 9).

- **How could you be sure about tumor extension before the MRI era**?
  From: William Enneking, University of Gainesville (Florida)
  In: ISOLS, 1995 Meeting, Firenze
  Answer: Sometimes we could not be sure, and so we used a modified surgical procedure.
  Before the advent of MRI, we used other imaging methods, such as, CT, scintigraphy, X-ray, and angiography when needed. In cases where we still found ourselves left with any doubt about whether the tumor was compromising the physis, we approached surgery with a variant of the usual technique. This variant has three surgical steps that enable us to inspect histologically the distracted margin (see Chap. 8). We believe that nowadays, owing to the accuracy of MRI, the three step variant is rarely necessary.

- **I believe that there is usually a high risk of local recurrence**; **how many of your patients had a follow-up longer than 2 years**?
  From: William Enneking, University of Gainesville (Florida)
  In: ISOLS, 1995 Meeting, Firenze
  Answer: Most of them.
  When Dr. Enneking put this question to us, he suggested that we had been lucky to have had no cases of local recurrence. We have been employing the technique since 1984, and so the first patient in our series now has 31 years of follow-up.

- **What happens if the distraction does not take place correctly**?
  From: Ulrich Exner, Zurich (Switzerland)
  Answer: Intra-epiphyseal osteotomy can still be performed.
  Although distraction is possible even in lytic tumors, in a couple of our patients, pathological fracture occurred during distraction. In these cases, we carried out an intra-epiphyseal osteotomy to remove the tumor. There were no complications, neither case suffered local recurrence, and function was good.

- **What happens to the femoralis trochlea or to the anterior tibial tuberosity in cases when epiphysiolysis cannot be done**, **and intraepiphyseal osteotomy is performed**?
  From: Seban Hopyan, Toronto, Canada
  Answer: In the distal femoral case, part of the epiphysis will be lost and the stability of the joint will be affected, the femoropatellar joint will also be affected. In the proximal tibia, it is necessary to reattach the patellar tendon to the graft. This is avoided with epiphysiolysis, because the whole anterior tibial tuberosity is retained.

- **Given the proven safety and the excellent results**, **why is this technique not more widely adopted**?
  From: Name unknown.
  In: ISOLS, 2007 Meeting, Hamburg
  Answer: Confidence in the technique requires very different types of specialist knowledge and experience. I think there are two main reasons why the technique has not been more widely adopted. First, orthopedic oncologists are not

necessarily accustomed to dealing with techniques such as external fixation, growth plate surgery, and lengthening procedures, because such surgeons concentrate primarily on tumor surgery. Without a clear understanding of how the growth plate breaks when distraction is slowly applied, a surgeon focused on resection may find it difficult to muster sufficient trust that epiphysiolysis can provide a safe margin of resection in bone sarcomas. Cañadell had a wide experience in pediatric orthopedics, external fixation, and many other fields of orthopedics, and it was perhaps this broad familiarity which enabled him to conceive of and develop his technique. Second, in many centers, the indications for amputation have only diminished very slowly during the last two decades; to stop amputating bone tumors requires considerable confidence in the efficiency of chemotherapy. Professor Cañadell was exceptional in his decision to stop amputating bone tumors once he knew of this efficiency. When he started this technique for preserving the joint, most people simply did not believe it was possible without diminishing the chances of survival. Nowadays, the technique is being used in many distinguished cancer centers around the world including centers in Seville, Barcelona, Madrid and Valencia (Spain), Zurich (Switzerland), Leiden (the Netherlands), Pernanbuco (Brazil), Istanbul (Turkey), Budapest (Hungary), Bologna (Italy), and Ji'Nan, He'Nan, TianJin, Xi'an (China).

Index

M. San-Julian (ed.), *Cañadell's Pediatric Bone Sarcomas: Epiphysiolysis before Excision*, DOI 10.1007/978-3-319-24220-0

MIX
Papier aus verantwortungsvollen Quellen
Paper from responsible sources
FSC® C105338

If you have any concerns about our products,
you can contact us on
ProductSafety@springernature.com

In case Publisher is established outside the EU,
the EU authorized representative is:
Springer Nature Customer Service Center GmbH
Europaplatz 3, 69115 Heidelberg, Germany

Printed by Libri Plureos GmbH
in Hamburg, Germany